Human Embryology

F. BECK
DSc, MD, ChB
Professor of Anatomy
University of Leicester

D.B. MOFFAT
VRD, MD, FRCS
Professor of Anatomy
University College, Cardiff

D.P. DAVIES
BSc, MB, DCH, DObst, FRCP
Professor of Paediatrics
The Chinese University of
Hong Kong

SECOND EDITION

BLACKWELL SCIENTIFIC PUBLICATIONS

OXFORD LONDON EDINBURGH

BOSTON PALO ALTO MELBOURNE

© 1973, 1985 by
Blackwell Scientific Publications
Editorial offices:
Osney Mead, Oxford, OX2 OEL
8 John Street, London, WC1N 2ES
23 Ainslie Place, Edinburgh, EH3 6AJ
52 Beacon Street, Boston
  Massachusetts 02108, USA
667 Lytton Avenue, Palo Alto
  California 94301, USA
99 Barry Street, Carlton
  Victoria 3053, Australia

First published 1973
Second edition 1985

Set by Setrite Typesetters, Hong Kong
Printed and bound in Great Britain

DISTRIBUTORS

USA
  Blackwell Mosby Book Distributors
  11830 Westline Industrial Drive
  St Louis, Missouri 63141

Canada
  Blackwell Mosby Book Distributors
  120 Melford Drive, Scarborough
  Ontario M1B 2X4

Australia
  Blackwell Scientific Publications
  (Australia) Pty Ltd
  107 Barry Street
  Carlton, Victoria 3053

British Library
Cataloguing in Publication Data

Beck, F.
  Human embryology.—2nd ed.
  1. Embryology, Human
  I. Title II. Moffat, D.B. III. Davies, D.P.
  612'.646 QM601

  ISBN 0-632-01041-X

Contents

Preface to the Second Edition

For its second edition, this book has been completely revised and largely re-written. Its change in title from 'Human Embryology and Genetics' to 'Human Embryology' reflects a considerable change in emphasis. Genetics is now normally taught as a separate course in most medical schools and there are many excellent text books suitable for undergraduates. This subject has, therefore, been largely deleted from the present volume although a basic account has been given in order to make intelligible the mode of inheritance of various congenital malformations and diseases. The other major change is that the embryological basis of congenital malformations has been covered in very much more detail than in the first edition and their clinical features are described and illustrated in the hope that the book will be of help to 'clinical' as well as 'preclinical' students. To this end, a clinician (D.P. Davies) has made a substantial contribution to the new edition, not only in respect of the pathology of the newborn baby but also of normal and abnormal growth and development.

It is our hope that this book will be an aid to the preclinical student in his study of this important subject and that it will dovetail helpfully with the later study of both obstetrics and paediatrics.

Inevitably, as in all books that attempt to cover a wide multidisciplinary field, the authors are deeply indebted to a number of friends and colleagues who have given valuable advice and assistance. We should like to mention particularly Professor J. MacVicar, Dr I. Young, Professor H.C. McGregor and Dr M.A. England.

Acknowledgements

We wish to thank Miss Margaret Reeve for typing and checking our manuscript. Her commitment has enabled us to produce this edition more quickly than we had dared to hope. We are also grateful to Miss Catherine Hemington and Mrs Angela Chorley for preparing the new illustrations included in this edition.

A number of the new illustrations are drawings from original photographs or are diagrams that have appeared in books or journals. We would like to express our thanks to the authors and editors for permission to publish the following:

Fig. 9.11 supplied by Dr. Ian Young

Figs. 10.21-10.24 from Congenital Abnormalities of the CNS by P.M. Davidson & D.G. Young (*British Journal of Hospital Medicine*, 1981, **26**, 222)

Fig. 17.9 from *Growth at Adolescence* by J.M. Tanner (Blackwell Scientific Publications, Oxford, 1962)

Fig. 17.11 from Revised Standards for triceps and subscapular skin folds in British children (*Archives of the Diseases of Childhood*, 1975, **50**, 12)

Figs. 17.12, 17.13, 17.16 and 17.18 from *Foetus into Man* by J.M. Tanner (Open Books Publishing Ltd) (17.12 is slightly modified)

Fig. 17.14 from Daily velocity, weight gain in infants over the first 5 months of life by M. Fujimura & F. Seryce (*Archives of the Diseases of Childhood*, 1977, **52**, 105)

Introduction —
Aids to the Study of Embryology

To the student studying embryology for the first time, the development of the various organs seems complex and sometimes difficult to follow. The latter is true even for professional embryologists and some of the processes of development are still imperfectly understood.

However, there are a number of general principles involved, knowledge of which will help greatly in the assimilation of embryological facts and figures. We suggest, therefore, that you read the following account carefully and refresh your memory from time to time as you study the development of the various organs.

(a) Cranio-caudal developmental gradient

There is frequently a cranio-caudal gradient of development, i.e. the most cranial part of the embryo, of a system, or of an organ, develops first and the process of maturation proceeds caudally, the cranial end of the system sometimes degenerating while the caudal end is still at an early stage of development. This gradient can easily be seen in the whole embryo when the mesodermal somites are developing and becoming differentiated into vertebrae, muscles etc. (Chapter 9). At the cranial end of the series the cervical somites may already be giving rise to the precursors of the vertebral bodies and early muscle cells (myoblasts) may be recognised. At the same time, the most caudal somites are still small and incompletely developed.

The aortic arches (Chapter 12) are never all present at the same time so that the 'Christmas tree' diagrams that are sometimes seen showing all five arches are misleading. The aortic arches develop sequentially but by the time the third arch is beginning to appear, the first is already breaking up. Later, the fourth arch develops but by this time the first arch has disappeared (apart from a few remnants) and the second arch is degenerating. Finally the sixth arch appears and only arches 3, 4 and 6 remain to play a major part in the development of the great arteries.

(b) Postnatal continuation of development

It should always be remembered that many organs are still not completely developed by full term and birth should be regarded only as an incident in the whole developmental process. Thus the lungs (Chapter 13) continue to develop new alveoli after birth and the kidneys (Chapter 14) develop new glomeruli and nephrons. The reproductive system, of course, does not complete its full development until puberty. The clinical importance of these observations will be referred to frequently in connection with the complications of prematurity.

(c) Development of organs lined by epithelium

The development of most organs and tissues that are covered by or lined by epithelium are very similar. To take the intestine as an example, it is first formed as a tube of endodermal cells. This is surrounded by *mesenchyme* (i.e., loose mesodermal tissue — the embryonic connective tissue) and it eventually pulls away from the dorsal body wall to form a mesentery. The endoderm differentiates to form the lining epithelium of the gut, with all its glands (see section (d)) while the surrounding mesenchyme becomes condensed and forms the smooth muscle, connective tissue and blood vessels of the gut wall. The surface layer of mesenchymal cells form a thin epithelium (a *mesothelium*) which is the visceral layer of peritoneum.

The ureter begins its life as a tube derived from mesoderm which is surrounded by mesenchyme. The mesoderm forms the transitional epithelium of the ureter, while the mesenchyme around it differentiates into smooth muscle, connective tissue and blood vessels.

(d) Development of glands

When, in the adult, a gland or organ A is connected to a lumen or a surface B, A almost always develops as one or more outgrowths from B, the number of outgrowths depending on the number of connecting ducts. Thus, the liver and gall bladder are connected to the duodenum (foregut) by the common bile duct and they develop as an outgrowth from the foregut. The outgrowth divides into two, one division forming the gall bladder and the other the common hepatic ducts, the bile duct system in the liver and the liver cells themselves.

The pancreas (usually) has two ducts — one main and one accessory — which connect it to the duodenum. The pancreas thus develops as two outgrowths from the foregut. The prostate is connected to the urethra by 15–20 ducts and it develops from 15–20 outgrowths from the embryonic urethra. Section (c) should also be applied to this form of development — in the case of the gall bladder, for instance, the endodermal outgrowth forms the columnar epithelium that lines the gall bladder, while the surrounding mesenchyme becomes condensed and forms the smooth muscle, connective tissue and blood vessels of the gall bladder wall.

Note however that there are a few exceptions to this general rule, the most important being the kidney and ureter. The collecting ducts, calices, pelvis and ureter develop from an outgrowth (the *ureteric bud*) not from the bladder but from a part of the mesonephric duct which will later form the trigone. The nephrons themselves develop from quite a different source (p.251).

(e) Migration

Be careful when describing 'migrations' of organs, which are often more apparent than real. In order to define a movement in any direction one needs a fixed point to which the movement can be related, and there are no such fixed points in a rapidly developing embryo. Thus, it is convenient sometimes to refer to the 'descent' of the diaphragm from the neck region, thus explaining the long course of the phrenic nerve from C3, 4 and 5 down to the midriff. In fact, when the diaphragm begins to develop, the embryo does not have a neck or thorax, and the descent of the diaphragm is really due mostly to growth of the thorax and neck away from it. The embryo may, in fact, be said to be 'sticking its neck out'.

The descent of the testis, too, is largely due to the growth in length of the posterior abdominal wall, the testis remaining almost stationary.

One must, therefore, be careful not to think of embryonic events in terms of adult anatomy. Students often picture the testis as developing high in the embryonic abdomen and slithering gracefully down a long slide to end up in the scrotum, so accounting for the long testicular vessels. In fact the posterior abdominal wall in the embryo is so short that the testis spends the whole of its intra-abdominal life very close to the deep inguinal ring. It is also difficult to picture the development of a horseshoe kidney (p.270) until one realises that when the metanephros first develops, it is only a fraction of a millimetre away from the metanephros of the opposite side, so that fusion can occur quite easily.

(f) Temporary embryonic structures

Remember that many structures in the embryo have only a temporary existence and soon degenerate or remain as vestigial remnants which may give rise to cysts in later life. Often such temporary structures, however, have a second-hand value and they may be used for other purposes. In the male mesonephros, for instance, there is a cranio-caudal gradient of development; the cranial mesonephric tubules functioning as excretory organs and then degenerating, their function being taken over by ever more caudal tubules until, with the development of the metanephros, the mesonephros becomes non-functional. Some of the tubules remain as remnants near the epididymis and may become cystic in later life. Others remain and take on a new lease of life to form the ductuli efferentia

There are many other such embryonic remnants in the adult. The thyroglossal duct (p.179), for example, may persist and give rise to thyroglossal cysts while the allantois, which normally degenerates in part to form the urachus, may persist *in toto* to produce a channel (*fistula*) from the bladder to the umbilicus, or, locally to produce a urachal cyst. Many other examples will be given in this book.

(g) Combined deformities

Congenital abnormalities tend to occur in 'clusters' rather than singly. Many of these combinations of deformities can be explained on embryological grounds. For example, since the differentiation of the local mesoderm to form nephrons depends upon the presence of an ureteric bud (p.251) it is obvious that an absent ureter must necessarily also mean the absence of a whole kidney. If both kidneys are absent or do not secrete the normal amount of urine, there will be a deficiency in the volume of amniotic fluid which, in turn, will result in the presence of other deformities such as Potter's syndrome (p.267).

In other cases, the connecting link is not so obvious but the deformities do form a well recognised pattern (*a syndrome*) and such groups of deformities often bear the name of the person who first described them. For example the combination of a ventricular septal defect, pulmonary stenosis, an overriding aorta and an enlarged right ventricle is called the *tetralogy of Fallot* (p.229) while *Marfan's syndrome* comprises abnormally long arms and fingers, defects of the arch of the aorta and other malformations of structures of mesodermal origin.

(h) Embryonic physiology

It should always be remembered that the embryonic organs and tissues may be carrying out important functions, even while they are developing and that you have to study developmental physiology as well as developmental anatomy. The embryonic heart, even in its earliest stage of development, is solely responsible for the circulation of the blood, including the fetal side of the placental circulation. The mesonephros is actively secreting a form of urine during its existence, and this is voided, making an important contribution to the amniotic fluid. Muscle contractions after the 5th month cause movements that can be felt by the mother, and these movements play an important role in the development of the synovial joints by modifying their shape. However, some organs in the embryo have a function different to that which they acquire later. The liver, for example, is an important haemopoietic organ during intra-uterine life, although it also produces bile which is responsible for the colour of the fetal faeces (*meconium*).

(i) Developmental age and developmental stages

Some variation exists in the rate at which individual human embryos and fetuses develop *in utero*. The post-fertilization age of a conceptus is, therefore, not an entirely accurate guide to its developmental stage and this should be borne in mind when consulting the sections on developmental stages given at the end of most chapters.

Some forty years ago G.L. Streeter, working at the Department of Embryology of the Carnegie Institution of Washington, used a very comprehensive collection of human embryonic material to construct a series of 'developmental horizons'. He described successive developmental stages in detail so that it became possible to correlate the state of individual systems with accuracy. Since then 'Streeter's Horizons' have been the most widely used system for classifying stages of human development.

Developmental horizons

Developmental Horizons in Human Embryos, description of age group XI, 13—20 somites and age group XII, 21—29 somites, G.L. Streeter, *Contr. Embryol. Carnegie Inst.* **30**, 211, 1942.

Developmental Horizons in Human Embryos, description of age group XIII, embryos about 4 or 5 mm long and age group XIV period of indentation of lens vesicle, G.L. Streeter, *Contr. Embryol. Carnegie Inst.* **31**, 27, (1945).

Developmental Horizons in Human Embryos, description of age groups XV. Being the 3rd issue of a survey of the Carnegie collection. XVI, XVII and XVIII, G.L. Streeter, *Contr. Embryol, Carnegie Inst.* **32**, 133, (1948).

Developmental Horizons in Human Embryos, description of age groups XIX, XX, XXI, XXII and XXIII. Being the 5th issue of a survey of the Carnegie collection, G.L. Streeter, *Contr. Embryol. Carnegie Inst.* **34**, 165, (1951).

Note: Developmental horizons I to X are not separately described. I = One cell egg. II = Segmenting egg. III = Free blastocyst. IV = Implanting ovum. V = Ovum implanted but still avillous. VI = Development of primitive villi and a distinct yolk-sac. VII = Branching villi, axis of germ disc defined. VIII = Development of Hensen's mode and primitive groove. IX = Stage of neural folds and elongated notochord. X = Early somites present.

Recently O'Rahilly has updated the staging of human embryos and included in his work much new material derived after Streeter's original publications. The table on p.xi is taken from his important review article in *Eur. J. Obstet. Gynec. Reprod. Biol.* (1979) **9**, 273—80.

Table I Developmental stages in human embryos. Early human development and the chief sources of information on staged human embryos. Courtesy of Professor R. O'Rahilly and the Carnegie Institution of Washington.

Carnegie stage	Pairs of somites	Length (mm)	Age (days)[1]	Age (days)[2]	Features
1				1	Fertilization.
2			1.5–3	2–3	From 2 to about 16 cells.
3			4	4–5	Free blastocyst.
4			5–6	5–6	Attaching blastocyst.
5		0.1–0.2	7–12	7–12	Implanted although previllous.
⌠5a		0.1	7–8		Solid trophoblast.
⎱5b		0.1	9		Trophoblastic lacunae.
⌡5c		0.15–0.2	11–12		Lacunar vascular circle.
6		0.2	13	13–15	Chorionic villi; primitive streak may appear.
⌠6a					Chorionic villi.
⌡6b					Primitive streak.
7		0.4	16	15–17	Notochordal process.
8		1.0–1.5	18	17–19	Primitive pit; notochordal and neurenteric canals.
9	1–3	1.5–2.5	20	19–21	Somites first appear.
10	4–12	2–3.5	22	22–23	Neural folds begin to fuse; 2 pharyngeal bars; optic sulcus.
11	13–20	2.5–4.5	24	23–26	Rostral neuropore closes; optic vesicle.
12	21–29	3–5	26	26–30	Caudal neuropore closes; 3 pharyngeal bars; upper limb buds appearing.
13	30–?	4–6	28	28–32	Four limb buds; lens disc; otic vesicle.
14		5–7	32	31–35	Lens pit and optic cup; endolymphatic appendage distinct.
15		7–9	33	35–38	Lens vesicle; nasal pit; antitragus beginning; hand plate; trunk relatively wider; cerebral vesicles distinct.
16		8–11	37	37–42	Nasal pit faces ventrally; retinal pigment visible in intact embryo; auricular hillocks beginning; foot plate.
17		11–14	41	42–44	Head relatively larger; trunk straighter; nasofrontal groove distinct; auricular hillocks distinct; finger rays.
18		13–17	44	44–48	Body more cuboidal; elbow region and toe rays appearing; eyelids beginning; tip of nose distinct; nipples appear; ossification may begin.
19		16–18	47.5	48–51	Trunk elongating and straightening.
20		18–22	50.5	51–53	Upper limbs longer and bent at elbows
21		22–24	52	53–54	Fingers longer; hands approach each other, feet likewise.
22		23–28	54	54–56	Eyelids and external ear more developed.
23		27–31	56.5	56–60	Head more rounded; limbs longer and more developed.

[1] Olivier, G. & Pineau, H. (1962) *C.R. Ass. Anat.* **47**, 573–576 for stages 11–23; miscellaneous for stages 1–10.

[2] Jirásek, J.E. (1971) *Development of the genital system and male pseudohermaphroditism.* Johns Hopkins Press, Baltimore.

1
Mitosis and Meiosis

The basic concept of the cell as the fundamental unit of biological structure stems from the work of Schleiden and Schwann who, in 1838, proposed that organisms are made up entirely of smaller units or cells and their products. In just over a century this idea has become commonplace and its extraordinary impact all but forgotten. Without it we could not begin to think of development in a meaningful way, but largely as a result of it we are able to divide embryological processes into three essential and to some extent interrelated processes. The first of these is *growth* which involves cell growth, cell division and the elaboration of extra-cellular materials. Conceptually this may be separated from *morphogenesis* which includes mass cell movements, allowing new cells to inter-react with each other as well as with extra-cellular structures such as basement membranes and results in the formation of discrete organs. *Differentiation* from the single fertilized egg to a multiplicity of adult cells and tissues performing specialized functions provides the third fundamental of development. Although these ideas will be further elaborated at various points in this book they should be borne in mind wherever any ontogenic process is being considered.

During embryogenesis a dividing cell must pass on its total genetic potential (or *genome*) to each of its daughter cells. It is true that differentiation implies that only restricted portions of the genome are allowed to function in each cell type but the balance of evidence points to the fact that the whole of the genome is represented in each nucleated cell.

In all but the simplest cells such as bacteria, the genetic material is contained (with some exceptions not pertinent to this argument) in a specialized cell nucleus in which it is present in organized structures known as *chromosomes*. The latter contain information in the form of a code which the cellular synthetic machinery can decipher to form its specific protein constituents and secretions. Biologists call each unit of information a *gene* and biochemists prefer to use the term *cistron*. Genes are arranged in a linear fashion along the length of chromosomes. Between divisions (the so-called *interphase*) the cell is concerned with making protein under the direction of its genes and its chromosomes are extremely elongated so that no known method of staining is able to demonstrate them individually. In growing tissues a cell, when it reaches an optimal size, undergoes division during which morphologically discrete chromosomes appear and divide longitudinally so that a full complement of new chromosomes (representing the whole genome) passes to each daughter cell. This process is known as *mitosis*.

The cell cycle

In some adult organs certain differentiated cells such as nerve cells *never* divide. Other organs in the same individual contain cells such as those of the liver parenchyma which divide only occasionally. This occurs when an extra functional load is put upon the liver so that its individual cells have either got to multiply or would have to increase their cytoplasmic mass to a point at which the nucleo-cytoplasmic ratio is such that they could not function optimally. A third category of cells continue to divide throughout life — for example, relatively undifferentiated cells in the skin, gut lining, nails, hair etc. are continually dividing to make good the mechanical wear and tear to which the structure is subject.

The interval between one cell division and the next in continually dividing cells is known as the cell cycle (Fig. 1.1). It consists of a G1 phase immediately following mitosis and characterised by active protein synthesis. This is followed by an S phase during which the DNA of the cell nucleus replicates but protein synthesis still continues; finally, another short phase of protein synthesis G2 is terminated by the onset of the next mitosis. Most adult cells, however, are not continually dividing and may remain for many weeks in interphase. Sometime during this period the cell may enter a transition phase which ends with a division signal so that after a lag period the doubling of its DNA content (at the S phase) begins. In embryonic tissues many (perhaps most) of the undifferentiated cells progress immediately from one cell cycle into the next. Sooner or later some

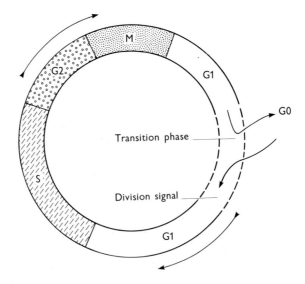

Fig. 1.1. Diagram to illustrate the cell cycle. See text for description.

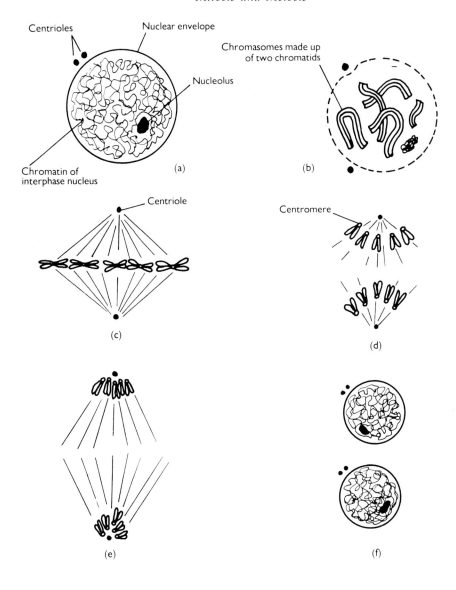

Fig. 1.2. The nucleus in mitosis:
(a) Interphase.
(b) Prophase.
(c) Metaphase.
(d) Anaphase.
(e) Telophase.
(f) Reconstitution of interphase nuclei.

of their progeny will cease to divide continually. At this stage they gradually take on specific tissue characteristics and are said to *differentiate* (Chapter 19). Some authors describe these cells as having passed into a so-called 'G0' stage of interphase. It should be remembered, however, that they can — as in the case of the adult liver — re-enter the division cycle if subjected to the appropriate division signal.

Mitosis

The first event relevant to cell division is the replication of deoxyribonucleic acid (DNA) which is the chemical code referred to above as being present in chromosomes and which forms the essential (though by no means the only) part of each of these structures. It is necessary to recall that DNA replication and therefore, in effect, chromosome duplication takes place during the S period of cell interphase when the chromosomes are not demonstrable as discrete units. In stained sections they are seen in the nucleus only as fine granular basophilic chromatin.

Mitosis is said to begin (somewhat arbitrarily) with the stage of *prophase* in which the chromosomes become visible as elongated threadlike structures still contained within the nuclear envelope (Fig. 1.2). Close inspection often reveals that each chromosome is made up of two strands known as *chromatids*. Soon the nuclear envelope disappears and this marks the onset of metaphase. Two small organelles known as *centrioles* which were closely associated with each other at one side of the nucleus during interphase become active and, as mitosis proceeds, one of these migrates to the opposite pole of the nucleus. A spindle made up of fibrous proteins in the form of microtubules is formed in which the tubules appear to be of two types. One form — the *continuous fibres* — runs between the centrioles while the other attaches the chromatids to the centrioles (*chromosomal fibres*).

The chromosomes which are now much shortened arrange themselves along the equator of the spindle and appear to become attached to the chromosomal fibres by a constricted region known as the *centromere* which also represents the only point of junction between the sister chromatids comprising each chromosome. There then follows the stage of *anaphase* at which the centromere of each chromosome divides and each member of a pair of chromatids begins to move along the spindle (centromere first) to opposite poles of the cell. The mechanics of this movement are not understood but result in each daughter chromatid — which may now be regarded as a chromosome in its own right — reaching opposite poles of the spindle at the final stage of nuclear division or *telophase*. The nuclear membrane is reformed at this stage and cytoplasmic division usually follows as the result (in animal cells) of a constriction of the cell membrane. The centriole associated with each of the two new nuclei now divides and the condensed chromosomes once again become the attenuated structures characteristic of interphase. Mitosis is diagrammatically represented in Fig. 1.2.

The normal human karyotype

Until 1956 it was believed that man had 48 chromosomes but in that year Tjio and Levan, using improved techniques, were able to demonstrate conclusively that the true number was 46. A variety of methods is now available for studying the human chromosome constitution of *karyotype* (*vide infra*) but all of these rely upon a number of common principles. First of all it is necessary to study a tissue in which a large number of cells are in mitosis and to this end the drugs colchicine or colcemid are usually added to cell cultures of the tissue because of their ability to arrest cell division at metaphase. It is thus possible to make preparations of a variety of tissues in which mitotic figures are very numerous. Secondly, the introduction of a chemical known as phytohaemagglutinin (and more recently a number of related compounds) has made it possible to perform much of this work on blood cultures. Phytohaemagglutinin has the dual effect of agglutinating red blood cells and stimulating cell division in the lymphocyte series of white cells; it is thus possible to karyotype individuals without resorting to cultures of red marrow obtained from sternal puncture, or of biopsies of skin unless the particular cells in these body regions are of interest.

Finally, treatment of cells in metaphase arrest with hypotonic solutions causes them to swell and by dropping them onto a wet slide followed by air drying, the chromosomes are spread by a quasi-explosive action, their resulting separation allowing individual morphological assessment. The usual practice is to photo-graph such a preparation (*the metaphase plate*) stained with a specific chromosome stain (Fig. 1.3) under oil immersion, to prepare a montage of the individual chromosomes by placing them in homologous pairs according to their morpho-logical characteristics and to assign each pair a number; this arrangement is called the karyotype. A widely accepted grouping of the chromosome pairs into seven groups A–G (each member of which, it will be remembered, is seen at metaphase as two chromatids joined by the primary constriction or centromere) now exists (Table 1.1). The groups of chromosomes are distinguished depending upon the position of the centromere which may be *median* (*metacentric*), *submedian* (*submetacentric*) or *subterminal* (*acrocentric*); chromosome size is also taken into

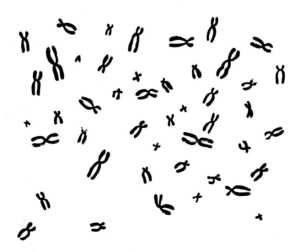

Fig. 1.3. The cell chromosomes prepared for karyotyping (a so-called *metaphase plate* preparation).

Table 1.1 Human chromosome groups.

Group	Pair Numbers	Description
A	1−3	Pairs 1 (metacentric) and 2 (submetacentric are the longest. Pair 3 (metacentric) are a little smaller.
B	4−5	Submetacentric. About the same size as pair 3.
C	6−12 (and X)	Pairs of submetacentric chromosomes of medium, but decreasing size
D	13−15	Acrocentric. Smaller than Group C. Often satellited.
E	16−18	Pair 16 are metacentric small chromosomes; 17 and 18 are submetacentric and a little shorter.
F	19−20	Small metacentric pairs.
G	21−22 (and Y)	Small, acrocentric. 21 and 22 are often satellited but Y is not.

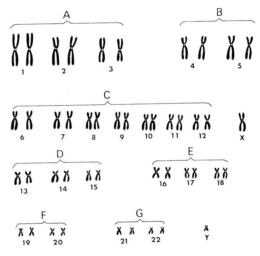

Fig. 1.4.(a) The male karyotype.

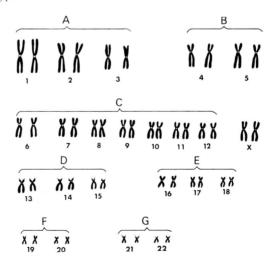

Fig. 1.4. (b) The female karyotype.

account, as is the presence of so-called *satellites* or masses of chromatin attached to the short arms of certain chromosomes.

In each cell, 44 of the chromosomes are known as *autosomes* (22 pairs) and the remaining pair as *sex chromosomes*. In the female, the latter are an identical pair of medium sized chromosomes with a submedian centromere called X chromosomes. The male possesses a single X chromosome together with a small acrocentric Y chromosome which has been supposed by some workers to contain male determining genes but 'maleness' is now known to depend upon a Y-linked antigen, which is further discussed in Chapter 15. Figs. 1.4a and b show the karyotypes of a normal male and female.

Within the chromosome groups the individual chromosomes are arranged in order of decreasing size. Using conventional staining methods it is often impossible to recognise individual chromosomes by number but various special methods of staining bands along the length of the chromosome have solved this problem. At first quinacrine mustard or quinacrine dihydrochloride was used to produce a fluorescent banding pattern. This is known as the Q staining method and the resulting stained Q bands are satisfactorily reproducible. A Giemsa dye-staining mixture produces G bands in an essentially similar pattern to the Q bands while the reverse staining Giemsa method gives R bands which are opposite in intensity to the G staining methods. Present day technology is thus sufficiently advanced to identify chromosomal abnormalities with confidence and much work is presently directed towards automating the whole system of routine karyotyping. Interested readers are referred to the 'Paris Conference' (1971) and to its 1975 supplement on Standardisation in Human Cytogenetics which present detailed diagrams and photographs of the individual bands found on each chromosome.

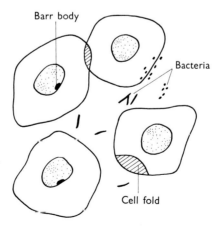

Fig. 1.5. Cells from a buccal smear from a female. Note the Barr bodies.

Sex chromatin

In 1949, after microscopists had been studying cells with quite sophisticated compound microscopes for over half a century, Barr and Bertram made the startling observation that the nuclei of male and female cells are morphologically distinguishable. They saw that a large proportion of interphase nuclei from female tissues (and the exact percentage varies with the techniques used) contained a characteristic small condensed mass of chromatin often lying against the nuclear membrane (Fig. 1.5). There is reason to believe that all female cells after early embryonic development contain this so-called *sex chromatin* (the Barr Body) at least at some stage during interphase and it is particularly easy to distinguish in certain human tissues. The most convenient method of examining Barr bodies in patients is by making preparations of stained epithelial cells from buccal smears. With experience, sex chromatin can be identified in over 20 per cent of cells from good smears of normal females, while practically none of the male cells show condensed chromatin which could be mistaken for sex chromatin by skilled workers. In polymorphonuclear leucocytes the sex chromatin looks rather like a drumstick (Fig. 1.6) which is identifiable in about 3 per cent of female polymorphonuclear leucocytes.

The significance of this mass of condensed chromatin characteristic of female cells is now becoming apparent. Figs. 1.4a and b show that the female karyotype contains two X chromosomes while the male contains a single X and a Y chromosome. Chapter 2 explains that many genes on the X chromosomes are concerned with the transmission of phenotypic characteristics not concerned with sex. Over 50 such traits are already known and there are no doubt many others. Furthermore, Chapter 2 also illustrates the untoward consequences of an excess of chromosomal material in conditions such as Down's syndrome. It has therefore been

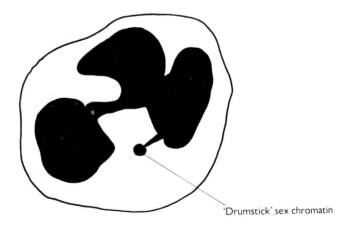

'Drumstick' sex chromatin

Fig. 1.6. The sex chromatin in a polymorphonuclear leucocyte.

suggested that the sex chromatin in normal female interphase nuclei represents much of one of the X chromosomes in a condensed, inactive form. As a result both sexes have a similar non-sexual genetic constitution and differ only in the possession of a Y chromosome by the male (which appears to be exclusively related to male sexual characteristics).

There is evidence that this explanation is an over-simplification; for example, an individual with an abnormal karyotype having only one X and no Y chromosomes (XO or Turner's syndrome) is not a phenotypically normal female (Chapter 2). Thus it may be that both sex chromosomes are active early during development, for the sex chromatin does not appear until later embryonic stages. It remains likely, however, that the Barr body represents some sort of dosage compensation for the excess of genetic material in the XX genotype. Interestingly enough, in individuals with abnormalities in the number of their sex chromosomes the number of Barr bodies in each nucleus is one fewer than the number of X chromosomes

The fluorescent Y chromosome

Recently it has been demonstrated that Y chromosomes in interphase nuclei can be visualized by staining with certain fluorescent dyes. Regions of some autosomal pairs can also be made to fluoresce under appropriate conditions. There is no question of dosage compensation here, but these powerful new techniques may add greatly to the number and flexibility of current cytogenetic techniques.

Meiosis

The human karyotypes shown in Fig. 1.4 make it clear that chromosomes can be separated into homologous pairs, one member of each pair being derived from each parent. The mammalian individual is therefore *diploid*, which implies that he carries 2n chromosomes in each cell. In the human, as we have seen, n is equal to 23, there being 22 pairs of autosomes and one pair of sex chromosomes. When sexual reproduction occurs, it is clear that the sex cells or gametes must halve their chromosome number to the *haploid* (n) condition. This is achieved by a process of *meiosis* or *reduction division* which also involves considerable *crossing over* (*vide infra*) of genetic material between homologous chromosomes. A significant heterogeneity is thereby achieved which allows the transmission of genetic material in a vast number of combinations. Inevitably this has considerable evolutionary significance.

Meiosis consists of two separate, but closely associated, cell divisions (Fig. 1.7) and, as in the case of mitosis, DNA duplication occurs before the morphological phenomena of cell division are manifest. In the first cell division the chromosome number is halved and this is followed by a modified mitotic division. The

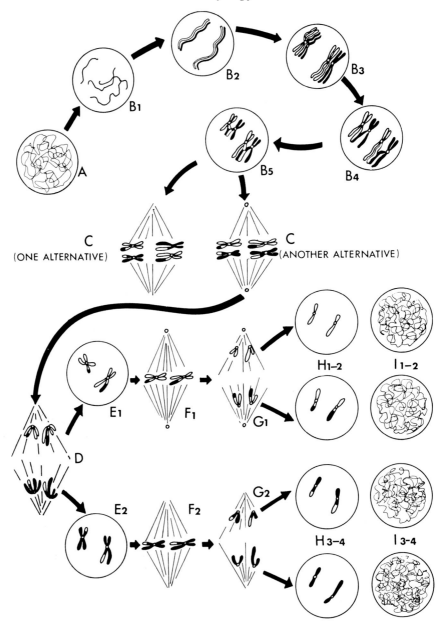

Fig. 1.7. Meiosis as it may affect two pairs of homologous chromosomes in man:

A Interphase	E1 Telophase I
B1 Leptotene	E2 Telophase I
B2 Zygotene	F1 Metaphase II
B3 Pachytene	F2 Metaphase II
B4 Diplotene	G1 Anaphase II
B5 Diakinesis	G2 Anaphase II
C Metaphase I	H1-4 Telophase II
D Anaphase I	I1-4 Interphase (haploid) germ cells

B1–B5 Prophase I

prophase of meiosis is prolonged and arbitrarily divided into 5 stages. It begins with *leptotene* when the chromosomes first become apparent as long thin strands and although their DNA content is double that of early interphase chromosomes (i.e. comparable to the DNA content of cells after the S phase of the cell cycle) each appears to be single, there being no morphological evidence of two chromatids at this stage. The following *zygotene* stage involves the pairing of homologous chromosomes in a very exact manner so that they match up precisely point for point; this is sometimes referred to as *synapsis*. The only exceptions are the X and Y chromosomes which are not homologous for most of their length and appear to show terminal association only. At the next or *pachytene* stage the chromosomes thicken and their centromeres are apparent. Each pair of chromosomes is now known as a *bivalent*. At the *diplotene* stage the bivalents begin to separate except at various points of residual contact known as *chiasmata* which mark the extremities of portions of chromatids exchanged between homologous chromosomes in a process known as 'crossing over' (Fig. 1.8). *Diakinesis* follows diplotene and is accompanied by further chromosome shortening; it leads to *metaphase 1* when the nuclear envelope disappears, a spindle forms and the centromeres of the bivalents arrange themselves one above and one below the equator. The bivalents are attached to the spindle in a random way so that the maternally or the paternally derived partner may be on either side of the equator (see p.18 for the consequence of this fact upon inheritance). *Anaphase 1* follows, at which the individual centromeres begin to move to the opposite poles of the spindle. The chiasmata are thus pulled apart and crossing over is completed. Each chromosome is clearly separated into two chromatids which are attached to each other only at the centromere. At *telophase 1* a nuclear membrane reforms and two cells with a

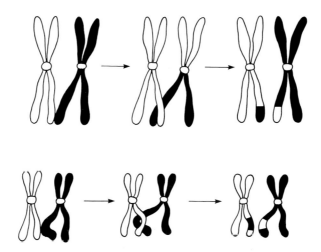

Fig. 1.8. Detailed diagram of chiasma formation followed by crossing over during diplotene (see Fig. 1.7, B_4, B_5 and C).

haploid number of chromosomes are formed. Their morphological nature is discussed in Chapter 3. Testicular material with cells in meiosis can be prepared for the visualization of chromosomes in a similar way to that described above for mitotic nuclei; such methods are of particular value in the study of various abnormal conditions such as the end-on attachment (*translocation*) of one chromosome to another as described in Chapter 2. *Metaphase II* and *anaphase II* which are essentially mitotic always follow the telophase of the first stage of meiosis although their nature and timing varies in the testis and in the ovary. New spindles are formed and the centromeres of the (now haploid) number of chromosomes divide allowing the chromatids to pass to opposite spindle poles. New cells reform and the net effect of meiosis is the formation of four haploid descendants of the original cell.

Further reading

Casperson, J. & Zech, L. (eds.) (1973) Chromosome identification, in: *Nobel Symposia on Medicine and Natural Sciences*. Academic Press, New York.

Ford, C.E. (1975) General mammalian cytogenetics, in: 'The Cell in Medical Science', Vol. II. (eds.) Beck, F. & Lloyd, J.B. Academic Press.

John, B. & Lewis, K.R. (1972) *Somatic Cell Division*. Oxford University Press.

John, B. & Lewis, K.R. (1976) *The Meiotic Mechanism*. Oxford Biology Readers. Oxford University Press.

Lewin, B. (1980) *Gene Expression*, Vol. 2, Eukaryotic chromosomes, 2nd edn., Chapters 4 and 7. Wiley, New York.

Nora, Jas. J. & Clarke Fraser, F. (eds.) (1981) The chromosomal basis of heredity, in: *Medical Genetics*, 2nd edn, pp. 10–35. Lea & Febiger.

Paris Conference (1971) Standardisation in human cytogenetics. *Birth Defects* 8:7. 1972. New York, The National Foundation: Report of the Standing Committee on Human Cytogenetic Nomenclature (1978) *Birth Defects* **14**:8, 1978.

Tjio, J.H. & Levan, A. (1959) A chromosome number in man. *Hereditas Lund*, **42**, 1.

2

Unifactorial and Multifactorial Inheritance, Mutations

It is appropriate to begin a section on unifactorial inheritance in man by defining a number of common genetic terms, many of which will doubtless be familiar to the reader but which are so frequently used (and misused) that their precise meaning becomes fundamentally important.

The sum of an individual's manifest physical, chemical and biological characteristics, i.e. those features revealed by appropriate physical and biochemical examination, is known as his *phenotype*. This is determined by the interaction of his genetic make-up with his past and present environment. The genetic make-up is called the *genotype* and consists of all usable or potentially usable genes, i.e. the total hereditary possibility. We have seen that the somatic cell is diploid (p.9), in other words that its nucleus contains 22 *pairs* of autosomes and a pair of sex chromosomes, one member of each pair being of maternal and the other of paternal origin. A gene situated on an autosome and coding for a particular characteristic or *trait* (for example, blood group M, p.16) will therefore be matched by a corresponding gene situated at an identical site or *gene locus* on the corresponding homologous chromosome. Such genes may be identical (i.e. the corresponding gene on the homologous chromosome may also code for blood group M), alternatively the second gene may produce *different* effects *on the same phenotypic characteristic* (as would be the case if one member of the gene pair coded for blood group M and the other for blood group N). When there is a possibility of two *or more* varieties of a particular gene occupying a specific gene locus on a pair of homologous chromosomes then these varieties are known as *alleles* or *allelomorphs*. When a choice of several alleles exists for an individual gene locus (as in the case of the ABO blood group system — *vide infra*) then we are dealing with what are known as *multiple alleles* though, of course, no more than two members of a series can be present in a single diploid cell. Mutation (p.22) of one member of an allelomorphic series to another, though very rare, is an important biological phenomenon.

An individual may bear the gene for blood group substance M on one chromosome and that for N on its homologue. The phenotype will then be MN and these alleles are said to be *codominant* (i.e. each is expressed in the phenotype even in the presence of the other). Under certain circumstances, however, only one gene of a contrasting pair is *phenotypically* manifest. This gene is then said to be *dominant* while its allele is *recessive*. The phenotype therefore does not give a complete picture of the genotype since a large number of genes will be denied obvious expression by their dominant alleles. The concept of dominance is a relative one and, in some cases, if one uses sophisticated techniques it is often possible to pick up the products of the so-called recessive gene or, put in another way, the effects of the polypeptide resulting from transcription and translation of the recessive cistron. There is therefore a gradation from almost complete recessivity through codominance to complete dominance. When an individual possesses an identical pair of genes at a given gene locus on homologous chromosomes he is said to be *homozygous* for the particular gene in question; if the genes differ he is *heterozygous*. From what has been said it is clear that a single (diploid) individual can only possess two alleles although a considerable number of variants can exist for a particular gene in the population at large.

Mendel's first law

This is also known as the law of purity of *gametes* i.e. germ cells (Chapter 3). It states that only *one* of a pair of alleles can be represented in a single gamete. Reference to the mechanics of meiosis (Chapter 1) makes it clear that the haploid germ cell only contains one set of chromosomes and, therefore, only one set of genes; fertilization will involve the combination of a paternal and a maternal set thereby re-creating the diploid condition and the presence of pairs of homologous genes in each genotype (see Tables 2.2−2.5 for examples).

Dominant and recessive inheritance

Dominant inheritance

The dominant inheritance of hundreds of human traits is well enough documented to be beyond doubt. They are easily identified if they produce a readily recognisable deviation from the normal. In such cases, however, the traits often produce such severe effects that affected individuals fail to reproduce. An example is

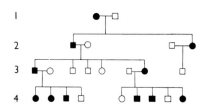

Fig. 2.1. A family tree showing dominant nystagmus:
● Affected female   ■ Affected male
○ Normal female   □ Normal male
(from Allen, M., *J. Hered.*, 1942)

achondroplasia (due to a gene affecting the skeleton and causing dwarfism) where about ⁷/₈ of all cases are the result of new gene mutations (*vide infra.* p.136). Other examples are of little clinical significance and here classical family trees with an average of 50 per cent of the offspring (of either sex) showing the dominant trait present in one parent are seen through many generations. An example is shown in Fig. 2.1 which illustrates the transmission of a condition known as hereditary nystagmus, a minor affliction of the eyes which exhibit involuntary jerking movements. One form of this condition is inherited as a dominant trait and in the example given one or more members of four generations are affected. A difficulty in the evaluation of hereditable human characteristics is that experimental matings cannot be done so that one has to rely upon carefully collected family data. One pedigree such as that shown in Fig. 2.1 is insufficient in itself to indicate the mode of inheritance beyond doubt, and accumulated data from several sources must be relied upon.

Even dominant genes may vary in *expressivity* i.e. the degree to which they are expressed in the phenotype. This is because genes do not work in isolation; their activity may be modified by the action of other genes or by the environment and by such means their phenotypic expression may be enhanced or diminished. Sometimes expressivity can be so reduced that a dominant gene may appear to have missed a generation, particularly if the individual bearing it is not examined closely. On the other hand, in conditions such as achondroplasia (*vide supra*) in which the dominant gene is expressed in all individuals who carry it, expressivity is said to be 100 per cent.

Other difficulties in making correct assessments of human inheritance exist, such as bias in sampling affected families. The *index case* or *reference* individual, i.e. the person in whom the trait is first recognised, is likely to exhibit it to a marked degree; when his pedigree is examined, his parents, grandparents etc. may have escaped earlier detection because they showed reduced expressivity and a spurious impression of progressive enhancement is thus created.

When two heterozygous dominants marry, approximately one offspring in every four will be homozygous for the dominant gene and about 3 out of 4 will have phenotypic evidence of its presence. This is illustrated in the checkerboard diagram shown in Table 2.1. When a dominant trait is deleterious it is frequently found that homozygous individuals express it to a degree that may be incompatible with life. Such a situation is found in the major deformities characteristic of homozygous achondroplastic fetuses; it clearly illustrates that the terms dominant and recessive are no more than convenient approximations to the facts.

Recessive inheritance

According to Mendelian principles mating between heterozygotes will produce an average proportion of one homozygous recessive, in which the recessive gene finds phenotypic expression and one homozygous dominant plus two heterozygotes in which it does not (Table 2.2).

Table 2.1. 'Checkerboard diagram' to illustrate a double heterozygote cross from which it will be seen that three out of four offspring show the dominant trait phenotypically (†). (Ā is the dominant allele. A is the recessive allele).

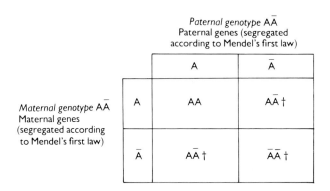

Table 2.2. 'Checkerboard diagram' similar to Table 2.1 of a double heterozygous cross to illustrate that the recessive gene will find expression in only one out of four offspring (†). B is the dominant allele. B̄ is the recessive allele.

Paternal genes	Maternal genes	
	B	B̄
B	BB	BB̄
B̄	B̄B	B̄B̄†

In practice the examination of brothers and sisters of homozygous recessives will result in a higher proportion of affected individuals than would be expected from the ratio of 3 unaffected to 1 affected. This is because a mating of 2 heterozygotes will be revealed only if they produce at least one affected child. The other heterozygous matings will be excluded from the sample.

The chances of producing homozygous recessives are increased in family pedigrees in which there is consanguineous mating (as, for instance, between first cousins). The rarer the recessive gene in question, the more important this factor becomes because the chances of two heterozygotes for the same gene marrying is slight for the population at large. On the other hand the chance of two unrelated heterozygotes marrying becomes greater with the frequency of the recessive allele in the gene pool of the population at large.

Codominance

This mode of inheritance is well illustrated by the transmission of the M and N

Table 2.3. 'Checkerboard diagram' similar to Tables 2.1 and 2.2 of a heterozygous cross between MN parents. Since the genes are codominant half of the offspring will be *phenotypically* MN.

Paternal genes	Maternal genes	
	M	N
M	MM	NN
N	NM	MN

blood group factors. Among the various antigens (i.e. specific substances capable of producing an immune response) present on the surface of red cells are two variants known as M and N. These are transmitted by allelic genes at the MN gene locus. The alleles in question are codominant so that cells from a heterozygous individual will stimulate the production of antibodies (i.e. serum proteins reacting with antigens) to both M and N if his blood is injected into (say) a rabbit. The situation is best illustrated by the double heterozygous mating shown in Table 2.3.

Recently it has been found that other (rarer) alleles at the MN gene locus exist (e.g. M_2, N_2, M^g, N^c) and that a gene locus coding for the blood groups S/s is so closely linked that crossover does not occur. This does not alter the fact that both M and N (in whatever allelic form they may be present) are *both* represented in the *phenotype* when they are present together.

X-linked inheritance

Genes on the sex chromosomes fall into a special category because the chromosomal constitution differs between males (XY) and females (XX), (Chapter 1). As on the autosomes, genes located on X chromosomes may be dominant or recessive but the unique quality of *X-linked inheritance* is that in the male a recessive gene located on the X chromosome is expressed phenotypically. This is because the male has only one X chromosome and consequently none of the genes on it can be masked by dominant alleles. In this connection the male is frequently referred to as *hemizygous*.

It is clear that X-linked traits cannot be transmitted from father to son (Table 2.4) because males transmit their X chromosomes only to daughters and Y chromosomes only to sons. By means of simple 'checkerboard diagrams' the reader will be able to work out for himself the results of various matings involving X-linked genes. It will be clear than an X-linked dominant gene will affect both males and females but, unlike autosomal dominant inheritance, affected fathers will transmit the trait to *all* their daughters but to *none* of their sons. X-linked recessive genes can also be phenotypically manifest in the female if they are present in the homozygous condition but this will only happen if a heterozygous female marries an affected male.

Table 2.4. Transmission of an X-linked trait (X̄) from an affected father to his offspring.
Note: Both daughters are 'carriers' of the condition if it is recessive but will exhibit it if it is dominant.
The father cannot transmit the trait to his sons.

Paternal genes	Maternal genes	
	X	X
X̄	X̄X	X̄X
Y	XY	XY

Over 50 X-linked genes have been demonstrated in man, the best known being that for classical haemophilia A, a recessive gene which has achieved fame by virtue of its presence in some of the royal families of Europe.

Reference to X-linked rather than to sex linked inheritance has been made in this section. The latter expression is often used but X-linked is considered more accurate since genes not associated with sexual characteristics have never been conclusively demonstrated on human Y chromosomes.

Sex limited characteristics

This is really a special form of variation in the expressivity of a gene in so far as the degree of expressivity is related to the sex of the individual. For example, pattern baldness (Fig. 2.2) a phenotypic trait of premature hair loss which runs in the males of certain families is carried by a dominant autosomal gene but, when heterozygous, is only expressed in the hormonal environment of the male. Hence, as a rule, only men will exhibit pattern baldness although phenotypically normal heterozygous women inherit the gene and transmit it to their offspring. If the gene is homozygous it is phenotypically manifest even in women whose hair becomes sparse — another example of the potentiation of effects when a dominant gene is homozygous. The crucial difference between sex-linked and X-linked inheritance is the fact that the former can be transmitted from father to son while the latter (as explained in the previous section) cannot. It is interesting that baldness can occur in a heterozygous female if the hormonal environment is changed as, for example, by a masculinising tumour.

Mendel's second law

This is the law of independent assortment of genes. It implies that, in gametes, either of a pair of alleles at one gene locus may be combined with either of another pair at *another* gene locus. The physical basis of this phenomenon is understandable when the mechanism of meiosis is reviewed (see Chapter 1). At Metaphase I, pairs of homologous chromosomes arrange themselves at the

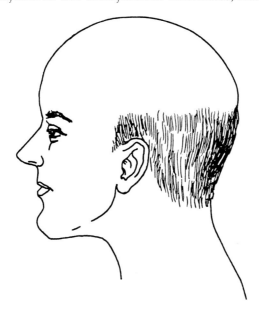

Fig. 2.2. Pattern baldness in the male.

equatorial plate of the meiotic spindle. If we consider just two pairs of homologous chromosomes it is obvious that two situations arise with equal frequency at the succeeding anaphase. This is illustrated in Fig. 2.3 where one homologous pair of chromosomes is called a and a' and the other b and b'. In example (i) chromosome a, represented by a continuous line, finds it way into the same cell as chromosome b, which is also represented by a continuous line. In example (ii) however, chromosome a is segregated with chromosome b', represented by a stippled line. For the sake of simplicity we have assumed that no crossing (see Chapter 1) has occurred.

Idealised matings between heterozygotes for *two* traits that assort independently (double heterozygote matings) will produce a phenotypic distribution of $9 + 3 + 3 + 1$ (Table 2.5a). This may also be expressed as $(3 + 1)^2$, 2 being the number of independently assorting characteristics. A double heterozygote mating with a double homozygous recessive (the so-called double back cross) will produce a ratio of $1:1:1:1$ (Table 2.5b). The examples given in Table 2.5 involve the dominant gene (T) representing an ability to taste phenylthiourea (a substance which to some individuals has a highly unpleasant taste but which to others is quite tasteless) under carefully controlled conditions. This gene assorts independently to another gene (Se) which in its dominant form, controls the ability to secrete the blood group substances ABO into various body fluids (e.g. saliva). The situation is naturally modified in other cases where dominance is incomplete.

A simple example of independent assortment is provided by Fig. 2.4 taken from an actual case history and illustrating that two rare variants of normal

Table 2.5a. The results of mating double heterozygotes having the ability to taste phenylthiourea (dominant, T; recessive, t) and the ability to secrete ABO antigens into the saliva (dominant, Se; recessive, se).

		Paternal genotype Tt/Sese Paternal genes (Produced in equal numbers)			
		T/Se	t/Se	T/se	t/se
Maternal genotype	T/Se	TT/SeSe	Tt/SeSe	TT/Sese	Tt/Sese
Tt/Sese	t/Se	tT/SeSe	tt/Sese	Tt/Sese	tt/sese
Maternal genes (produced in equal	T/se	TT/Sese	Tt/Sese	TT/sese	Tt/sese
numbers)	t/se	Tt/Sese	tt/Sese	Tt/sese	tt/sese

Results: 9 tasters and secretors,   non-tasters and secretors,
           3 tasters and non-secretors and 1 non-taster and non-secretor.
           9:3:3:1.

Table 2.5b. The results of a back cross mating between a double heterozygote (able to taste phenylthiourea and to secrete blood ABO antigens into the saliva) and a homozygous non-taster, non-secretor.

			Paternal genotype Tt/Sese Paternal genes (Produced in equal numbers			
			T/Se	t/Se	T/se	t/se
Maternal genotype tt/sese	Maternal genes (All of one type only)	t/se	Tt/Sese	tt/Sese	Tt/sese	tt/sese

Results: One taster and secretor.
          One non-taster and secretor.
          One taster and non-secretor.
          One non-taster and non-secretor
          1:1:1:1.

haemoglobin (haemoglobin S and haemoglobin Hopkins 2) are inherited independently. Not surprisingly the variants are due to changes on different chains of the haemoglobin molecule since these are coded on different cistrons. Haemoglobin S is due to a change in the β-chain while haemoglobin Hopkins 2 is a variation in the α-chain. Gene loci coding for the α and β chains are therefore not linked (*vide infra* for explanations of linkage).

Linkage

The reader will no doubt have appreciated that Mendel's second law requires qualification when the gene loci in question lie relatively close to each other on the same chromosome. Such genes are said to be *linked* and will usually segregate

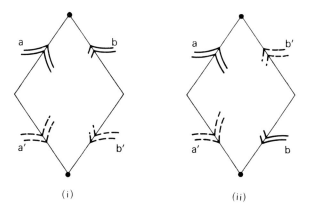

Fig. 2.3. For explanation see text.

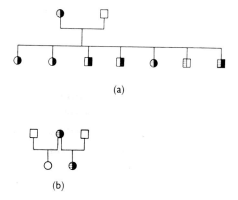

Fig. 2.4. Two parts of a family described by Bradley, Boyer & Allen (1961), ('Hopkins-2-haemoglobin: A revised pedigree with data on blood and serum groups.' *Bull. Johns Hopkins Hospital*, **108**, pp. 75–9. The Johns Hopkins Press) showing that the gene for haemoglobin S and that for haemoglobin Hopkins 2 assort independently. In (a) a doubly affected female has passed both traits to two of her offspring while in (b) a doubly affected female has had one daughter with both traits and one with neither:

⊞ ◕   Male and female with haemoglobin Hopkins 2

◼ ◑   Male and female with haemoglobin S

together. An example is provided by the nail-patella syndrome. This dominant syndrome of congenital malformations consisting of defective nails, dislocation of the radial heads, small patellae and horn-like projections from the iliac bones is determined at a gene locus which is present on the same chromosome as the ABO blood group locus. *Provided no crossing over takes place* the nail-patella syndrome will always be inherited with the same blood group locus. This is illustrated in Fig. 2.5. A complication is introduced by the phenomenon of 'crossing over'

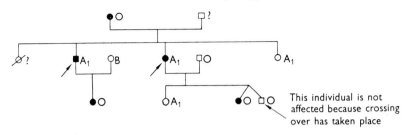

Fig. 2.5. Part of a family described by Renwick & Lawler (*Ann. Hum. Genet. Lond.*, 1955) showing inheritance of the nail-patella syndrome consistent with linkage to blood group O. The example illustrates the phenomenon of linkage masked by dominance because the individuals marked ↗ must have had the phenotype AO. Thus in this family although nail-patella allele is present on a chromosome bearing the gene for blood group O, two blood group A phenotypes manifest the condition.

Ø stillbirth   ■ affected male
                  ● affected female
                  □ normal male
                  ○ normal female
                     dizygotic twins
The blood group phenotype is written beside each individual.

during meiosis (Chapter 1); this is a process in which portions of chromatids from homologous chromosomes are exchanged in the prophase of the first meiotic division (Fig. 1.8). As a result linked alleles may become separated and *recombinant* genotypes result. By the laws of chance, crossing over will become more frequent the further apart two gene loci are on the chromosome. If they are near each other they are said to be closely linked and a measure of their proximity may be obtained by calculating the amount of crossing over which takes place.

These calculations are the basis of chromosome mapping which is beyond the scope of this volume. Suffice it to say that 1 per cent crossing over means that the two gene loci are one so-called 'map unit' apart. When loci are separated by large distances in long chromosomes, crossing over may reach the 50 per cent level in which case the genetic results are effectively those of true independent assortment as postulated by Mendel's second law.

Mutations*

Mutations are of two types, *point mutations* and *chromosome mutations*. The former term is applied to an alteration at a single gene locus. This frequently has no effect on adjacent genes although, as will be seen below, it may have a profound effect on the phenotype. Chromosome mutations, on the other hand, involve the addition, deletion or rearrangement of whole or large parts of chromosomes. It will be appreciated that while chromosome mutations can be recognised from a study of the karyotype, point mutations produce no visible change in the chromosomes.

*In this and subsequent sections a basic knowledge of functioning of the genetic code is assumed (see 'Further reading' — *Molecular Biology of the Cell*).

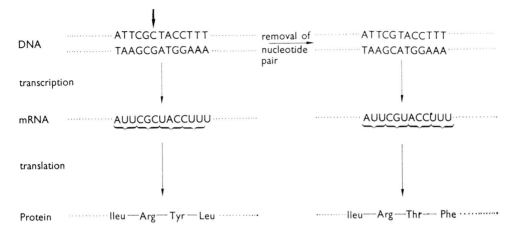

Fig. 2.6. Effect on the amino acid sequence specified of deleting one DNA nucleotide pair (at ⬇)
Note that, in this case, because of the degeneracy of the genetic code, translation of the codon
containing the deletion is unchanged. Beyond this point the amino acid sequence will be quite
different from that for the original form.

Point mutations

Theoretical considerations

Nucleic acids, although stable molecules, are not completely resistant to chemical
change and a number of agents are known that induce specific modifications in
DNA under experimental conditions. First we shall attempt to classify the various
types of change theoretically possible and deduce, from what is known about the
genetic code, their effects upon protein synthesis.

The effect of removing a single nucleotide from a strand of DNA is shown in
Fig. 2.6. The frame of reading, set by the *initiation triplet* (which begins the reading
of a cistron) will be shifted, so that an entirely different polypeptide sequence will
be specified beyond the point at which the nucleotide was removed. A similar
result is obtained if an additional nucleotide is inserted at a point in the DNA
sequence. Mutations of this type, caused by addition or deletion of nucleotides are
termed *frameshift* mutations. Unless they occur at the distal end of a cistron, so
that only a few amino acids are affected, they change the nature of the protein
produced so completely that the gene is effectively silenced.

Another type of mutant is the *base-substitution*. Here one nucleotide pair in
DNA is replaced by another. Where a purine nucleotide in one chain is replaced
by the alternative purine nucleotide (or a pyrimidine by a pyrimidine) the
mutation is further classified as a *transition*; where purine replaces pyrimidine (or
vice versa) the term *transversion* is used. The effect of a base-substitution mutation
does not alter the frame of reading of a polynucleotide, merely the translation of
one codon (i.e. a triplet of bases which selects for one amino acid). The effect on

the protein specified is, therefore, limited to one amino acid. Certain base-substitutions, because of the degeneracy of the code (i.e. the fact that one base in a codon may in certain cases have the same effect in the selection of amino acids as another one) would not even do that. Altering one amino acid in a sequence in many cases has no significant effect on the function of a protein. If, however, the amino acid in question is important in determining a protein's three-dimensional structure or forms parts of a reacting site of an enzyme the effect may be profound.

Origin of spontaneous mutations

The origin of base-substitution mutations may be found in errors made during replication. One suggested mechanism, to explain transition mutations, proposes that the bases of DNA may in their tautomeric forms base-pair with the 'wrong' nucleotide. Thus thymine could specify guanine and similarly cytosine could specify adenine. Since the bases exist only to a very minor extent in their tautomeric forms, mistakes are comparatively rare.

As already stated spontaneous mutations are sometimes of the transversion and frameshift types. The mechanisms responsible are not known, although a number of ingenious hypotheses have been advanced.

Human point mutations

Many rare human diseases are caused by the absence of a single enzyme. The defective or absent gene is presumably due to a mutation (frameshift or base-substitution) that alters the properties of the specified polypeptide sufficiently to rob it of its characteristic enzymic activity. Whether the useless polypeptide is actually produced is often not known. A heterozygote bearing one normal and one mutant gene will exhibit enzymic activity so that such conditions are inherited as recessive (autosomal or sex linked) with only individuals who are homozygous for the ineffective gene afflicted. However, heterozygotes for conditions caused by defective or absent enzymes, e.g. galactosaemia (*vide infra*), are frequently found to have markedly lower levels of the relevant enzyme than have homozygous normals. Thus rather surprisingly there is a gene dosage effect showing that the mechanisms that control gene expression cannot compensate for the absence of half of the normal quantity of genetic material. This is a very useful finding as, in an increasing number of inborn errors of metabolism, it makes possible the detection of heterozygotes.

The metabolic consequences that may result from an absent enzyme are predictable: the accumulation of the enzyme's substrate and the absence of its product. However, the presence of alternative metabolic pathways in many cases modifies these effects. The classic example of such a disease is *phenylketonuria*, in which phenylalanine hydroxylase activity is absent. Phenylalanine, unable to

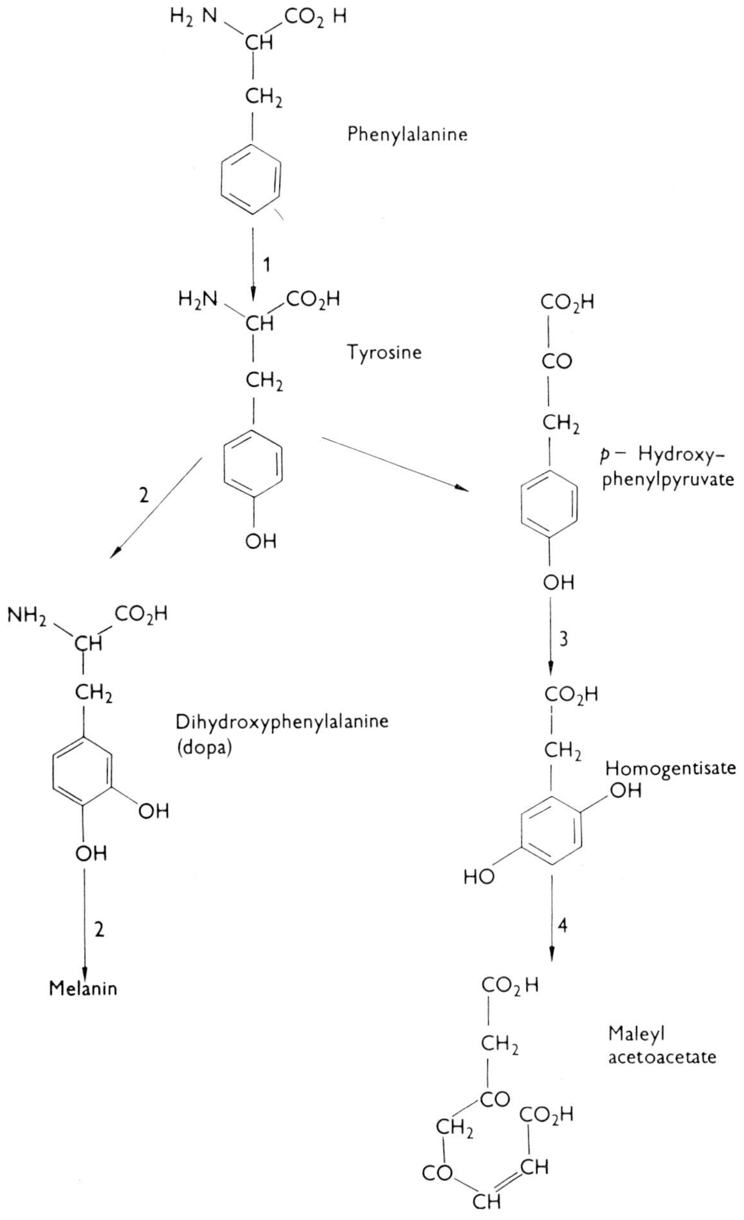

Fig. 2.7. Genetic defects in phenylalanine and tyrosine metabolism, each caused by absence of a single enzyme. 1, phenylketonuria, lack of phenylalanine hydroxylase; 2, albinism, lack of tyrosinase; 3, tyrosinosis, lack of *p*-hydroxyphenyl-pyruvate oxidase; 4, alcaptonuria, lack of homogentisate oxidase.

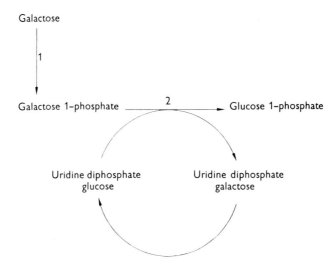

Fig. 2.8. Genetic defects in galactose metabolism. 1, galactokinase deficiency; 2, galactosaemia, lack of galactose-1-phosphate uridyl transferase.

oxidise to tyrosine, accumulates in the tissues and plasma and is in part converted to phenylpyruvic acid. The latter is not a normal constituent of plasma or urine and its presence is a key diagnostic finding. There is no significant depletion of tyrosine in phenylketonuria, because tyrosine is a normal constitutent of food protein. The pathways of phenylalanine and tyrosine metabolism are affected by a number of absent-enzyme conditions (see Fig. 2.7). So also are the pathways of galactose metabolism (Fig. 2.8). Classical *galactosaemia* is due to the absence of galactose-1-phosphate uridyl transferase while another condition has been described more recently in which galactokinase is absent. In both conditions plasma galactose is elevated.

Similar examples could be drawn from many metabolic pathways. However, those enzymes whose absence would be incompatible with the survival of the cell are exempt. This point is well illustrated by comparing the enzymes of the mitochondria and of the lysosomes. The *mitochondria* contain the enzymes of fatty acid oxidation, the tricarboxylic acid cycle and the electron transport chain; these reactions are essential to the life of the cell and a metabolic block could not be tolerated. *Lysosomes* on the other hand are concerned with the breakdown of macromolecules that accumulate as a result of the normal turnover of cell constituents. They accomplish this by their numerous hydrolytic enzymes which, between them, are able to break down most of the constituents of animal cells. Absence of any one of a number of such enzymes will result in the accumulation of undegraded macromolecules. Examples are glycogen storage disease type II (absent α-glucosidase) and Tay–Sachs disease (absent β-galactosidase). In these diseases macromolecules of various types accumulate progressively in the lysosomes, but this usually has no apparent effect upon cell function until engorged lysosomes fill virtually the whole of the cytoplasm. As a result, these diseases only have serious repercussions in long lived cells such as those of muscle and nerve.

We now turn to mutations that result in the synthesis of a slightly modified version of the normal protein. Sickle cell anaemia is the best documented example; the basic defect is in the gene coding for the β-chain of haemoglobin. In normal haemoglobin (HbA) the N terminus of this chain begins Val-His-Leu-Thr-Pro-Glu-Lys-Ser-Ala-Val...; in sickle cell haemoglobin (HbS) valine replaces glutamic acid at the sixth amino acid position. The condition is due to a transversion mutation. Many other variants of the haemoglobin molecule are known and, as might be expected, their effects on the molecule's function differ widely. Some, like HbS, are responsible for a recognisable pathology; others are chemical variants of no clinical importance. Comparison of the amino acid sequence of haemoglobin from different animal species reveals many homologies. Human and horse haemoglobins, for example, differ at only 17 out of 141 amino acid positions in the α-chain and 25 out of 146 in the β-chain. These differences presumably represent the accumulation of point mutations during separate evolution from a common ancestor. The two chains of normal haemoglobin are themselves closely related in structure. It is believed that in the distant past a gene coding for some ancestral protein underwent duplication, possibly as part of a chromosome mutation (*vide infra*). Each gene later underwent further modification by point mutation and present-day haemoglobin comprises the polypeptide products of both. This phenomenon of gene duplication is thought to explain the existence of certain isoenzymes, many of which are multimeric structures in which two or more polypeptides are combined in different proportions. Thus lactate dehydrogenase, the enzyme that interconverts pyruvate and lactate in anaerobic glycolysis, exists as five distinct isoenzymes, each a tetramer composed of different combinations of two polypeptides. If the polypeptides are termed A and B, the five isoenzymes will have the composition: A_4, A_3B, A_2B_2, AB_3 and B_4.

Chromosome mutations

Sufficient has been said about human point mutations to make it clear that profound changes in cellular metabolism can be effected by no more than the absence or modification of a single key polypeptide. Because only a single gene locus is affected the resultant phenotype frequently does not involve widespread somatic changes. A far larger effect results from chromosome mutations. In these cases changes affect whole chromosomes or large segments of them and the results are usually incompatible with life. Early abortion of such conceptuses is the rule. Occasionally, however, the sum total of the effects is not lethal; the result is an individual with a very large number of relatively minor abnormalities of gene function — a situation in which widespread physical anomalies are commonly seen.

Chromosome mutations usually take the form of reduplication or deletion

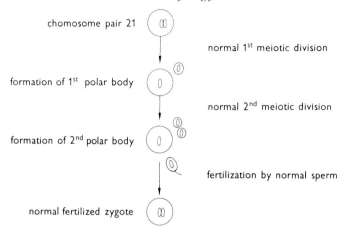

Fig. 2.9. Diagram of the normal behaviour of chromosome pair 21 during germ cell formation and subsequent fertilization.
Note: In this and subsequent diagrams the first polar body is not shown as dividing (see Fig. 3.6).

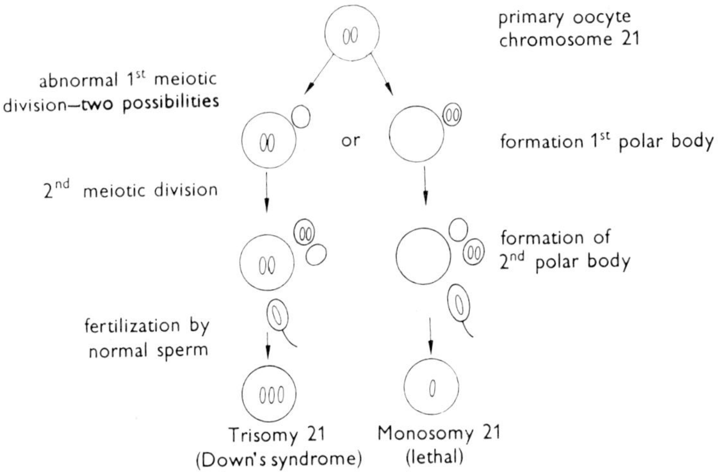

Fig. 2.10. Non-disjunction of chromosome pair 21 during the first meiotic division, cf. Fig. 2.9
Note: Non-disjunction during the second meiotic division would also cause Down's syndrome.

(absence) of a part or the whole of a chromosome though more subtle changes (for example the inversion of a chromosome segment) may occasionally produce an effect. Abnormalities of karyotype are most frequently the result of non-disjunction of chromosomes during cell division. In this condition, the members of a chromosome pair fail to separate, usually in the first or second division of meiosis (i.e. during germ cell formation). The result, after union of the abnormal with a normal gamete, is an individual with either *trisomy* (3 chromosomes of a particular number) or *monosomy* (1 chromosome only of the particular number

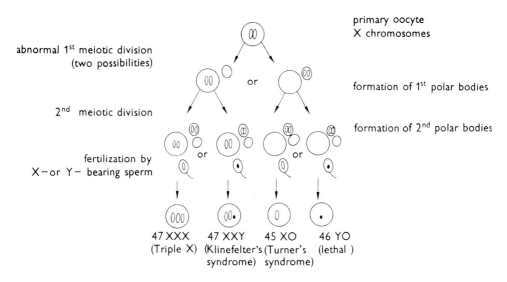

Fig. 2.11. Non-disjunction of sex chromosomes during meiosis (the number given before the sex chromosome constitution refers to the total number of chromosomes present).

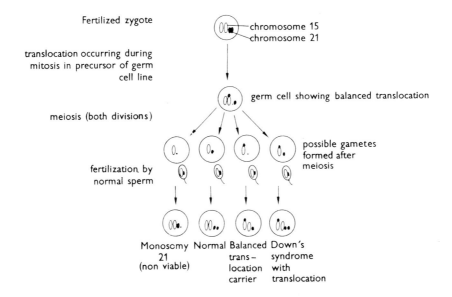

Fig. 2.12. Effects of 15/21 translocation in the precursor of the germ cell line. *Note:* This is merely a particular example. Translocation may occur at other stages of embryonic development.

involved) (compare Figs. 2.9 and 2.10).

Variation in chromosome number is best tolerated among sex chromosomes because in the later stages of development and postnatally all X chromosomes in excess of one are inactive during interphase and appear in the form of discrete masses of sex chromatin (p.8). Fig. 2.11 gives an example of how numerous types of abnormalities of the sex chromosomes may arise following non-disjunction of the X chromosomes in the female (the reader may work out himself the possible consequences of XY non-disjunction during sperm formation). *Triple* X females are designated by the formula (47XXX) which indicates that there are 47 chromosomes of which 3 are X chromosomes — they appear physically normal and often pass unnoticed; occasionally, however, they have irregular menses and there is an overall reduction in intelligence and fertility. Two Barr bodies are present. *Klinefelter's syndrome* (47XXY) presents as a sterile male with some feminisation of physical features (possibly female type development of the breasts, sparse beard and body hair) and usually some reduction in intelligence. A single Barr body is demonstrable. Females with *Turner's syndrome* (45XO) have a single X chromosome and no Y chromosome and are sterile; they have a characteristic 'webbing' of the neck, are short in stature and have underdeveloped secondary sexual characteristics. Regional narrowing or *stenosis* (*coarctation*) of the aorta is present in some cases. No sex chromatin is present. About 95 per cent of all cases of Turner's syndrome are aborted but the abortion rate in the sex chromosome triploidies is no higher than in pregnancies without apparent chromosome defect.

Non-disjunction among autosomes will lead to trisomic and monosomic individuals (Fig. 2.10). The latter do not survive embryonic life and even the former have a very large intra-uterine mortality. Though trisomies of the large autosomes exist it is interesting that only those of group G (i.e. members of the smallest chromosome group, presumably containing the least amount of active genetic material) survive infancy with any frequency. They constitute the commonest form of *Down's syndrome*, a condition in which severe mental deficiency is the rule. Patients are usually short and usually exhibit characteristic palm prints; the eyes appear slanted and a typical skin fold at the medial angle of the eye gave rise to the old name of *mongolism*. Congenital malformations of the heart are frequently present. There is (as in many other chromosome mutations) a sharp rise in the frequency of the condition with increasing maternal age.

As well as arising during meiosis, non-disjunction occasionally complicates mitosis. Sister chromatids fail to separate and, in addition to normal somatic cells, two distinct cell lines or clones (i.e. groups of cells derived from a single ancestor) arise. When this happens early in development it has widespread effects even if only one of the two abnormal cells formed survives and reproduces itself. Individuals with autosomal trisomy, others with anomalies of the sex chromosomes and yet others composed of a mixture of cell lines (*mosaics*), have all been described; the possible variations are legion.

Chromosomal anomalies may also result from chromosome breaks during meiosis. Usually the breaks reunite with no loss of chromosomal material or with perhaps an exchange of chromosomal material between homologous chromosomes. Occasionally, however, reunion occurs in an abnormal manner. Inversion of chromosome segments may occur or sometimes *translocation* of one chromosome onto another by union of their 'raw' ends takes place. The best known example is a translocation in which chromosome 21 becomes attached to chromosome 15 which is therefore longer than usual. The way in which this translocation is transmitted is shown in Fig. 2.12. The offspring with Down's syndrome has 46 chromosomes but one of the chromosomes 15/21 has an extra chromosome attached to it. The genetic material of three 21 chromosomes is, therefore, present in the karyotype. The balanced 15/21 translocation carrier has only 45 chromosomes; one of the 21 chromosomes is attached to a chromosome 15. These individuals are clinically normal but the cells of their germ cell line all have a balanced translocation and will give rise to one of four possible gametes. On fertilization the zygote will have one of four karyotypes (i) 45 chromosomes with 21 monosomy (this is non-viable); (ii) normal 46 chromosomes; (iii) 45 chromosomes with balanced 15/21 translocation and (iv) 46 chromosomes with Down's syndrome (unbalanced 15/21 translocation). The individual with a balanced translocation is, therefore, a carrier of the translocation type of Down's syndrome and classically this form is familial and shows no increasing tendency to occur in the offspring of older mothers.

Chromosome anomalies are very common and probably as many as one zygote in ten is affected. Fortunately most of these are aborted so that only 0.5 per cent of liveborn children have a chromosome mutation. The examples given above illustrate some of the commoner forms but many others have been described and the reader is referred to specialist textbooks for an account of these.

Polygenic inheritance

If a phenotype trait is the result of genes present at a single gene locus only, Mendel's laws are easily demonstrable with respect to the effects of those genes. This is clear from what has been said in the earlier part of this chapter. Difficulties in recognising simple unifactorial inheritance are relatively few and include partial expressivity, co-dominance and multiple alleles.

Simple unifactorial inheritance in man is, however, the exception rather than the rule. Most recognisable characteristics are determined by multiple genes which are often not closely linked. Each gene individually obeys Mendel's laws but the overall phenotype effect resulting from the summation of the action of many genes is complex. This phenomenon is known as *polygenic* inheritance and its fundamental characteristic is that the trait in question is continuously variable in the population. Although the matter is still further complicated by assortative mating, typical polygenic inheritance is characteristic of the genetic basis of height, intelligence and blood pressure. Of less clinical importance but better worked out than the above examples are the ways in which dermatoglyphics (skin markings on hands and feet) are inherited. The particular advantage here is that their inheritance is not greatly subject to the disturbing influences of assortative mating.

We have considered the effects of unifactorial and multifactorial inheritance in this chapter because, without a basic knowledge in this field, the biological basis of clinically important congenital malformations could not be understood (see Chapter 18). Most deformities are, in fact, multifactorial in origin. That is to say that they have a polygenic origin on the one hand and probably result from the interaction of many environmental factors on the other. Their analysis in terms of causation, therefore, presents considerable difficulty.

We have seen that in unifactorial inheritance the result is often that a certain trait is either present or absent. Paradoxically this may also be the case resulting from the multifactorial causation of some congenital malformations such as cleft palate. The explanation for this, which involves a 'threshold' phenomenon, is given on p.352. Such 'all or none' cases of defect do not follow the simple Mendelian rules of unifactorial inheritance.

In concluding this and the previous chapter it is necessary to point out that neither is intended as substitute for texts in genetics, biochemistry or cell biology. They merely present the minimum required for an understanding of human embryology and the student is advised to read them from the point of view of a summary designed to obviate repeated reference to other text books while studying embryology.

Further reading

Alberts, B., Bray, D., Lewis, J., Raff, M., Roberts, K. & Watson J. D. (1983) *Molecular Biology of the Cell*, pp. 98–111. Garland Publishing Inc., New York and London.
Carter, C.O. (1976) *An A B C of Medical Genetics*. Lancet.
Emergy, A.E.H. (1983) *Elements of Medical Genetics*, 6th edn. Churchill-Livingstone.
McKusick, V. (1969) *Human Genetics*, 2nd edn. Englewood Cliffs, London.
Nora, J.J. & Fraser, F.C. (1981) *Medical Genetics. Principles and Practice*, 2nd edn. Lea & Fabiger. Philadelphia. Section 1: Heredity and Disease.

3
The Germ Cells

Germ cell production cannot be considered in isolation because the testis and ovary have functions other than the production of the germ cells. The interstitial (Leydig) cells of the testis produce a group of sex hormones known as *androgens* (principally testosterone) but small quantities of *oestrogenic hormones* are also produced. The spermatozoa are formed by division and differentiation of the cells which line the seminiferous tubules (*vide infra*); these structures form the main bulk of the testis. The ovary, in addition to producing the germ cells in the form of mature ova, also produces *oestrogens, progestogens* and small quantities of *androgens*. The control of the production of hormones and their functions in the reproductive cycle will be discussed further in Chapter 4.

Before describing the germ cells themselves, it will be necessary to give a brief outline of the genital system in order that the sequence of events may be followed.

The male reproductive system

The testes are normally situated in the scrotum, into which they descend during the 7th or 8th months of intra-uterine life. Each testis is about 4cm in length and consists of a series of lobules, the whole being enclosed in an outer fibrous sheath, the *tunica albuginea* (Fig. 3.1). Each lobule consists of between one and four highly convoluted *seminiferous tubules*, which communicate by means of a number of terminal straight tubules with a plexus of fine tubules known as the *rete testis*. The latter lies in a posterior fibrous septum of the gonad known as the mediastinum testis (Fig. 3.1). From this, about a dozen *efferent ductules* leave the upper pole posteriorly and enter the beginning of a long extremely convoluted tubule which is applied to the posterior aspect of the testis and forms the *epididymis*. As may be seen in Fig. 3.1, this consists of a head (caput), body and tail (cauda), the efferent ductules entering the head. At the tail of the epididymis, the tubule becomes continuous with the *ductus deferens* (or vas deferens). This is a long, relatively thick walled muscular tube which ascends in the spermatic cord passing through the inguinal canal to enter the abdomen. The spermatic cord also conveys, along with other less important structures, the testicular artery and the pampiniform plexus of veins to and from the testis respectively. The ductus deferens then runs to the base of the bladder where it joins the duct of the corresponding *seminal vesicle* to form the *ejaculatory duct*. The seminal vesicle is a convoluted tubule

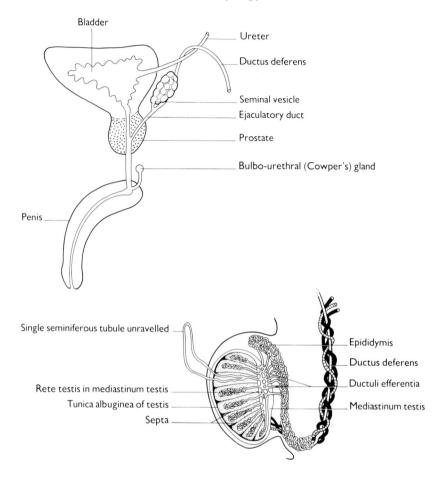

Fig. 3.1. A diagram of the male genital organs.

which secretes a viscid component of the semen into the ductus deferens. The
ejaculatory duct passes through the prostate gland and enters the prostatic urethra
just to one side of the midline. The *prostate* itself consists of a mass of glandular
tissue from which 15–30 excretory ducts arise and open into the prostatic urethra.
The whole is enclosed within a fibro-muscular capsule. The *bulbo-urethral*
(Cowper's) glands are a pair of glands each about the size of a pea which lie in the
deep perineal pouch, a potential space positioned distal to the prostate gland
which opens by means of a duct into the bulbous part of the urethra. Other small
glands are found in the urethral lining itself.

Spermatogenesis

In describing the processes of spermatogenesis and oogenesis and the relation
between these processes and the level of circulating hormones, it is important to

remember that there are important species differences in the behaviour of the reproductive system. For obvious reasons, the majority of histological and experimental studies have been performed upon animals rather than upon human subjects and, although it is likely that many findings in animal experiments can be extrapolated to apply to man, some caution is necessary. The following account deals with the state of affairs in the human subject except when stated otherwise.

The active production of spermatozoa begins at puberty; before that time the seminiferous tubules of the testis are virtually filled by rather spherical cells known as *spermatogonia*. At puberty, these cells begin to divide actively and they continue to do so throughout life, some of the daughter cells forming *primary spermatocytes* while others remain as spermatogonia to continue the process of division. The primary spermatocytes move away from the basement membrane towards the lumen and the amount of cytoplasm increases until each undergoes further division to form a pair of *secondary spermatocytes*. This is an extremely important stage in development since this division is the first of the two that constitute meiosis. It gives rise to secondary spermatocytes which contain the *haploid* number of chromosomes (p.9). The significance of this, and of the process of 'crossing over' which may take place between the chromosomes, has been described in Chapter 1. Each of the secondary spermatocytes very rapidly divides again to form a pair of *spermatids*, each of which therefore also carries the haploid

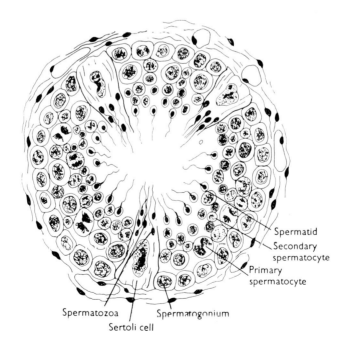

Spermatid
Secondary spermatocyte
Primary spermatocyte

Spermatozoa   Spermatogonium
Sertoli cell

Fig. 3.2. A seminiferous tubule, to show the cells involved in spermatogenesis.

number of chromosomes. The spermatids, without further division, develop tails and become transformed into *spermatozoa* by a process called *spermiogenesis* which calls for a great reduction in the amount of cytoplasm present. The excess cytoplasm during this process is, in fact, cast off.

The process of spermatogenesis is illustrated in Fig. 3.2 which represents the appearance of a typical part of a seminiferous tubule in man. The appearance may, however, differ in different tubules. In many animals the developmental stage reached by the sperm during spermatogenesis follows a variable gradient along the length of the seminiferous tubules; this is not so in man where different stages of spermatogenesis may often be seen in a single cross section of the seminiferous tubule. The explanation for the synchronous development of sperm in circum-scribed areas of the seminiferous tubules is not well understood. A plausible explanation is that in all but the earliest spermatogonial divisions cell division is incomplete so that eventually very large numbers of spermatids embedded in the apical cytoplasm of the *Sertoli cells* (*vide infra*) remain connected by *cytoplasmic bridges* which may well regulate their maturation. Individual sperm are only separated on release from the Sertoli cells. In addition to the cells which are destined to form spermatozoa, other rather large conical cells which, by light microscopy, appear to have indistinct margins are present in the seminiferous tubules, their bases being applied to the basement membrane. These are *Sertoli cells* and their apices are closely related to the developing spermatids, which occupy deep invaginations of their apical cytoplasm. The Sertoli cells provide support for the maturing spermatids, may be involved in their nutrition and are involved in the utilisation of androgens (p.39). Recent observations with the electron microscope in animals have shown that the head of the spermatozoon is gradually extruded from the invagination in the Sertoli cell cytoplasm into the lumen, almost all of the residual cytoplasm remaining embedded in the Sertoli cell.

In the final stage, the fully developed spermatozoa are released from the Sertoli cells into the lumen of the seminiferous tubules about 64 days after the division of the original spermatogonium. In many animals the outermost cells of the semini-ferous tubules appear to have contractile powers but this does not appear to be so in primates where secretion of sperm into the epididymis seems to be a con-sequence of raised intratesticular pressure inside an unyielding fibrous *tunica albuginea*. In somewhat simplified terms each spermatozoon is seen, under the electron microscope, to consist of a *head*, which contains the nucleus, and a *tail*. The latter is further subdivided into a *neck*, *middle piece*, *principal* (or main) *piece* and *end piece* (Fig. 3.3). The total length of the human spermatozoon is a little more than 50 microns. The head is rather flattened and consists mostly of the nucleus. There is also an *acrosomal cap* which is derived from the Golgi apparatus of the spermatid, but this is relatively inconspicuous in the human spermatozoon, although it is very prominent in many animals. At the base of the head is a *centriole*. The neck is short and connects the head to the middle piece. The middle piece is the 'engine room' of the spermatozoon since it contains a helically

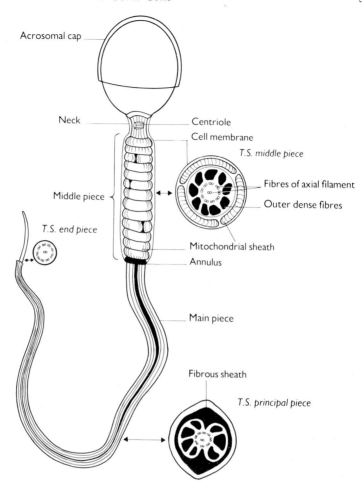

Fig. 3.3. A somewhat simplified diagram of a mature spermatozoon.

arranged covering of mitochondria which provide the enzymes necessary for the production of some of the energy required by the sperm. The mitochondria seem to be prevented from slipping distally by the development of an annulus between the middle piece and the principal piece. They are arranged around an axial filament consisting of a pair of central fibrils surrounded by a circle of nine paired fibrils. An outer circle of nine single but stouter filaments is present just outside the peripheral ring of nine fibrils. In the principal piece a fibrous sheath appears consisting of continuous dorsal and ventral longitudinal columns connected by circumferential ribs. The outer dense fibres 3 and 8 terminate in these longitudinal columns but the remainder of the dense fibres and the fibrous sheath continue to the end piece (Fig. 3.3). The end piece consists only of the axial filament and of covering cell membrane.

Not all spermatozoa are normal and giant forms as well as conjoined forms and forms having two nuclei or two tails are not uncommon. Occasionally in normal semen and frequently in some pathological conditions a thin membranous 'cap', apparently detached from the head, is found and this has been called the *galea capitis* on the assumption that it represents a distinct structure. Electron microscopy, however, indicates that this is not so, the 'galea' presumably being one or more of the normal components of the head which have become detached.

The normal position of the testes in the scrotum and a countercurrent heat exchange system between the testicular artery and the pampiniform plexus ensure that they are maintained at a temperature lower than that of the body, this being essential for normal spermatogenesis. Undescended testes (p.273) are unable to produce mature spermatozoa.

Seminal fluid

The spermatozoa pass from the testis into the epididymis. At this stage they are still non-motile and are carried along by contraction of the smooth muscle of the wall of the epididymis. Their passage along the twenty feet or so of coiled tubule which forms the epididymis takes a number of days, or perhaps weeks, and it is in this tubule that they are stored and undergo partial maturation. During coitus they are rapidly propelled along the ductus deferens by contraction of its muscular wall and enter the urethra. The seminal vesicles and prostate also contract and add their secretions to the semen which passes into the posterior penile urethra. The whole mass is then ejaculated by the contraction of the bulbo-spongiosus muscle, the secretion of the bulbo-urethral glands and other small glands being added in the urethra.

The average volume of the ejaculate is 3.5 ml and this contains 50 to 100 million spermatozoa per ml. The seminal fluid has a neutral pH. It is made up of a small amount of liquid secretion originating in the testis and epididymis together with the major secretions of the seminal vesicles, prostate, bulbo-urethral glands and small glands in the wall of the urethra. Fructose from the seminal vesicles and citric acid from the prostate are major chemical components and sperm probably use fructose as their major source of energy. Enzymes responsible for the clotting of semen have been identified and, in man, the semen coagulates within one minute of ejaculation and liquefies again after 20 minutes. Human semen also contains *hyaluronidase* which may facilitate the passage of sperm through the cervical mucous by liquefying it. *Prostaglandins* E_1, E_2 and $F_{2\alpha}$ are present in high concentration and these fatty acids are probably of great importance. In particular prostaglandin $F_{2\alpha}$ by stimulating smooth muscle contraction may accelerate sperm transport in the female tract. Substances with similar physiological action (e.g. gangliosides) are also present. The spermatozoa first become motile during their passage along the epididymis but their motility and potential fertilizing power increases as they pass into the female tract (see p.65 for *capacitation*). Sperm which are not ejaculated in semen are either voided in the urine or subjected to phagocytosis in the epididymis.

Germ cells are very susceptible to poisons though Sertoli and interstitial cells are less so. Many general infectious diseases, alcoholism and dietary deficiencies affect spermatogenesis as does local inflammation. Mumps, particularly in adults, is especially dangerous. X-rays also produce degeneration and abnormal sperm. In the majority of cases in all the above conditions recovery occurs because some spermatogonia frequently remain so that complete sterility need not result.

Spermatogenesis continues into old age in the male but seminiferous tubules do undergo progressive involution with age. An important fact to remember is that the process of *normal* sperm formation is an extremely complex and inefficient one. It appears that *up to 90 per cent* of spermatogonia *fail* to produce spermatozoa and degenerate (see p.70 for infertility).

The endocrine functions of the testis

Steroid hormones are produced by the *interstitial cells* (Leydig cells) of the testis which lie between the seminiferous tubules. Their principal secretion is the androgen, *testosterone*, but they also produce some oestrogen. Beside controlling spermatogenesis, testosterone is also responsible directly or indirectly for the development and function of the accessory sexual organs, the secondary sexual characteristics and much of man's sexual behaviour.

Testosterone secretion is dependent upon luteinizing hormone (LH) secreted by the anterior lobe of the pituitary gland (Chapter 4) and prolactin, also from the anterior pituitary, acts synergistically with LH in producing steroids. The sequence of events appears to be that LH (a glycoprotein) is taken up by specific receptor molecules on the surface of the interstitial cells. The intracellular release of adenyl cyclase and subsequent formation of cyclic AMP (the second messenger) then occurs and cAMP acts on an inducer protein which causes the formation of biologically active steroids from cholesterol precursors. Some authorities also believe that LH may affect Sertoli cells.

Once formed, the steroids have a variety of actions (see above) which are achieved by penetration of the target cell nucleus and presumably by modulation of the genome. 5α-Dihydrotestosterone (DHT) is even more potent than testosterone (particularly in maintaining the prostate) and large amounts of 5α-reductase are present in most androgenic target tissues suggesting that testosterone may only be a circulating precursor for DHT. Androgen receptors are present on the Sertoli cells as well as perhaps on spermatogonia and spermatocytes and testosterone is, in fact, essential for spermatogenesis and spermiogenesis. It acts on the Sertoli cells by causing them to secrete an androgen-binding protein into the seminiferous tubule lumen which has a high affinity for DHT.

Sertoli cells are only able to mature under the action of follicle stimulating hormone (FSH) which is also of anterior pituitary origin.

A process such as spermatogenesis dependent upon a highly ordered series of endocrinological events obviously has to be regulated by a sophisticated feed-back mechanism. The subject is discussed further in Chapter 4. Here it suffices to say that the balance of evidence is now in favour of the fact that LH and FSH (p.60) are released in response to the same releasing hormone (GnRH) (p.57) from the hypothalamus via the hypothalamo-pituitary portal system. Prolactin release is principally controlled by the hypothalamic prolactin inhibitory factor (PIF), which has now been identified as dopamine, acting on the anterior pituitary. Both LH and LRF are under the control of negative feed-back mechanisms from the testis. Testicular testosterone can act directly on the hypothalamus and there is evidence of androgen receptor sites situated in the hypothalamus as well as the enzyme 5α-reductase. Feed-back loops may also directly alter the sensitivity of the anterior pituitary to GnRH.

The female reproductive system

The general arrangement of the female genital organs is illustrated in Fig. 3.4. The *uterus* consists of a body and cervix, the lower part of the latter normally projecting downwards and backwards into the vagina. The wall of the body of the uterus consists of an extremely thick layer of smooth muscle, the *myometrium* and a lining

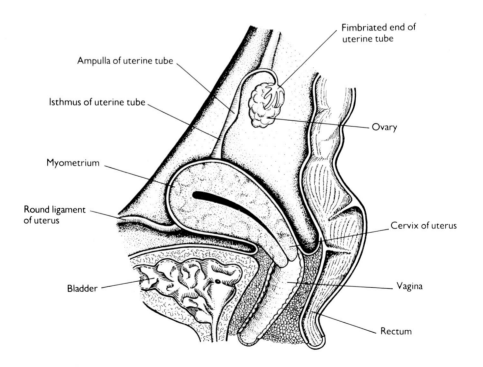

Fig. 3.4. A diagram of the female genitalia. The ostium at the fimbriated end of the tube is not visible.

mucous membrane, the *endometrium*, which undergoes a series of changes during the menstrual cycle. These are described in Chapter 4.

The *uterine (Fallopian) tubes* pass laterally from each side of the uterus and each ends in close proximity to an ovary, the ends of the tubes being fimbriated (p.64) and expanded to form the *infundibulum*. The main part of the tube is known as the *ampullary part*, medial to which lies the narrower *isthmus*. Finally the uterine part of the tube passes through the substance of the myometrium. The *broad ligament* is a curtain-like double fold of peritoneum in whose free border the uterine tube lies and which also contains the uterine and ovarian vessels and certain embryological remnants (Chapter 15).

The ovary

In order to understand the process of ovulation and the endocrine functions of the ovary it will be necessary to describe its structure in some detail. The adult ovary is about 3 cm in length, is flattened from side to side and its surface has a rather irregular appearance owing to the presence of follicles, corpora lutea and scars (*vide infra*). It is tethered to the postero-superior surface of the broad ligament by a mesentery known as the *mesovarium*. The ovary is covered with a layer of low columnar epithelium, continuous with the peritoneum, which is known mis-leadingly as the *germinal epithelium* for it was once thought that germ cells were budded off from this throughout life to form new ova. The epithelium is separated from the stroma of the ovary by a fibrous *tunica albuginea* which is, however, much thinner than the corresponding layer in the testis.

Oogenesis

The germ cells are derived from specially segregated cells in the mesoderm of the yolk sac (see Chapter 15) which, well before birth, migrate to the ovary (or the testis in the male) and form *oogonia* (corresponding to the spermatogonia in the male). They undergo mitotic division to form *primary oocytes* or primordial ova of which a very large number, perhaps two million, are present in the ovary at birth so that no further such primordial ova need be produced; in fact the vast majority of them undergo only partial maturation and then atresia; many die even before birth.

After puberty, in the normal course of events, only one ovum completes its maturation each month. The process is as follows. The primary oocyte, which is about 30 μm in diameter, lies in the cortex of the ovary and is surrounded by a single layer of squamous *follicular cells*, which are derived from the ovarian stroma. The whole complex is known as a *primordial follicle*. As the primary oocyte grows larger, the follicular cells divide and produce several layers of cuboidal *granulosa cells* which become separated from the oocyte by a rather thick homo-genous membrane, the *zona pellucida*. This actively developing mass of cells is

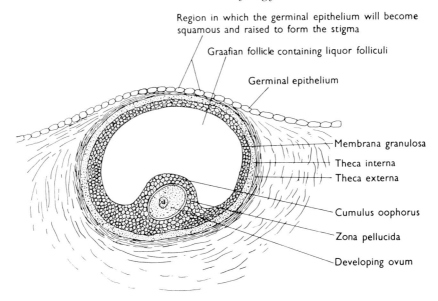

Fig. 3.5. A Graafian follicle which is beginning to form a surface elevation on the ovary.

now known as a *primary follicle* and with further increase in size, a cleft, the *antrum*, appears in the granulosa cells in which the *liquor folliculi* accumulates. At this stage the primary follicle becomes a *secondary follicle.* The liquor increases in amount until there is so much present that the follicle has a diameter of about 1 cm so that it is easily visible to the naked eye. It is now called a *Graafian follicle*, named after de Graaf who first described it although he believed the follicle to be the ovum itself and since it is obviously too large to enter the uterine tube, he was disbelieved. The structure of the Graafian follicle is seen in Fig. 3.5. The oocyte is surrounded by the zona pellucida and by an accumulation of granulosa cells which form the *cumulus oophorus.* The large cavity of the follicle which is filled with liquor folliculi, is lined by a further layer of cells which are known as the *membrana granulosa.* Outside this, the cells of the ovarian stroma produce a well vascularized layer known as the *theca interna*, while the whole follicle so compresses the surrounding tissue by its growth that an outer-most connective tissue layer, the *theca externa*, is formed around the follicle. By the time ovulation is ready to occur the oocyte undergoes its first meiotic division (see p.9). This differs from the similar process in the testis in that, in the latter, two similar secondary spermatocytes are produced whereas, in the ovary, although the chromatin is shared between the two secondary oocytes, nearly all the cytoplasm remains with one of the daughter cells, the other remaining very small and being known as a *polar body.* The secondary oocyte therefore possesses a dis-proportionate amount of cytoplasm. The second division (corresponding to the division of the secondary spermatocyte to form spermatids in the male) begins almost immediately after the first but is not completed until, and unless,

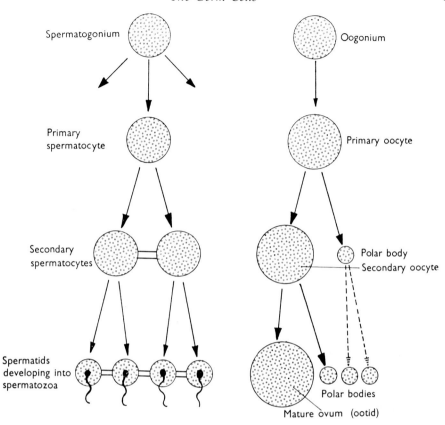

Fig. 3.6. A diagram to illustrate the production of the mature germ cells. Note how, in the case of the ovum, the cytoplasm is conserved to form one large cell. The cytoplasmic bridges connecting the male germ cells (p.36) are shown diagrammatically.

fertilization occurs. In this division, too, the bulk of the cytoplasm remains with only one of the daughter cells, the other forming another polar body. A comparison between the developing germ cells of the male and female is shown in Fig. 3.6.

As stated above a very large number of oocytes never reach maturity. Many, however, form follicles which fail to ripen and eventually shrink and become *atretic*. Although, therefore, they do not develop completely they are most important since, each month, the oestrogenic hormones produced by the numerous follicles which are destined to become atretic play an indispensible part in activating the uterine endometrium.

Ovulation

Just before ovulation occurs, the cumulus oophorus with its contained oocyte separates from the membrana granulosa and floats free in the liquor folliculi. The

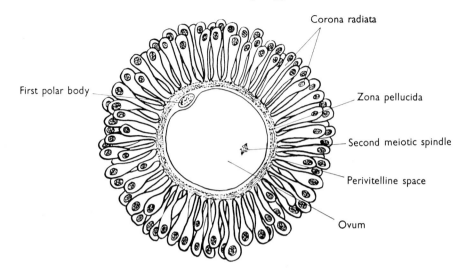

First polar body

Corona radiata

Zona pellucida

Second meiotic spindle

Perivitelline space

Ovum

Fig. 3.7. An ovum which has just been shed from a ripe Graafian follicle. The cells of the cumulus oophorus now form the corona radiata. The final, maturation division is taking place.

projecting surface of the follicle now breaks down (the follicle does not suddenly burst like a balloon) and the ovum is released with the liquor folliculi, usually passing straight into the fimbriated end of the Fallopian tube. The mature ovum, which contains very little yolk, is just visible to the naked eye, having a diameter of 100–150 μm. It is surrounded by the zona pellucida, within which also lies the first polar body. The whole is surrounded by cumulus cells, which often radiate from the oocyte and are known collectively as the *corona radiata* (Fig. 3.7). Ovulation and the transport of the released ovum will be discussed in more detail in Chapters 4 and 5.

Corpus luteum

When ovulation has taken place, the wall of the follicle collapses inwards and forms a series of folds. At the same time there is usually a little haemorrhage from the surrounding blood vessels so that the collapsed follicle is often filled with blood. Occasionally ovulation is slightly painful; this is the so-called *Mittelschmerz* of which some women are aware about half-way between successive menstruations. The granulosa cells proliferate and form a large yellow mass of lipid-filled cells, often called *granula lutein* cells. The cells of the theca interna also proliferate to some extent (*theca lutein cells*) and the whole, large yellowish body forms the *corpus luteum*. The mass of cells is invaded by an ingrowth of blood vessels from the theca. The corpus luteum has a diameter much the same as that of the original Graafian follicle and it consists of a large mass of polygonal, clear cells with a number of blood vessels so that it resembles an endocrine gland which, in fact, it is. If pregnancy occurs, the corpus luteum becomes still larger, reaching a size of 2—3 cm, but otherwise it diminishes in size, degenerates in 14 days and eventually forms a mass of scar-like tissue known as a *corpus albicans*. After the menopause (p.60) almost all the remaining follicles become atretic and disappear, as do the primordial ova, but corpora albicantes can still be recognised.

The endocrine function of the ovary

The ovary, under pituitary control (p.54), produces a number of steroid hormones which are of closely related structure. These are the *oestrogenic hormones, progesterone* and other related hormones often known collectively as *progestogens*, as well as some *androgenic hormones*, particularly testosterone. The source of the oestrogenic hormones — 17β-oestradiol and oestrone — is mainly the theca interna cells and perhaps the interstitial cells of the ovarian stroma. The latter are presumably the source of oestrogens before puberty. Progesterone is secreted by the cells of the corpus luteum. The interstitial cells and/or the collection of cells in the hilus of the ovary (*'hilus cells'*) are the source of the androgenic hormones. The androgens are produced only in small amounts and may be considered by-products in the production of oestrogens.

Function of the ovarian hormones

The functions of the ovarian hormones are difficult to define exactly, since there are so many types of related hormones which are produced elsewhere and have certain actions similar to those of ovarian hormones, In general, however, it may be said that the oestrogens are responsible for the development and maintenance of the female secondary sexual characters during and after puberty, for the control (together with progestogens) of the menstrual cycle (Chapters 4 and 17) and for the 'feedback mechanism' which controls the output of gonadotrophic hormones from the pituitary gland. They stimulate mobility of the uterus and uterine tube and also stimulate growth of the uterine muscle and its vasculature during pregnancy. Furthermore, they play a part in the preparation of the duct system of the breasts during pregnancy in preparation for subsequent lactation. They have other, more general, effects on metabolism such as the retention of salt and water, which will not be further mentioned here.

The action of progesterone is closely related to that of the oestrogens since it acts largely on tissues which have already been primed by oestrogens. Progesterone is important in producing the secretory phase in the endometrium (see Chapter 4) and it reduces the excitability of the myometrium. It also slightly raises the body temperature, which is a useful phenomenon in investigation of the menstrual cycle. The body temperature is taken immediately on waking and this basal temperature is plotted each day throughout the cycle. If ovulation has occurred, the production of progesterone by the corpus luteum leads to a rise in temperature. The temperature usually rises 1—2 days after ovulation and this hyperthermic phase normally lasts for 12—13 days. A hyperthermic phase of less than 10 days may be associated with infertility. In addition, progesterone acts, together with oestrogens, to stimulate the growth of the glandular tissues of the breasts during pregnancy.

The ovarian cycle

In view of the enormous number of animal experiments which are performed in investigating the action of the sex hormones, it should be realised that there are extremely important differences between the reproductive cycles of animals and man. In most mammals the peak of oestrogen production produces cornification of the vagina and the onset of *oestrus* or 'heat' — the period when the female will accept the male. In the human female oestrus does not occur, although slight cornification of the vagina can often be recognised at one stage of the menstrual cycle (Chapter 4). Secondly in the human female ovulation occurs spontaneously and usually regularly, whereas it may be induced by various outside factors in many animals. In the rabbit, for instance, it occurs only after coitus. A true *menstrual cycle* occurs only in man and higher primates.

In the human ovary as a rule only one follicle ripens at intervals of approximately 28 days although, as has been mentioned already, many more each month undergo varying degrees of maturation. The exact timing will be described later (Chapter 4) but here it may be said that during the first 14 days of the cycle follicles are enlarging and ripening so that ovulation normally occurs at about the 14th day. The follicular phase of the cycle is variable in duration, only the luteal phase being constant. The time of ovulation is, therefore, related accurately to the time of onset of the *next* menstrual period and not to the previous one. This has an important bearing on the 'safe period' method of contraception (Chapter 5). Following ovulation the corpus luteum develops and persists for 14 days when, if fertilization has not occurred, it begins to degenerate. Using radioimmunoassay methods, the level of oestrogens in the circulating blood is found to reach a peak at, or just before, the time of ovulation (14th day) and it then falls, but rises again to produce a secondary peak at about the 21st day, i.e. in the mid-luteal phase. Progesterone levels show a relatively low level during the follicular (oestrogenic) phase of the cycle, with a rise beginning at about the time of ovulation which continues to reach a peak at the mid-luteal phase. The level then gradually falls (Fig. 4.2).

The ovarian cycle is primarily responsible for changes in the endometrium which constitute the menstrual cycle. As in the case of the testis (p.60) the ovary is controlled by the pituitary which, in turn, is primarily influenced by the hypothalamus (see Chapter 4). Thus the distensibility of the wall of the Graafian follicle seems to be due to LH from the pituitary combining with specific receptors on the surface of the follicle cells. This stimulates formation of cyclic AMP in the affected cells and leads to progesterone output by these cells. The progesterone (via the stimulation of a collagenase) lowers the breaking strength of the follicle and rupture follows.

It also appears to be the case that subtle interactions occur below the level of the pituitary. Thus various hormones may affect the number of receptors on a particular tissue. For example, FSH stimulates the production of more FSH receptors on the granulosa cells and, therefore, progressively increases sensitivity to its own action. Oestrogen and FSH in combination stimulate LH receptor production and consequently prepare the follicle for the LH surge which causes its rupture (see Chapter 4).

Further reading

Austin, C.R. & Short, R.V. (eds.) (1982) *Reproduction in Mammals, Vol. 1: Germ cells and fertilization.* Chapter 2: Oogenesis and ovulation (Baker, T.G.); Chapter 4: Spermatogenesis and spermatozoa (Setchell, B.P.).

Fawcett, D.W. (1970) A comparative view of sperm ultrastructure. *Biol. of Reprod.,* Suppl. **2**, 90.

Fawcett, D.W. & Bedford, J.M. (1979) *The Spermatozoon.* Urban & Schwarzenberg, Baltimore.

Peters, H. & McNalty, K.P. (1980) *The Ovary.* Paul Elek, London.

Setchell, B.P. (1978) *The Mammalian Testis.* Paul Elek, London.

Zuckerman, S. & Weir, B.J. (1977) *The Ovary.* (Vols. 1, 2 & 3) (2nd edn). Academic Press, New York and London.

4

The Histology of the Female Genital Tract, Menstruation and its Control

The uterus and uterine (Fallopian) tubes

The general structure of the uterus and the uterine tube has been described in Chapter 3. The muscle coat is thickest in the region of the isthmus (p.41) and the fertilized ovum is temporarily held up in this region during its passage to the cavity of the uterus. The mucous membrane of the tube is thrown into folds, particularly in the ampullary portion. The epithelium is ciliated columnar but, as well as the ciliated cells, at least one other type of cell is present. These are secretory cells which show cyclical changes during the menstrual cycle and may aid nutrition of the ovum as it passes along the tube. Their secretion is discharged into the lumen of the tube after ovulation, at which time the smooth muscle in the walls of the tube becomes more active.

The wall of the body of the uterus consists of an extremely thick mass of smooth muscle fibres which form interlacing bundles and run in various directions. They are supported by a framework of connective tissue and are traversed by blood vessels. The mucous membrane that lines the uterus — the *endometrium* — shows very marked changes during the menstrual cycle so that separate descriptions have to be given of its appearance at different stages of the cycle. The cycle normally lasts about 28 days but wide variations occur. The first day of the cycle is defined as the first on which menstrual bleeding occurs, since this is normally an easily recognised and accurately timed occurrence. It is more convenient here, however, to begin the description of the endometrium at about the time of ovulation; this takes place most frequently between the 12th and 15th days of the cycle. For accurate timing, however, the 'LH surge' (*vide infra*, p.56) provides a more easily recognised and convenient base line for the study of the menstrual cycle. The cyclical changes in the endometrium are illustrated diagrammatically in Fig. 4.1.

At about the time of ovulation, the endometrium is nearing the end of the *proliferative phase*; this is also known as the *follicular phase*, since it is controlled by the oestrogens (principally oestradiol) produced by the maturing Graafian follicle, probably from the cells of the theca interna and membrana granulosa of the theca folliculi. The level of oestrogen production rises to a peak shortly before the LH surge (which itself precedes ovulation by 24–36 hours); it then falls, and rises again in the post-ovulatory period (Fig. 4.2). During the proliferative phase

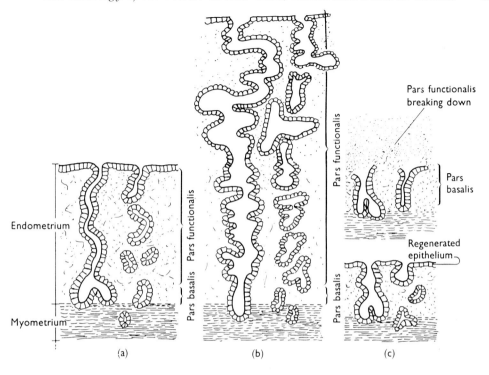

Fig. 4.1. The changes which take place in the endometrium during the menstrual cycle. (a) Proliferative phase; (b) Secretory phase; (c) Menstruation; (d) Regeneration and beginning of another proliferative phase.

the endometrium is repaired after the previous menstruation and is then built up to the stage of complete development when it reaches a thickness of 2–3 mm. It consists of an endometrial stroma into which extend numerous long tubular uterine glands which open into the cavity of the uterus and secrete a small quantity of serous fluid. The lining epithelium consists of columnar secretory cells, some of which bear cilia. The glands, too, are lined by a similar epithelium and it is probable that the cilia in the glands beat towards the lumen while those on the surface beat downwards towards the cervix. The cytoplasm of the epithelial cells contains much RNA and granular endoplasmic reticulum, indicating the synthesis of protein. Mitotic activity is a conspicuous feature. At this stage of the cycle, the glands are slightly tortuous and they extend through the whole thickness of the endometrium. Some of them branch in the deepest part of the endometrium and the tips of the glands may be partly embedded in the myometrium. The stroma consists of a very loose type of connective tissue resembling Wharton's jelly (p.100) in that it consists of a copious ground substance containing glycosaminoglycans in which are found scattered stellate cells as well as leucocytes and macrophages. The endometrium has a rich blood supply. The arteries, after passing through the uterine muscle wall (*myometrium*) enter the endometrium and give a number of straight branches to the deepest layers which form the *pars basalis* (*vide infra*). The main vessels then pass towards the lumen of the uterus; in this part of their course they are known as *spiral arteries*. Because of this arrangement, in histological sections each artery is represented by a number of lumina. The spiral arteries do not, at this stage, extend to the most superficial layers of the endometrium since they break up into branches before reaching this level.

During the proliferative phase the cervical mucus becomes less viscous and more alkaline in reaction. It reaches its lowest viscosity at ovulation and, if at this time it is smeared on a slide with a little saline, it dries in a characteristic pattern resembling the fronds of a fern.

As ovulation approaches, the uterine glands become even more tortuous and the arteries form tighter spirals until the endometrium approaches the beginning of the *secretory* or *luteal phase*. As has been seen in Chapter 3, after ovulation, the cells of the follicle itself and — to some extent — those of the tunica interna of the theca folliculi proliferate to produce the corpus luteum. The secretory phase in the endometrium results from the action of progestogens (principally progesterone) produced by the corpus luteum (Fig. 4.2), together with the action of oestrogens. At the beginning of this phase there may be a little extravasation of blood into the lumen of the uterus which, rarely, may produce a small amount of intermenstrual bleeding at the time of ovulation.

As the corpus luteum matures, the endometrium, under the influence of the oestrogens and the luteal hormones, increases still further in thickness and eventually enters upon a fully developed *secretory phase*. During this period the thickness of the endometrium reaches 5–6 mm, although much of this increase is due not to further proliferation of the endometrial components but to swelling and oedema of the stroma which becomes paler in colour. The cells of the surface and glandular epithelium now secrete glycosaminoglycans and glycogen freely, but may become less tall and are often cuboidal rather than columnar in shape due to the stretching of the surface which occurs. The secretions are poured into the cavity of the uterus and into the lumina of the glands, the latter becoming dilated and tortuous and — in the later stages of this phase of the cycle — sacculated. Two distinct zones may now be distinguished in the endometrium. These zones can be made out in the follicular phase but with the increase in size of the glands in the secretory phase, they become much more easily recognized. In the deepest parts of the endometrium, the bases of the glands do not become particularly dilated or sacculated and this region is known as the *pars basalis*; this part remains after menstruation and serves as an active zone from which regeneration can occur. The remainder of the endometrium is known as the *pars functionalis*, being the portion which is shed during menstruation (Fig. 4.1).

The blood supply to the endometrium becomes more extensive and complex during the secretory phase. The spiral arteries increase greatly in length and become very convoluted. They extend further towards the surface than they do in the follicular phase and, ultimately, reach the superficial parts of the endometrium where they break up into capillaries. The whole endometrium thus forms a thick,

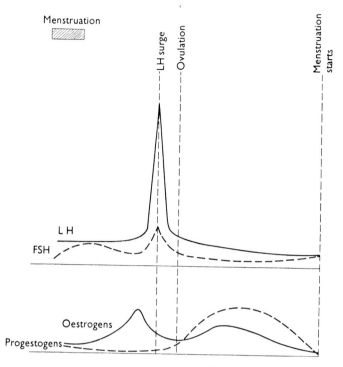

Fig. 4.2. A diagram to illustrate the varying blood levels of hormones during the menstrual cycle. The LH surge is considerably more marked than the FSH surge but, otherwise, the curves are not meant to be quantitative.

water-logged, highly vascular lining to the uterus, rich in glycogen and mucin and ready for the reception of the fertilized ovum. It is now said to be in the *progestational stage*.

Menstruation

If fertilization does not occur, the levels of the circulating oestrogen and progesterone both fall (Fig. 4.2) and with the withdrawal of their maintaining and stimulating effect, the endometrium begins to regress a day or two before menstruation is due to commence. The thickness decreases owing to water loss, the glands become less saccular and the blood flow through the spiral arteries diminishes. Finally, the spiral arteries undergo marked constriction and the superficial layers of the endometrium become ischaemic. This leads to necrosis of the surface cells and when, later, the arteries relax once again, blood is lost into the lumen of the uterus and menstruation commences. Bleeding is accompanied by the gradual loss of the pars functionalis of the endometrium so that the menstrual discharge consists of altered blood, which is largely arterial in origin and which normally does not form large clots, together with the degenerating endometrium and its secretions. The arteries in the deepest layer (pars basalis) of the endometrium do not undergo contraction so that this region remains unaffected by menstruation.

During the premenstrual period, various general symptoms may occur including headaches, tenderness of the breasts and undue fatigue and irritability. When these symptoms occur in an exaggerated form the condition is known as *premenstrual tension* and may require treatment.

The duration of the menstrual period varies from individual to individual; an average time is 4–5 days. As was described above, the onset of the menstrual period seems to result from the fall in the levels both of oestrogens and of progesterone; an analagous form of bleeding may be produced artificially by the administration, with the appropriate timing, of the two hormones followed by their withdrawal (p.70). If pregnancy occurs, the corpus luteum persists and continues to secrete progesterone (p.110). No menstruation therefore occurs and, in fact, the endometrium continues to grow in thickness, as will be described in Chapter 8. Menstruation is thus a confession of failure to produce a fertilized ovum; it has been described as 'the weeping of a disappointed uterus'.

By the time menstruation has ceased, a number of new follicles will have started to develop in the ovary (one of which will normally reach maturity) and the level of oestrogens will gradually be rising. As a result of this, a new proliferative phase begins even before the process of menstruation is complete; the cells remaining in the glands of the pars basalis rapidly begin to grow out and form a new epithelial lining for the uterus (Fig. 4.1) and the endometrium then increases in thickness building up to the stage at which ovulation occurs, when it reaches a thickness of 2–3 mm once again.

The cervix of the uterus (Fig. 3.4)

The mucous membrane of the cervix is 2–3 mm thick and differs from that of the uterus in that it is not shed during menstruation. Most of the cervix is lined by columnar mucus-secreting cells, as are the cervical glands which branch in a complicated fashion and are found in the upper two thirds of the cervix. Towards the external os the columnar epithelium gives way to stratified squamous epithelium which extends over the vaginal surface of the cervix. In the upper one third, the mucous membrane undergoes some changes during the menstrual cycle but otherwise the only definite cyclical change involves the mucus, which is increased in amount and decreased in viscosity around the mid point of the cycle. The mucus is more easily penetrated by spermatozoa when it is in this condition (p.62). During pregnancy, the cervix becomes enlarged, is softer to the touch and secretes a great deal of thick viscid mucus which plugs the cervical canal.

The vagina

The vagina (Fig. 3.4) is lined by a thick stratified squamous epithelium and is devoid of glands. At puberty the vaginal epithelium becomes thickened under the influence of oestrogens and its glycogen content increases. The glycogen is converted into lactic acid by bacterial action so that the pH of the vagina falls to about pH 4. Only slight cyclical changes are seen in the vagina and, at the time of ovulation, there is no stage of intense cornification such as is seen in some animals during the period of oestrus. Nevertheless, examination of vaginal smears may be of value in estimating oestrogenic activity in human subjects. At the menopause (*vide infra*) the vaginal epithelium undergoes some degree of atrophy. Glycogen is no longer present and consequently vaginal acidity is lost.

Anovulatory bleeding

Uterine bleeding mimicking menstruation can occur without ovulation taking place. This is a very common occurrence at the time when menstruation is just beginning round about the age of 13 years (*vide infra*) but it can also occur later in life. Confirmation of ovulation is, therefore, an essential part of the investigation of female infertility. The endometrium undergoes a proliferative phase under the influence of oestrogens but, in the absence of ovulation, no corpus luteum can be formed and no secretory phase develops. At regular or irregular intervals, however, a fall in the level of circulating oestrogens due to progressive follicular atresia leads to a form of *'withdrawal bleeding'*. If it is necessary to confirm the absence of ovulation, a biopsy taken just before the expected day of 'menstruation' will show that the endometrium is still in the proliferative phase.

Confirmation of ovulation

In the absence of pregnancy, ovulation can only be directly confirmed by recovering the already shed ovum by washing out the tube or uterus. Diagnosis of ovulation in practice depends on monitoring the activity of the corpus luteum. Certainly, if the menstrual cycles are regular, normal in amount and timing and particularly if they are accompanied by the systemic manifestations of menstruation (such as headaches and breast tenderness) it may be assumed that ovulation has taken place. Methods for the confirmation of luteal function involve daily temperature recordings (p.45) and vaginal cytology, examination of endometrial biopsy to confirm the presence of a secretory phase, the estimation of pregnanediol (the excreted form of progesterone) in the urine and the loss of the ferning pattern in the cervical mucus (*vide supra*). More sophisticated techniques are the serial estimations of plasma levels of progesterone or gonadotrophins, particularly the LH surge (p.56). The most useful observations are the rise in body temperature that follows ovulation and serum progesterone levels in the third week of the menstrual cycle but, in many cases, use of all the available investigations may be necessary.

Control of reproductive rhythm

We have seen how, in the human, the endometrium of the uterus undergoes regular cyclical changes during the course of which its lining becomes prepared for pregnancy every month and, in the absence of fertilization, is equally regularly shed leaving only a very thin pars basalis from which the remainder of the epithelium regenerates. Some idea of the hormonal control of these changes has been given. It will now be necessary to describe the control in more detail and also the control of the release of the hormones themselves. In the greatly simplified discussion that follows, it must be remembered that most of the research work on this subject has been done on animals (principally the rat and the monkey), that hormonal control differs from one species to another and that the results can only be applied to man with the greatest caution. Furthermore, the large amount of research work in this developing field means that changes in our ideas occur frequently and it is likely that additional control mechanisms will be elucidated in the next few years.

As has been seen, the cyclical changes in the endometrium depend on the regularly varying levels of oestrogens and progestogens in the blood, these hormones having been produced mainly by the ovary. The ovarian cycle is not a primary rhythm, however, since the release of the ovarian hormones is itself governed by the action of circulating hormones which are produced by the pituitary gland. These hormones, in turn, are released by the action of yet another hormone which is transported to the anterior lobe of the pituitary by the hypo-physio-portal system of vessels from the hypothalamus. The 'timekeeper' is in the hypothalamus (the so-called *hypothalamic clock*) but this may not be the initiating factor responsible for the LH surge; it certainly acts as a metronome, however, as will be seen later. In any case, the metronome can be over-ridden by emotional or psychological effects and by other factors, such as suckling, which usually stop it. It also appears to be affected by the circulating level of oestrogens and proges-terone. In order to follow this complicated pattern of events it will first be necessary to describe the relevant anatomy of the pituitary gland and hypothalamus.

The anterior lobe of the pituitary gland is developed from an ectodermal upgrowth from the stomatodeum (the primitive mouth) which also forms various other parts of the gland. The posterior lobe develops as a downgrowth from the forebrain to which it remains attached by the pituitary stalk (p.149). It will readily be understood, therefore, that the adult posterior lobe has direct nervous con-nections with the hypothalamus which are lacking in the case of the anterior lobe. There is, however, a direct vascular connection between the brain and the anterior lobe by means of the *hypophysio-portal system*. The vessels that supply various nuclei in the hypothalamus break up into a primary capillary plexus and then reunite in the region of the base of the pituitary stalk and the area surrounding it (i.e. the infundibulum and median eminence) to form a leash of hypophyseal portal vessels which pass down on the surface of the pituitary stalk and again break up to supply the anterior lobe. Numerous nerve fibres end in close relation to the primary capillary plexus in the hypothalamus. Chemical transmitter substances produced in the hypothalamus (p.57) can thus pass directly to the anterior pituitary via the hypophysio-portal vessels.

The hypothalamus forms the floor and lower part of the lateral walls of the third ventricle, lying just behind the optic chiasma. It contains numerous nuclei, but these will not be discussed in detail since the importance of different nuclei varies from species of species. Non-myelinated peptidergic neurones from the hypothalamic nuclei terminate in the vicinity of the vessels on the median eminence where the releasing hormones that they have synthesised are passed into the vessels for transport to the anterior pituitary. Other neurones coming from outside the hypothalamus end in the hypothalamic nuclei and modulate their activities.

The hormones of the anterior lobe of the pituitary

Gonadotrophins

The anterior lobe of the pituitary gland possesses a number of different types of cell and produces numerous hormones. The most important of these from the point of view of the control of ovulation, and thus of the menstrual cycle, are the *follicle stimulating hormone (FSH)* and the *luteinizing hormone (LH)*. These two hormones are known collectively as *gonadotrophins* since they exert a direct stimulating effect on production of hormones in the gonads — the ovary in the female and the testis in the male. In the female, their effects on the endometrium are entirely secondary and are produced as a result of the secretion of the ovarian hormones only, just as in the male, the gonadotrophins exert their effects on the secondary sexual organs only through the medium of the hormones of the testis. FSH, as its name implies, stimulates the secretion of the liquor folliculi so that under its influence the primary follicle grows in size until it is a fully developed Graafian follicle.

It must be stressed again that many of these ideas are based on animal experiments and it is possible that, in man, corpus luteum development may be autonomous once rupture of the follicle has occurred. Some animal experiments have suggested that a *luteotrophic hormone (LTH)*, which has been shown to be identical to *prolactin* and is produced by the pituitary, has a part to play in the output of luteal progestogens but its role in the human cycle is uncertain. There is some evidence that it may act on granulosa cells to promote their full maturation. A further important function of both FSH and LH, acting synergically, is the production of oestradiol by the theca and granulosa cells. The follicular fluid contains an increasing concentration of oestradiol as the follicle develops; this hormone plays an important role in a feedback mechanism (*vide infra*).

The gonadotrophins are difficult to prepare in a pure state and efforts are currently being made to separate and characterize them. They are glycoproteins composed of α and β peptide chains with a carbohydrate component containing sialic acid.

One of the difficulties which arises in using gonadotrophins for research or therapy in the human subject is that, unlike some of the other anterior pituitary hormones, the gonadotrophins tend to be species specific. Human FSH can, however, be prepared from the urine of post-menopausal women but it is always contaminated to a greater or lesser degree by LH. A gonadotrophin having a luteinizing action similar to that of LH is produced by the placenta (see Chapter 7) and this *human chorionic gonadotrophin (HCG)* may be prepared from the urine of pregnant women.

It can thus be seen that the two pituitary gonadotrophin hormones act together to produce maturation of the follicle, ovulation and formation of a corpus luteum and they thus indirectly control the menstrual cycle (Fig. 4.3). Assays of gonado-trophin in the serum show that FSH levels rise in the first part of the follicular phase, but then fall again towards mid-cycle as a result of negative feedback acting on the pituitary and possibly the hypothalamus (*vide infra*). The level rises again to reach a peak shortly before ovulation after which it subsides. The LH level rises slowly in the follicular phase and, shortly before ovulation, there is a sudden and abrupt rise to very high levels (*the LH surge*) before an equally sudden decline occurs (Fig. 4.2). The mid-cycle surge of LH is a great deal more marked than that of FSH. The cause of the surge will be discussed later.

The LH surge reduces oestradiol production in the ovary, possibly by inhibit-ing androgen production but stimulates the luteinization of the granulosa cells which hypertrophy and eventually form the corpus luteum which itself produces progesterone. Ovulation follows so soon after the LH surge that it is likely the two events are linked in some way, but the mechanism is uncertain. One theory, which is backed by a good deal of experimental evidence, suggests that the LH surge stimulates the production in the follicles of prostaglandins (PGE_2 and $PGF_{2\alpha}$) and that the prostaglandins are responsible for ovulation, possibly by inducing contraction of the theca externa cells. A hormone, *inhibin*, found in the mature follicle, may also help to control FSH production.

Neuro-endocrine control of gonadotrophin secretion

We have seen how the uterine cycle is controlled by ovarian hormones and how the ovarian hormones are, in turn, controlled by the gonadotrophins. It is next necessary to discuss the control of the gonadotrophins by the hypothalamus, this being (as far as is known at present) the first step in the cascade (if one excepts the neural control of hormone release).

It was long believed that the hypothalamus produced two gonadotrophic releasing hormones — one for the control of LH and the other for FSH. It is now recognized that a single releasing hormone from the hypothalamus is able to promote the release of both gonadotrophins but the release is primarily of LH; a

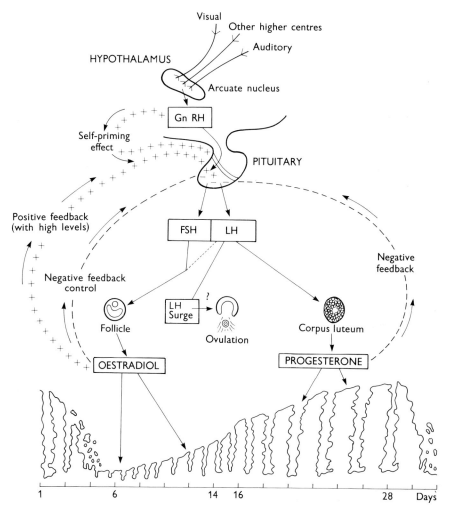

Fig. 4.3. A diagram to illustrate the hormonal control of menstruation. Note the many tiered hierarchy of control. The endometrium is shown at the bottom, then the ovarian control, next the pituitary control of the ovary and, finally, at the top, the hypothalamic control of the pituitary. The hypothalamus itself is subject to influences from higher centres.

more prolonged exposure of the pituitary to the hormone is necessary to release FSH, so that its LH releasing potency is about 5 times that of FSH. For this reason, the hormone is often referred to as an LHRH (*luteinizing hormone releasing hormone*) but, since under normal conditions some FSH release also occurs, the term GnRH (*gonadotrophic releasing hormone*) is more commonly used.

GnRH is released at the endings of the peptidergic neurones in the arcuate nucleus (at least in the monkey) and is transported to the anterior pituitary via the hypophyseal portal system. Throughout most (and possibly all) of the cycle the release of the hormone is pulsatile, the pulses occuring approximately one to two hourly in the human, hence our use of the term 'hypothalamic metronome' (p.54).

Other extra-hypothalamic neurones that form synapses with the peptidergic neurones come from various other parts of the nervous system so that visual and auditory stimuli can affect the output of GnRH. These are of varying importance in different species. For example, oestrus in the ferret is brought about by reflex stimulation of the optic pathway. In the human subject it is important to realise that impulses from the higher centres may also affect the menstrual cycle, as may alterations to the normal circadian rhythm — hence menstrual irregularities may occur as the result of worry, fear of pregnancy and other stressful situations. Nurses and other workers on night duty may also experience disturbance of the normal cycle.

The mechanism of production of the pre-ovulatory LH (and FSH) surge is not fully understood but it is likely that the sharp rise in plasma oestradiol levels that occurs just before the surge (Fig. 4.2) is the initiating factor. In the earliest part of the cycle, the increasing production of oestradiol by the ripening follicle has an inhibiting effect on the release of gonadotrophic hormones (*negative feedback*) but when sustained high levels of oestradiol are attained, the effect on the pituitary and hypothalamus is reversed and the release of hormones stimulated (*positive feedback*). This effect is enhanced by the so-called *self-priming effect* of GnRH, i.e. this hormone not only stimulates release of gonadotrophins but also increases the sensitivity of the pituitary to further doses of GnRH (Fig. 4.3). Thus the mutually enhancing effect of oestradiol and GnRH have the effect of stimulating the pituitary to produce the LH surge. The LH surge therefore depends primarily on the rise of oestradiol output by the ovary (the '*pelvic clock*') and this explains why, in the male, no LH surge occurs. According to some research workers, this mechanism is sufficient to explain the cycle, in some animals at least, but there is also a great deal of evidence that an independent surge of GnRH released from the hypothalamus is responsible for the LH surge by its action on the sensitized cells of the pituitary.

Summary of the menstrual cycle
(Fig. 4.3)

Beginning at the first day of the menstrual period, the thick progestational endometrium breaks down as a result of ischaemic changes and, at the same time, FSH and LH levels begin to rise in the blood. A number of eligible primary follicles in the ovary begin to enlarge, although usually only one completes the course, the others gradually dropping out to form *corpora atretica*. These follicles begin to produce oestrogens (particularly oestradiol) by the combined action of FSH and LH on their theca and granulosa cells. As more and more oestradiol is produced it passes into the follicular fluid along with FSH so that the granulosa cells are exposed to a high concentration of the two hormones. They respond by increasing the output of follicular fluid and oestradiol still further so that the follicle gradually matures. Prostaglandins probably facilitate the migration of the successful follicle towards the surface of the ovary. LH receptors develop on the granulosa cells ready for the LH surge and the luteal phase.

Although the plasma level of FSH is initially prevented from rising too rapidly because of a negative feedback effect, prolonged exposure of the pituitary and hypothalamus to high levels of oestradiol finally elicits a positive feedback response and the GnRH surge from the hypothalamus along with the increased responsiveness of the pituitary produce the LH and FSH surges. The LH surge, probably with the aid of prostaglandins, triggers off ovulation which is followed by the proliferation and luteinization of the lining cells of the follicle. Thus the corpus luteum is formed and the progesterone levels rise, inhibiting further follicles from developing. Another negative feedback operated by progesterone then leads to a rapid fall in FSH and LH levels.

The positive feedback mechanism develops rather late in puberty, so that the first few cycles after menarche may be anovulatory (p.61) since no LH surge occurs.

Artificial induction of ovulation

In many parts of the world infertility in women is commonly caused by pelvic sepsis with consequent blocking of the uterine tubes but attention is increasingly being directed to endocrine causes. Failure to ovulate may be due to obvious disease of the ovaries, pituitary or hypothalamus (such as tumours in these situations) but, when these have been excluded, ovarian function may be investigated by serial estimations of oestradiol and progesterone in the plasma or by administering progesterone for a period of time and then observing the presence, or absence, of withdrawal bleeding which can only occur if the endometrium has been primed with oestrogens. In some cases, more elaborate investigations involving the estimation of FSH, LH and other hormones may be needed. Occasionally it appears that there is a defect in the negative feedback system so that circulating oestradiol has an exaggerated inhibiting action on the pituitary secretion of gonadotrophins. Anti-oestrogen drugs, such as clomiphene which antagonises the inhibitory effect of oestrogens on GnRH, will often raise the concentration of FSH and LH and lead to ovulation, as long as the positive feedback mechanism is intact and can produce an LH surge. In other cases follicular maturation may be induced by by-passing the pituitary and administering exogenous gonadotrophins extracted from human pituitaries or from the urine of post-menopausal women (*menotrophin*). When one or more follicles are ripe (this may be checked by ultrasound examination) human chorionic gonadotrophin (HCG), which is rich in LH, may be used to induce ovulation. The treatment is sometimes too successful and multiple births are likely to occur, so this treatment is only carried out in specialised centres. It is possible that, in the future, the administration of GnRH may be used but this treatment is still in the experimental stage.

Gonadotrophins in the male

In the male, hormones identical to FSH and LH are produced by the pituitary in response to stimulation by GnRH from the hypothalamus but although release of the latter is pulsatile, as in the female, no LH surge occurs in the male because there is no 'pelvic clock' and the two gonadotrophic hormones act together as a complex. FSH acts on the seminiferous tubule, particularly on the Sertoli cells, stimulating the production of spermatozoa. LH acts on the interstitial cells to produce testosterone which, in turn, is necessary for the normal functioning of the Sertoli cells as well as being responsible for the stimulation and maintenance of the accessory structures in the male reproductive system. As in the female, the secretion of gonadotrophins is affected by a negative feedback mechanism from the testicular output of hormones — principally testosterone. Chorionic gonado-trophin (HCG) can be used to replace deficient LH activity. It is given, with or without FSH, in certain cases of infertility and is also used to induce descent of the testis (p.275).

Sex hormones common to both sexes

The accounts given above of the male and female reproductive systems may give the impression that only oestrogens are present in the female and only androgens in the male. In fact, the sex hormones have a very similar chemical make-up and conversion of one to the other can, and does, occur. For example, the Sertoli cells in the male can aromatize testosterone to oestradiol while, in the female, LH stimulates androgen production by the thecal cells and FSH interacts with granulosa cell receptors to produce enzymes that convert androgens to oestradiol. Androgens are also produced by the ovarian stroma and these, too, are converted to oestrogens.

Finally, it must be said that the above account is a very simplified and incom-plete summary of the enormous amount of experimental work which has been done on man and on animals and it has omitted to mention numerous other hormones, some of which may prove to be of fundamental importance.

Menarche and menopause

The age of onset of menstruation (menarche) varies in different populations. In Great Britain it occurs between 10 and 16 years, the average age at the present time being 13.1 years. Menarche is but one event in the onset of puberty and is by no means the first, although it is the most dramatic. The first sign is usually the early development of the breast, with elevation of the nipple and areolar enlargement. The breasts enlarge and pubic, and later axillary, hair appears. The labia majora and minora enlarge, the female distribution of subcutaneous fat develops, the internal genitalia mature and the whole process is accompanied by the adolescent growth spurt with the peak rate of height increase occurring about a year after the beginning of breast development. Since puberty occurs in the female earlier than in the male, girls of this age group tend to be taller than boys of the same age (see Chapter 17).

A rise in FSH levels occurs during childhood but the output of LH does not begin to rise appreciably until early puberty and it is at this time, too, that the output becomes pulsatile. Oestradiol levels rise during puberty but progesterone stays low for some time, even though an LH surge may occur. In spite of the rise in oestradiol levels, the positive feedback mechanism develops rather late in puberty and the first few menstrual cycles may be anovulatory.

The menopause, when menstruation ceases, usually occurs between 45 and 55 years, the average being 48. Its onset is essentially due to a gradual failure of ovaries regularly to produce the ovarian hormones (particularly oestrogens) rather than to an insufficiency of follicles awaiting maturation. Diminution in the negative feedback mechanism leads to an elevated FSH level. Oestrogen production continues to fall and loss of the positive feedback mechanism leads to loss of the LH surge; anovulatory cycles occur or the cycles may become irregular. With cessation of ovulation, LH levels rise and finally menstruation ceases. Occasional ovulation may occur later, however, so that menstruation may recur even after a relatively long cessation. The endometrium becomes thin and atrophic although, even many years after the menopause, oestrogen levels may still be high enough to maintain a reasonably active-looking endometrium. Cyclic changes in the vagina also cease and the epithelium may become atrophied. The menopause is accompanied by systemic symptoms, such as hot flushes, insomnia and depression. If the symptoms are sufficiently severe, oestrogen therapy with natural or synthetic oestrogens, may be very helpful. Vaginal administration has a local effect in increasing the thickness of the epithelium and is particularly indicated in the senile vaginitis that occurs late after the menopause.

Further reading

Fink, G. (1979) Neuroendocrine control of gonadotrophin secretion. *Brit. Med. Bull.*, **35**, 155−160.

Henderson, K.M. (1979) Gonadotrophin regulation of ovarian activity. *Brit. Med. Bull.* **35**, 161−166.

Johnson, M. and Everitt, B. (1984) *Essential Reproduction*, 2nd edn. Blackwell Scientific Publications, Oxford & London.

Knobil, E. (1980) The neuroendocrine control of the menstrual cycle. *Recent Progress in Hormone Research* **36**, 53−88.

Lincoln, G.A. (1979) Pituitary control of testicular activity. *Brit. Med. Bull.*, **35**, 167−172.

Page, E.W., Villee, C.A. & Villee, D.B. (1981) *Human Reproduction*, 3rd, edn. W.B. Saunders, Philadelphia.

Reiter, E.O. & Grumbach, M.M. (1982) Neuroendocrine control mechanisms and the onset of puberty, *Ann. Rev. Physiol.*, **44**, 595−613.

5
Fertilization, Cleavage and Ovum Transport

Blastocyst formation

In common with all higher vertebrates, human insemination is internal. The site within the female reproductive tract at which ejaculation by the male takes place varies in different mammals. In the human, semen is deposited in the immediate vicinity of the external uterine os and from here the spermatozoa must find their way to the outer third of the uterine tube where fertilization of the ovum takes place; the journey must be accomplished within 24–48 hours for there is good evidence to suggest that the sperm cannot live longer than this. They probably have a diminished fertilizing power for some time before loss of motility.

Sperm transport

The coagulation of human semen within a minute of ejaculation and its sub-sequent liquefaction about 20 minutes later has already been mentioned (p.38). This probably facilitates the retention of sperm for a critical period during which they can penetrate the cervical mucus. The alkaline semen raises vaginal pH from pH 3–4 to pH 7.2 for a time and, although this temporarily reduces the barrier to infection, it allows the sperm to become motile. At pH 3–4 their movement would be completely inhibited.

The cervical mucus through the greater part of the menstrual cycle provides an effective barrier not only to infection but also to the passage of sperm but, due to the rise in oestrogen level that precedes ovulation, its chemical and physical characteristics change abruptly. Microscopically an 'open' structure with gaps between the mucus fibrils forms and the glycoprotein molecules become arranged in parallel micelles along which actively swimming spermatozoa are guided upwards. Proteolytic enzymes are present in the ejaculate and endogenous protein inhibitors normally present in the cervical mucus fall to low levels at mid-cycle.

Another important characteristic of the cervical mucus at the time of ovulation is that its molecular lattice is so constituted that it allows sperm whose tail beat frequency is within normal limits to traverse it but delays or stops abnormal forms and other particulate matter. This is because of the frequency of its well developed thermal oscillation, i.e. the cervical mucus as a whole has a 'beat frequency' which can be measured by nuclear magnetic resonance.

The uterus, like the vagina, does not provide a very congenial place for sperm to exist and they rapidly pass to the utero-tubal junction (*vide infra*). The utero-tubal junction acts in the same way as the mid-cycle cervix to provide a 'reservoir' for sperm and releases a steady stream proximally towards the Fallopian tubes. Both the muscular contractions of the uterine tube and the proven tendency of spermatozoa to move *against* the ciliary stream, which causes intraluminal tubal fluid to move towards the uterus, result in the arrival of sperm at the site of fertilization within a short time of coitus. They have been isolated from the inner part of the tube a few *minutes* after ejaculation.

The passage of sperm to the uterine tube thus depends partly upon the active motility of the sperm itself and partly on other factors such as the contraction of uterine musculature. The sperm are, in general, carried passively but sperm motility is an important factor in passing through the mucous barrier present in the cervix, in traversing the utero-tubal junction and in penetrating the corona radiata and zona pellucida of the ovum. Various agents have been suggested as having an effect upon muscular contractions in the female genital tract though their relative importance awaits further study. Thus it has been shown that physiological concentrations of certain prostaglandins, secreted into the semen by the seminal vesicles, increase the motility of uterine musculature *in vivo* at certain stages of the menstrual cycle and may, therefore, facilitate the transport of sperm from the vagina to the uterine cavity. Uterine contractions occur during orgasm and may also result from the release of posterior pituitary hormones during coitus.

The unanswered questions concerning sperm transport are numerous but it is believed that no more than a few hundred spermatozoa reach the general region of fertilization compared with an average of 210 million present in the ejaculate. The great excess of sperm secreted is understandable if one considers that perhaps a majority of them are probably not capable of fertilising the egg. Furthermore, the concentrations found are required because the chances of a fertile sperm reaching the ovum appear to be entirely a matter of chance. Natural selection has no doubt resulted in a number being produced which maximises the chances of successful coitus to the level required.

Ovulation and egg transport

As previously described (p.41) a number of Graafian follicles approach maturity at mid-cycle but usually only one of these releases its contained ovum. A great accumulation of fluid occurs within the antrum and a portion of the follicular circumference becomes superficial, separated from the peritoneal cavity by little more than a much thinned membrana granulosa and an attenuated ovarian epithelium (Fig. 3.5). Ovulation occurs through a small opening which forms in a region at which the ovarian epithelium thins still further and becomes elevated to form the *stigma*. The aperture enlarges and the ovum, together with the surrounding cells of the cumulus oophorus which now form the *corona radiata*, are expressed with the follicular fluid over a period of 1–2 seconds (Fig. 3.7).

Expulsion is the result of intrafollicular pressure and possibly also of contraction of ovarian smooth muscle in the theca externa as a result of stimulation by prostaglandins (see Chapter 4), but it is a gentle process rather than the explosive one previously envisaged. Within a few minutes of ovulation the ovum leaves the peritoneal cavity and enters the ostium of the uterine tube. This is because the outer end of the tube is prolonged into a series of finger-like processes called *fimbria* (p.41) which almost completely embrace the ovary and which are lined by a ciliated epithelium. Furthermore, the surface of the ovary also has ciliated areas and the newly shed ovum thus almost invariably comes into contact with a ciliary field. The latter transports it to the ostium which is sufficiently relaxed to allow unimpeded entry to the funnel shaped outer part of the Fallopian tube which is known as the *infundibulum* (Fig. 3.4).

The infundibulum is the trumpet-shaped distal portion of the uterine tube and this leads to the longest portion of the tube — the *ampulla* which is about 5–8 cm long. The lumen of its outer end has a diameter of 1 cm narrowing to 1–2 mm at its junction with the *isthmus*. The isthmus has the narrowest lumen of any segment in the tube (100 μm–1 mm) as well as the thickest wall. It connects the ampulla with the *intramural part* of the uterine tube at the *utero-tubal junction*. The total length of the uterine tube is about 11–12 cm; its epithelium contains both ciliated and secretory cells and these vary in histology and function during the various phases of the ovarian cycle.

Human ova pass rapidly through the infundibulum but there is a prolonged period of arrest in the ampulla which lasts for about 72 hours. The ampulla is also the site of fertilization. There follows a rapid passage through the isthmus so that ova reach the endometrial cavity roughly 80 hours after rupture of the follicle. There is no evidence of delay at the utero-tubal junction or in the intramural part of the tube.

It is obvious, therefore, that the various parts of the uterine tube are physiologically distinct and act together in a co-ordinated fashion in order to arrange for the fertilized ovum to reach the uterus at the optimum time.

Because of the complex nature of the tube, operations to reconstitute it after its interruption for contraceptive measures are — more often than not — unsuccessful. Many factors have been putatively associated with ovum transport; they include muscle contractility, adrenergic innervation, the role of the mucosa (especially the epithelium) at various stages of the cycle and the role of the ampullary isthmic junction. In our present state of knowledge all that can be said is that no single factor is predominant.

The premature delivery of the fertilized egg into the uterus may still be associated with pregnancy and, therefore, attempts at achieving contraception by causing rapid expulsion of the tubal egg do not at present seem to constitute a very promising approach.

The mechanism of fertilization

The freshly ovulated ovum is described in Chapter 3. It is at the spindle stage of the second meiotic division (i.e. a dividing secondary oocyte) having already extruded the first polar body. Surrounding it (and its polar body) is a thick, non-cellular capsule, the *zona pellucida*, outside which lies the *corona radiata* formed from the cells of the cumulus oophorus (p.44). Once ovulated the human egg must be fertilized within 24 hours or else it undergoes degenerative changes and becomes incapable of normal development. Since only low numbers of sperm (about 200) manage to find their way to the outer part of the uterine tube it is not unnatural to suspect that they may be attracted in some specific way to the immediate vicinity of the ovum. If fact, simple mechanical factors may well channel the gametes to the same region of the tube and the evidence for a chemically mediated attraction between them is unconvincing. An antigen—antibody type of reaction has been demonstrated in the sea urchin and it has recently been suggested that similar mechanisms may play a part in mammalian reproduction. No final judgement on this issue can yet be made.

Freshly ejaculated sperm are incapable of fertilizing the ovum and normally require to undergo *capacitation* in the female genital tract. This phenomenon usually seems to depend upon intimate contact between spermatozoa and the epithelial lining of the uterus and takes about 8 hours in the human. Capacitated sperm show no morphological change but they become more active and are now capable of penetrating the egg coverings. The exact nature of capacitation is unknown; it may be due to the removal of glycoproteins (decapacitating factors) which are present on the sperm surface while it is in seminal fluid. Capacitation is followed by changes in, and eventual shedding of, the anterior part of the acrosomal cap. This is known as the *acrosome reaction* which is associated with the sequential release of acrosomal enzymes. The first of these is *hyaluronidase* which is capable of breaking down certain mucopolysaccharides (glycosaminoglycans) and probably helps to dissociate the cells of the corona radiata. It thus facilitates their penetration by sperm which must next pass through the zona pellucida. Exactly how this is achieved is not completely understood though attachment of the sperm to the zona pellucida and release of low concentrations of the protease *acrosin* present in the acrosome are probably involved. The human zona pellucida is rich in sialic acid. *Neuraminidase*, which is next released from the acrosome, breaks this down. It makes the zona more resistant to further action of proteolytic enzymes such as acrosin and thus to penetration by further sperm. The precise means by which the sperm head penetrates the plasma membrane of the ovum, which underlies the zona pellucida, probably differs in various mammalian species; on reaching the egg surface the sperm is tangentially orientated and it seems possible that the egg and post-acrosomal sperm cell membranes fuse (cf. diagram of sperm Fig. 3.3). The fused areas then disappear and (posterior part first) the sperm head thus comes to lie in the egg cytoplasm.

Blockage to polyspermy

For obvious reasons the head of only one sperm must be allowed to fuse with the female pronucleus. To this end mechanisms are developed to prevent the penetration of the ovum by more than one sperm. Thus a reaction in the zona pellucida appears to be initiated by contact with the first spermatozoon; the function of this reaction is to prevent penetration by other sperm. The zonal reaction is only partially effective in the human and supernumerary sperm are sometimes seen in the substance of the zona though rarely deep into it or in the egg cytoplasm. A second, and probably more important reaction is initiated by penetration of the plasma membrane of the egg by the fertilizing sperm. As a result of this, rapid changes occur in the cortical region of the ovum which include the breakdown of cortically located granules, a shrinkage in the size of the ovum and the appearance of a space between the plasma membrane of the egg and the zona pellucida. Once the cortical changes have taken place no more sperm are able to penetrate the egg. Basically similar cortical changes in invertebrate eggs include the raising of a 'fertilization membrane' from the surface of the egg.

The union of nuclei

Minutes after penetration of the tubal ovum (i.e. the secondary oocyte, see Chapter 3) by a spermatozoon, activation occurs and a second polar body is formed; the ovum is now called an *ootid* (cf. spermatid), the term zygote being reserved for the stage at which fusion of the male and female pronuclei has occurred.

Shortly after penetrating the ovum the sperm loses its tail and middle piece while its head forms the male *pronucleus* by enlarging, migrating towards the centre of the egg and forming numerous somewhat atypical nucleoli together with a dispersed chromatin network. Similar changes occur in the ootid nucleus which now becomes known as the female pronucleus or *germinal vesicle*. Within 12 hours of fertilization the pronuclei meet near the centre of the ovum and their nuclear membranes fuse; the nucleoli disappear and it has been tentatively suggested that ribosomal precursors may escape into the cytoplasm at this stage in development.

In its passage towards the female pronucleus, the sperm head rotates through 180°. It was, at one time, thought that the male centriole divided to form the first cleavage spindle but this now appears to be doubtful and the female centriole is believed to perform this function; the chromosomes of both pronuclei arrange themselves on the spindle and each is seen to consist of two chromatids. DNA duplication (at least in the rabbit) has been shown to occur between 3 and 6 hours after fertilization. The chromatids pass to opposite poles of the spindle, as they would in normal mitosis, and the nuclear membranes are reconstituted. A circumferential furrow appears opposite the equator of the spindle and deepens, thus completing the first cleavage division of the human ovum. This occurs within

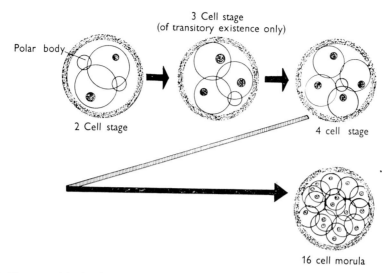

Fig. 5.1. Cleavage of the fertilized ovum and the formation of the morula just before entry into the uterus. Often one or both polar bodies are not visible (e.g. compare 2 cell stage with 3 and 4 cell stages).

24 hours of fertilization. The polar bodies eventually disintegrate within the space between the plasma membrane of the egg and the zona pellucida.

Parthenogenesis

Sperm penetration of the ovum not only restores the diploid chromosome number but also activates the egg biochemically; this then leads on to cleavage. Under certain circumstances the ovum may be activated and begin to divide without sperm penetration. In contrast to what has been found in many lower vertebrates, it is very unlikely that such development has ever led to the production of live mammalian offspring although parthenogenetically-induced rabbits have been reported. It has been estimated that, on average, man carries between 3 and 8 lethal equivalents; that is, numerous genes each with a slightly deleterious effect equivalent to 3 to 8 recessive genes which, if homozygous, would result in death before reproduction. Since diploid parthenogenetic individuals formed by fusion of the ootid with the second polar body would be homozygous for every genetic characteristic one would imagine the chances of survival would be slight.

Contraception

In the middle of the nineteenth century world population estimates were around 1,000 million. By 1967 it had increased to 3,420 million and it has been forecast that between 6,000 and 7,000 million people will be alive at the turn of the present century. Obviously there is a limit to such an increase and, seen in this context, contraception as a method of population control becomes a sociological and demographic as well as an individual issue. Many methods varying in reliability, safety, cost, ease of use and aesthetic acceptability are available and naturally the method chosen (if any) depends upon local circumstances. Quite apart from ethical and legal considerations, abortion is not a medically acceptable alternative to effective contraception.

The principal techniques of contraception in common use are the following:

Coitus interruptus

This term is applied to withdrawal of the penis before ejaculation. It is an unreliable and psychologically unacceptable method.

The so-called safe period

This is based upon the fact that ovulation takes place around the middle of the menstrual cycle (p.46). Unfortunately, although the period of time which elapses between ovulation and subsequent menstruation (i.e. the luteal phase of the cycle) is fairly constant at 14 days, there is considerable variation in the length of the interval between menstruation and subsequent ovulation. For this reason avoidance of coitus for a week or ten days centred upon the middle of the cycle cannot be said to be an effective means of contraception.

Spermicidal agents

The use of spermicidal agents introduced into the vagina before coitus. These usually act by altering the local pH but they are rarely used alone because they are of limited efficacy.

Physical barriers

Protective devices for use by the male, such as condoms or sheaths covering the penis, are available; alternatively, various types of rubber diaphragm stretched on springs and fitted to occlude the cervical os after being covered with spermicidal jelly may be used (Fig. 5.2a and b). Either method is reasonably effective but may be aesthetically unacceptable.

Intra-uterine devices

The insertion of intra-uterine coils or springs prevents pregnancy either by inhibiting sperm migration to the uterine tubes or (more likely) by causing the uterine environment to be hostile to the implantation of the blastocyst. The method is particularly valuable to women who have previously had children.

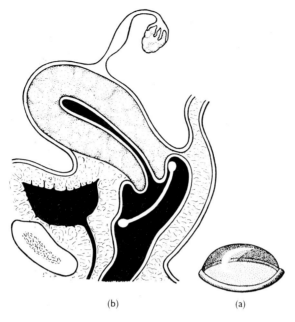

Fig. 5.2. (a) A contraceptive diaphragm (b) The diaphragm *in situ.*

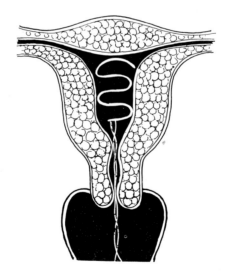

Fig. 5.3. An intra-uterine coil which has been introduced through the cervix.

Contraceptive pills

Pills containing various combinations of oestrogens and progestogens abolish ovulation by inhibition of gonadotrophin secretion (negative feedback — see Chapter 4) but the content of oestrogens must be kept low to avoid undesirable side effects. Pills are usually taken between 5 and 25 days of an artificial cycle, they are then stopped and withdrawal bleeding occurs; on the fifth day of bleeding the treatment is repeated. There are unwanted side effects however, and though occurrence of fatal blood clotting (thrombosis) is an extremely rare one, some women experience other troublesome symptoms such as headaches, depression, weight change and other common accompaniments of sex hormone therapy such as raised blood pressure. Since oestrogens are probably responsible for the serious side effects of combined pills, pills containing progesterone only are sometimes used. This form of contraception probably still allows ovulation to occur but the hormone acts on the endometrium, the cervical mucus and the uterine tubes to produce a reasonable contraceptive effect. It is, however, markedly less effective than the combined pill. These tablets are taken every day throughout the cycle. A post-coital contraceptive measure is available in emergency but not for routine use. Ovarian hormones taken in large doses after coitus but before implantation can prevent pregnancy. Two doses of 100 mg of ethinyl-oestradiol are taken 12 hours apart. The first dose should be taken as soon as possible after coitus and in any case within 72 hours. There is sufficient risk of failure to make the method unsuitable as a routine measure.

Voluntary sterilization

This is a simple procedure in the male, consisting of ligature and cutting the ductus (vas) deferens outside the inguinal canal. From a practical point of view it is important to note that sterility does not immediately result from this operation and the patient must continue to practise adequate contraception for about two months. In the female, occluding the uterine tubes, though a more extensive operation, is frequently practised. These methods are the most effective of all and are used when there is an overwhelming medical necessity to prevent further pregnancies. Unfortunately, they are largely irreversible.

Other methods

Various contraceptive methods not in general use yet are being intensively studied. They include experimental work on the non-hormonal prevention of spermatogenesis and sperm maturation and the stimulation of immune responses to spermatozoa.

Infertility

Up to 40 per cent of infertile, or subfertile, couples are unable to conceive because of unsatisfactory spermatogenesis. The testis will not produce sperm if it has not descended into the scrotum (most probably because it is subject to a relatively high intra-abdominal temperature) although the interstitial cells are active and libido is unimpaired. Non-descent, or maldescent, of the testes is therefore a common cause of sterility but, in other cases, normally situated testes do not produce normal numbers of actively motile sperm. Opinions differ considerably but repeated sperm counts of less than 30−40 million/ml are usually considered to be associated with sub-fertility and individuals with counts of less than 5 million/ ml hardly ever conceive. In addition to sperm concentration and numbers, sperm motility as well as morphology are important though, in a man with a high count, the presence of relatively large numbers of abnormal forms is comparatively unimportant. Anatomical abnormalities of the male genitalia, such as hypospadias (p.273) may, of course, also lead to infertility.

Abnormalities or disease of the female reproductive system also account for many cases of infertility. Congenital anatomical abnormalities are relatively rare but diseases affecting the reproductive organs are far more common and lead to secondary anatomical defects, such as blockage of the uterine tubes, following infection or the inability of the uterus to sustain a pregnancy as a result of the presence of a large benign fibrous tumour known as a *fibroid*.

A small number of women do not ovulate spontaneously and, in these cases, the artificial induction of ovulation (p.59) has lead to dramatic results. Unfortunately, the effects are not entirely predictable and multiple births may, therefore, occur when this therapy is used.

Apart from an inability to conceive due to lack of potency which may be basically a psychological problem, a number of marriages remain childless even though investigation of both partners gives normal results. No adequate explanation of these cases is forthcoming though a number of factors are currently under investigation. Among them may be mentioned the ability of the sperm to survive in the female genital tract, and particularly their ability to penetrate the cervical mucus (p.62); immunological incompatibility based upon sensitization of the female to her partner's semen has also been suggested as a factor in causing sperm death in infertile couples.

In view of what has been said above, the investigation of a case of infertility involves first of all taking a careful history, particularly of the menstrual cycle, and examination. The male is next investigated since this is easy and rapid. Finally, the hormonal changes during the menstrual cycle are studied with particular reference to the presence, or absence, of ovulation (see Chapter 4).

Extra-corporeal fertilization

In certain cases of sterility, particularly those due to blockage of the uterine tube, attempts at extra-corporeal fertilization of the ovum followed by implantation of the fertilized ovum into the uterus have begun to meet with some success. The method clearly has enormous potential besides being of great medical interest. A number of factors have been of importance in its development:

1 Freshly ejaculated sperm are capacitated *in vitro*. The previously held assumption that sperm had to be collected from the female tract has been abandoned although seminal fluid is still removed from the ejaculate, the sperm being 'cleaned' by gentle centrifugation and re-suspension of the spermatozoa in culture serum;

2 Simple salt solutions containing pyruvate, albumin and perhaps glucose are used as media in which fertilization takes place. Careful attention to osmolality is essential (280–290 mosm kg) and the pH is kept at between 7.2 and 7.3. Reduced oxygen tension compared to air is optimal and the temperature is adjusted to just over 37°C;

3 Concentration of spermatozoa between 10^5 and 10^6 ml^{-1} are used in the fertilization droplets. This is very important because higher concentrations lead to polyspermy and resultant aneuploidy while lower levels result in loss of fertilizing capacity;

4 Oocytes are removed from the ovaries at laparoscopy 20–24 hours after the initiation of the LH surge as estimated by urinary hormone levels. Eggs are taken from mature follicles and the practice of inducing ovulation hormonally is commonly used;

5 At the 8–16 cell stage the embryo is inserted into the female reproductive tract through the cervical canal. Timing is critical and it seems that success is much more likely if the egg is replaced in the evening. Clearly there must be synchrony between the uterine cycle and embryonic development. It seems possible that a longer incubation before insertion may lead to better results;

6 A successful outcome may be helped by progesterone therapy after placing the fertilised eggs in the uterus but essentially the body's own hormonal response is paramount. It is for this reason that synchrony is essential. The egg obtained at laparoscopy is placed with the fertilization droplet within two minutes of its removal;

7 If pregnancy occurs it must clearly be carefully monitored. Congenital defects are rare but the possibility of chromosomal defect resulting perhaps from polyspermy is present. Amniocentesis followed by karyotyping of fetal cells is essential even though most aneuploidies are spontaneously aborted. At the same time the other usual test on amniotic fluid (such as determination of levels of alphafetoprotein) are performed. Ultrasound investigations and careful repeated checks of maternal hormone levels are essential.

Cleavage

Male and female pronuclei meet near the centre of the ovum within 12 hours of fertilization and fuse, converting the ootid into a zygote. Almost immediately the first cleavage spindle is formed and each chromosome, at this stage, is seen to consist of 2 chromatids since DNA replication in each pronucleus has taken place some hours earlier. The stage is thus set for the first cleavage division of the zygote and this is completed 24 hours after fertilization. Penetration of the sperm stimulates a great deal of metabolic activity in the egg as seen in experimental studies in which labelled amino acid incorporation and oxygen consumption are greatly increased.

Cleavage consists of repeated mitotic divisions of the zygote *which is still contained within its zona pellucida* with the consequent formation of an increasing number of cells called *blastomeres* but without an increase in total cytoplasmic mass. In the uncleaved egg, which it will be remembered is some 100−150 μm in diameter, the amount of cytoplasm is greatly in excess of that present in a normal somatic cell. As a result of segmentation the nucleo-cytoplasmic ratio is gradually increased to only a little less than the average for diploid human cells (Fig. 5.1). There is now considerable evidence that the formation of immediately active messenger RNA is absent during early cleavage. When substantial gene transcription is re-initiated the nuclei have a much smaller amount of cytoplasm to deal with and the functional genes on the chromosomes are thus able to produce sufficient RNA to control the cells efficiently. An obvious effect of cleavage is the partitioning of zygote cytoplasm among the blastomeres. There is evidence that in some sub-mammalian species the nuclei of individual cells come to lie in quantitatively and qualitatively different cytoplasmic environments and the initial circumstances for cellular differentiation could be created. Furthermore, the blastomeres of the future inner cell mass (*vide infra*) are able to move with respect to one another; the ground-work for the *morphogenetic movements* of gastrulation are therefore laid and the possibility of *inductive cellular interaction*, resulting from the acquisition of a new micro-environment by an individual cell, is established. The blastomeres are morphologically distinct until about the 8 cell stage. They are held together by interdigitations of their microvilli rather than by tight junctions. At about the 16 cell stage the *morula* enters the uterus and a process known as *compaction* occurs as a result of which the blastomeres become less distinct. At this stage the cells on the outside of the morula become adherent by means of gap junctions and a topographical difference is established between the surface cells and those inside them. It is possible that this is the stage at which a restriction of blastomere totipotency first begins. Work done on the mouse embryo suggests that the outer cells *under the influence of the inner cell mass* form the *trophectoderm* which will finally form the fetal membranes while the inner cells (the *inner cell mass*) will form the embryonic cells and will perhaps also contribute to the extra-embryonic membranes. Certainly the outer cells very quickly develop functional differences and acquire the morphological appearances characteristic of specific activity (such as large quantities of granular endoplasmic reticulum, organised cell organelles, etc.) which those of the inner cell mass lack. Nevertheless, there is still no unanimity of opinion regarding the restriction of inter-changeability between the two types of cells and, therefore, the degree to which the embryo is able to 'regulate' its development at this stage.

While undergoing cleavage the ovum is, as previously explained, passed along the uterine tube by a combination of currents in the mucus created by the ciliary action of its lining epithelium and by muscular contraction. It moves somewhat erratically towards the medial, or uterine, end of the ampulla but its passage along the isthmic portion of the tube is probably fairly rapid and the conceptus is thought to reach the uterine cavity about 3 or 4 days after ovulation. At this stage it is known as a *morula* from its resemblance to a mulberry.

The nutritional requirements of the fertilized tubal ovum are slight; they are provided in part by the sparse yolk granules of the egg but chiefly they come from the tubal secretions. Different regions of the uterine tube each provide a different environment and this is probably important for normal development. The fact that the zona pellucida is freely permeable to gases and low molecular weight substances is demonstrated by the requirement of an exogenous source of lactate or pyruvate for the second cleavage (but not for subsequent divisions) in mouse ova. It seems, therefore, that cleaving eggs are metabolically active and to some extent dependent upon their surroundings; they incorporate labelled amino acids into their proteins even in the presence of Actinomycin D, a drug which stops DNA-dependent RNA synthesis. This fact has been interpreted as showing that at least some of the restricted protein synthesis occurring during cleavage has been 'programmed' in the unfertilized ovum and normally begins to function only as a result of activation by fertilization.

Formation of the blastocyst

Between 4 and 6 days after ovulation the morula imbibes uterine fluid which passes through the zona pellucida and eventually forms a confluent *blastocyst cavity*. This separates the inner cell mass from the trophoblast except over the so-called *polar trophoblast* which overlies the inner cell mass (Fig. 5.4).

During blastocyst formation the conceptus increases from 150 μm to 300 μm in diameter while the zona pellucida thins and eventually disappears though the

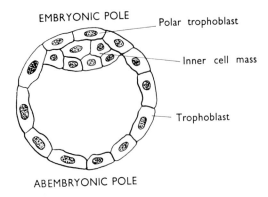

Fig. 5.4. Diagram of the human blastocyst.

precise mechanism of its shedding is not entirely clear. The cells of the blastocyst are now exposed and the polar trophoblast becomes adherent to the uterine wall most commonly high up and posteriorly. Next, the blastocyst becomes implanted in the endometrium and the fetal membranes differentiate rapidly. We shall take up this subject again in Chapter 7 but, in order to understand it fully, we must first turn our attention to the further development of the inner cell mass.

Developmental stages

1 Fertilization — within 24 hours of ovulation.
2 Passage through the isthmus — 72 hours after ovulation.
3 Entry into uterus — over 80 hours after ovulation.
4 Blastocyst formation — 4–6 days after ovulation.
5 Implantation — circa. 7 days after ovulation.

Further reading

Aitken, R.J. (1979) Contraceptive research and development. *Brit. med. Bull.*, **35**, 199–204.

Bedford J.M. (1982) Fertilization In: *Reproduction in Mammals*, 2nd edn. Book 1, Chapter 6, eds. Austin C.R. & Short, R.V. Cambridge University Press.

Blandau, P.J. (1968) Gamete transport–comparative aspects. In: *The Mammalian Oviduct*, eds. Hafeg, E.S.E. & Blandan, J. University of Chicago Press.

Edwards, R.G. (1980) *Conception in the Human Female*. Academic Press, London & New York.

El Badrawi, H.H. & Hafez, E.S.E. (1982) Factors and mechanisms affecting success of *in vitro* fertilization and embryo transfer. In: In vitro *Fertilization and Embryo Transfer*, eds. Hafez, E.S.E. & Semm, K. M.T.P. Press, Lancaster.

Fridhandler, L. (1968) Gametogenosis to implantation. In: *Biology of Gestation*, Vol. 1. ed. Assali, N. Academic Press, New York & London.

Hafez, E.S.E. (ed.) (1976) *Human Semen and Fertility Regulation in Man*. The C.V. Mosby Co, St Louis.

Hogarth, P.J. (1978) *The Biology of Reproduction*, Chapter 3. Blackie, Glasgow & London.

Moghissi, K.S. & Hafez, E.S.E. (eds.) (1972) *Biology of Mammalian Fertilization and Implantation*. C.C. Thomas, Springfield, III.

6

Formation of Germ Layers (Gastrulation) and Early Development

The formation of the amnion, yolk sac and bilaminar disc

During the early stages of the implantation of the blastocyst into the uterine endometrium, i.e. about the 6th to 8th day after ovulation, the inner cell mass begins to undergo a process of differentiation which will eventually result in the formation of a complete embryo. At first the deepest cells, those facing the blastocyst cavity, become cuboidal and form a single layer of primary *embryonic endoderm*. The remainder of the inner cell mass then gradually forms a layer of columnar cells which constitutes the precursor of the *embryonic ectoderm* and will also later give rise to the *embryonic mesoderm* (p.81). The *amniotic cavity* appears between these columnar cells and an overlying layer of cells forming the *amniotic ectoderm* derived from the deep aspect of the polar trophoblast (Fig. 6.1). The cells of the future embryo, i.e. the inner cell mass, thus form no more than a *bilaminar embryonic disc* and the whole of the remainder of the conceptus goes on to form the fetal membranes (Chapter 7). The earliest implanted human embryo, described by Rock and Hertig, is approaching this stage of development; it is believed to be not more than 7½ days old.

While the amniotic cavity is being formed the blastocyst cavity becomes lined by cells of *extra-embryonic endoderm*. The details of this process have not been observed in man and the earliest available specimens of this stage of development already have a blastocyst wall made up of three layers (Fig. 6.2). These consist of a thick outer trophoblast (the *extra-embryonic ectoderm*), a loose reticular layer of *extra-embryonic mesoderm* and an inner squamous layer of *extra-embryonic endoderm*. The trophoblast itself can be subdivided into an inner layer of discrete cells, the *cytotrophoblast* giving rise to a thick *syncytiotrophoblast* layer on its outer aspect (Figs. 6.1, 6.2, etc.). As the name suggests, plasma membranes are absent between the individual cells of the syncytiotrophoblastic cells. The extra-embryonic endoderm, in continuity with the cuboidal layers of primary embryonic endoderm of the bilaminar embryonic disc, forms the wall of the *yolk sac* (Fig. 6.2). The origin of extra-embryonic endoderm is in some doubt; in man it may well have formed *in situ* from the inner layer of the extra-embryonic mesoderm.

In a localised area of the roof of the yolk sac the cuboidal cells become columnar and form the *prochordal plate*. This change takes place at the cranial end of the future embryo and confers bilateral symmetry upon the bilaminar embryonic disc (Figs. 6.3., 6.4., and 6.5). The prochordal plate will form the endodermal constituent of the buccopharyngeal membrane (Fig. 6.7). Meanwhile the extra-embryonic mesoderm, which in any case consists of a loose network of cells,

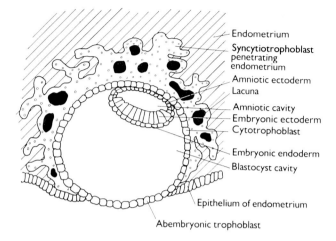

Fig. 6.1. An almost completely implanted conceptus. The inner cell mass has formed a bilaminar embryonic disc and an amniotic cavity. The trophoblast has formed cytotrophoblast and syncytiotrophoblast over most of the surface of the conceptus.

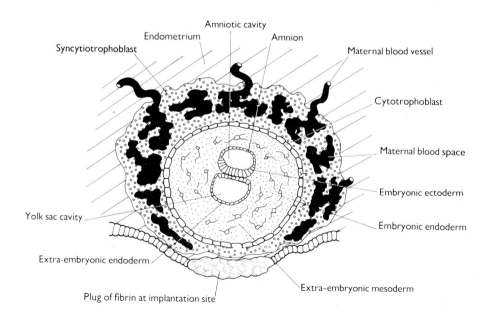

Fig. 6.2. The conceptus is now completely implanted in the endometrium. The original cavity of the blastocyst is filled with loose, cellular extra-embryonic mesoderm.

begins to develop fluid-filled spaces. These become confluent and a large cavity is
formed which surrounds the whole of the yolk sac and the amnion (except for a
circumscribed mesodermal *connecting stalk*). This is the *extra-embryonic coelom*
which largely splits the extra-embryonic mesoderm into 'visceral' and 'parietal'

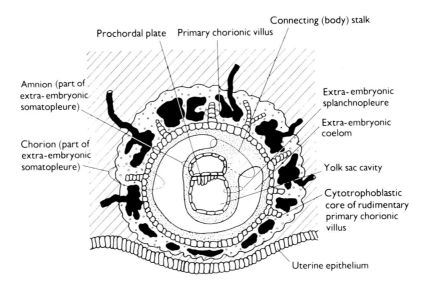

Fig. 6.3. Chorionic vesicle in which the extra-embryonic mesoderm has broken down, except in the
region of the connecting stalk, to form the extra-embryonic coelom. Note the prochordal plate which
confers a bilateral symmetry on the embryonic disc.

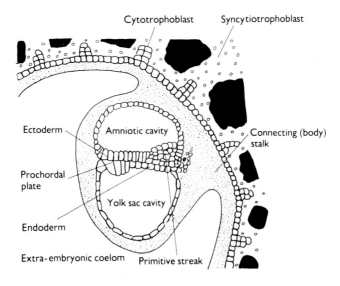

Fig. 6.4. Embryonic region on the inner aspect of the chorionic vesicle. The anterior (cranial) end of the
embryonic disc is marked by the prochordal plate and the caudal end by the primitive streak.

layers and separates the amniotic and yolk sac cavities from the outer wall of the conceptus (Fig. 6.3).

The endoderm of the yolk sac, together with its covering of extra-embryonic mesoderm, is known as the *extra-embryonic splanchnopleure* while the extra-embryonic ectoderm (both trophoblastic and amniotic) and the adjacent mesoderm form the *extra-embryonic somatopleure*. The trophoblast and its underlying mesoderm (i.e. the whole of the somatopleure except that of the amniotic ectoderm and overlying mesoderm which, together, constitute the *amniotic membrane* or — more simply — the *amnion*) is called the *chorion* and forms the outer wall of the *chorionic vesicle* (Fig. 6.3).

The primary germ layers

We have introduced the terms 'ectoderm', 'endoderm', and 'mesoderm' into the foregoing account and have differentiated between their embryonic and extra-embryonic portions. At this point it is worthwhile considering the implications of distinguishing between various tissues of the conceptus. Ectoderm, endoderm and mesoderm are known as the three *primary germ layers* and during the normal course of development they give rise to specific organs and tissues.

Embryonic ectoderm, as its name implies, forms the outer covering of the embryo; this includes the outer layers of the skin and its derivatives (p.128) as well as of the mucous membrane at the cranial and caudal extremes of the digestive tract (p.278). The central and peripheral nervous systems (including the retina) are also ectodermal in origin (p.138) as is part of the iris of the eye. A comprehensive list of all structures of ectodermal origin will not be given here since the most important are dealt with in appropriate sections but it is worth stating that, except for the nervous system, ectodermal derivatives generally form epithelial tissues in the adult. This fact has no real biological significance and, indeed, there are exceptions (as in the case of the musculature of the iris (p.156)). It is important, therefore, to distinguish clearly between epithelial tissues (i.e. an histological type which may be derived from any of the germ layers) and ectodermal tissues (derivatives of a primary germ layer).

Embryonic endoderm forming, as we have seen, the lower layer of the embryonic disc (Figs. 6.2., 6.3., 6.4., 6.6 and 6.7) gives rise to the epithelial lining of the alimentary tract between its ectodermally derived cranial and caudal extremities, as well as to the parenchyma of its associated glands (such as the liver and pancreas). Derivatives of the gut including the pharyngeal pouches (p.176), the epithelial lining of the respiratory system (p.237) and most of the epithelium of the bladder and urethra (p.254) are also of endodermal origin. Endodermally-derived structures are epithelial.

So far we have only noted the emergence of extra-embryonic mesoderm; in the next section it will be observed that embryonic mesoderm becomes interposed between the ectodermal and endodermal layers of the embryonic disc (Figs. 6.5

and 6.6). The derivatives of this germ layer may give rise (like those of the ectoderm and endoderm) to adult epithelial structures including the coelomic epithelium (sometimes, therefore, known as a mesothelium (p.234)), the lining of the uterine tubes and uterus (p.261), the epithelial tissues of the kidney and the ureteric lining (p.251). However, certain parts of the embryonic mesoderm lose their epithelial characteristics early in embryonic life (for example, the cells of the sclerotome (p.119)) and form an embryonic connective tissue known as *mesenchym*.

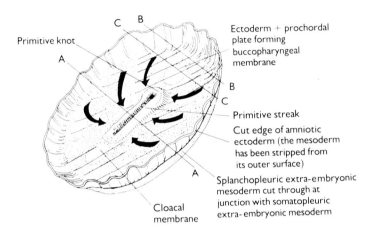

Fig. 6.5. A diagrammatic representation of the embryonic disc, revealed by cutting away most of the amniotic ectoderm and all of the extra-embryonic mesoderm covering it. Intra-embryonic mesoderm is stippled; the ectoderm is represented as transparent. The arrows indicate the migration of cells towards the primitive streak. Sections through the embryonic disc at A, B and C are shown in Fig. 6.6.

The latter has important supporting functions similar to those of adult connective tissue but, in addition, its loosely arranged fusiform and stellate cells are phagocytic and serve to eliminate dying cells. Among other structures, the mesenchyme gives rise to all the adult connective tissues (including cartilage and bone), to smooth, striated and cardiac muscle and to the lymphatic system and the cardio-vascular system including the cells of the blood. Some of its cells, for example the cells lining the blood vessels, therefore revert to an epithelial form.

Clearly there is no fundamental distinction in the histological nature of the ultimate derivatives of primary germ layers. Ectoderm, endoderm and mesoderm may all form epithelial structures and in restricted regions (such as in the iris) ectodermal structures form smooth muscle, a tissue that otherwise arises largely from mesenchyme. Thus, tissue differentiation is not the same as germ layer formation. In fact, division of the early embryo into three primary germ layers is, to some extent, one of descriptive convenience.

The extra-embryonic tissues (*fetal membranes*) are derivatives of the wall of the blastocyst and form structures necessary for the intra-uterine maintenance of the embryo and fetus. They do not contribute to the fetus proper but are shed at birth. Like the embryonic tissues they are made up of ectoderm, endoderm and

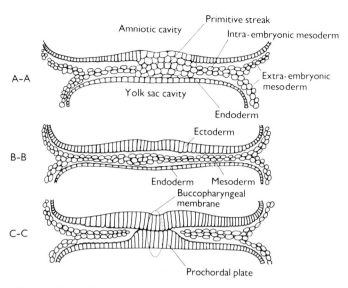

Fig. 6.6. Sections through the embryonic disc, now trilaminar throughout most of its extent, at levels A, B and C in Fig. 6.5.

mesoderm. We have already seen that the yolk sac lining consists of extra-embryonic endoderm while the trophoblast and amniotic lining are extra-embryonic ectodermal tissues. Between them lies the extra-embryonic mesoderm (Fig. 6.2) which eventually surrounds the extra-embryonic coelom (Fig. 6.3).

The formation of the trilaminar disc

Shortly after the delineation of the bilaminar embryonic disc (p.76) the *trilaminar embryonic disc* is formed by the interposition of notochord and mesoderm (the so-called *chorda-mesoderm*) between embryonic ectoderm and endoderm. The process begins about 15 days after fertilization with the heaping up of cells in the upper layer of the bilaminar disc towards the posterior part of the midline to form a structure known as the *primitive streak* (Fig. 6.4). The effect is chiefly due to a backward and medial migration of actively proliferating ectodermal cells (Fig. 6.5). Once within the primitive streak, the cells lose their columnar characteristics, become rounded and spread laterally and forward between the ectoderm and endoderm as *intra-embryonic mesoderm*. At the lateral extremity of this migration the mesodermal cells reach the lateral border of the embryonic disc and become continuous with the extra-embryonic (splanchnopleuric) mesoderm covering the yolk sac and with the extra-embryonic (somatopleuric) mesoderm covering the amnion (Fig. 6.6 A—A). Anteriorly, the embryonic mesodermal cells of each side become continuous across the midline in front of the prochordal plate (Fig. 6.6 B—B) though, in the region of the prochordal plate itself, ectoderm remains in contact with endoderm to form the *buccopharyngeal membrane* (Fig. 6.6 C—C). As

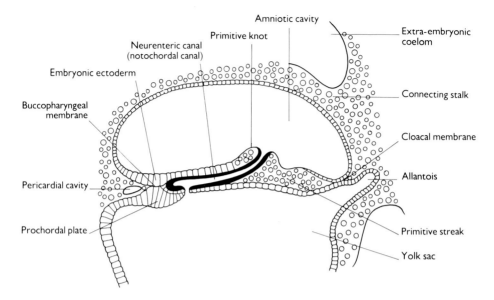

Fig. 6.7. A longitudinal section through the centre of the embryonic disc. For clarity, the notochord and neurenteric canal are shown larger than they should be.

the embryo grows, the primitive streak takes the form of a cellular thickening with a linear depression along its summit marking the site at which ectodermal cells are being invaginated to form mesoderm. It elongates by addition of cells to its posterior extremity and, when the whole embryonic disc is viewed from above, the primitive streak is seen in its posterior part (Fig. 6.5). The endoderm in the roof of the yolk sac behind the primitive streak remains adherent to the overlying ectoderm to form the *cloacal membrane* but some of the intra-embryonic mesoderm migrates backwards from the streak to surround this structure. It then mingles with, and contributes to, the extra-embryonic mesoderm of the connecting stalk (p.78) from which it is morphologically indistinguishable (Fig. 6.7).

Shortly after the first appearance of the primitive streak as a line on the surface of the embryonic disc a further heaping up of cells takes place at its anterior extremity. This is the *primitive knot* and, from it, an elongated *notochordal process* extends forward to the posterior edge of the prochordal plate. The notochordal process undergoes a series of changes which include a stage when the process becomes hollowed out to form a canal called the *notochordal canal* (Fig. 6.7). The ectoderm overlying the notochordal process and the region immediately anterior to it becomes thickened to form the *neural plate*; this later becomes a broad neural groove (Fig. 6.8) which will eventually give rise to the *neural tube* and thus to the brain and spinal cord (see Chapter 10).

As the embryonic disc grows the notochordal process elongates and the primitive streak shortens. At this stage the embryonic disc is elongated with the primitive streak in its narrower posterior part (Fig. 6.9). For a while the noto-

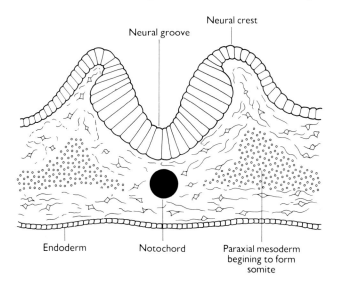

Fig. 6.8. The neural plate beginning to sink below the general ectodermal surface to form the neural groove. The mesoderm on either side of the midline (paraxial mesoderm) is beginning to form somites (p.84).

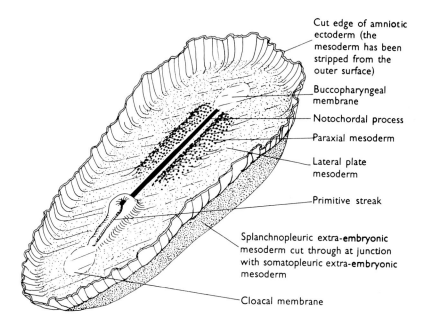

Fig. 6.9. A more advanced stage of development than that shown in Fig. 6.5. The notochord is greatly elongated and the paraxial mesoderm is heaped up on either side of the midline as the somites begin to form cranially, from paraxial mesoderm.

Human Embryology

chordal canal connects the posterior extremity of the neural groove with the yolk sac cavity and is now known as the *neurenteric canal* (Fig. 6.7). Its rare persistence leads to a congenital malformation in which the spinal canal is connected to the gut lumen and may give rise to maldevelopment of the vertebral bodies. Later the notochordal process loses its lumen and becomes a solid rod of cells — the notochord proper (Fig. 6.8).

The mesoderm on either side of the definitive notochord becomes thickened to form two longitudinal strips of *paraxial mesoderm* (Fig. 6.9). These will eventually become segmented cranio-caudally to form about 44 blocks of mesoderm known as *somites* (Chapter 9). No somites are formed in front of the anterior tip of the notochord although mesoderm extends forward to the anterior limit of the embryonic disc (Fig. 6.9). Lateral to the paraxial mass the intra-embryonic mesoderm forms a thinner layer of *lateral plate mesoderm* (Fig. 6.9) and it is this layer that is continuous with the extra-embryonic mesoderm at the edges of the disc (*vide supra* and Fig. 6.6). Connecting the lateral edges of the paraxial mesoderm and the main bulk of the lateral plate mesoderm is a longitudinal tract of *intermediate mesoderm* (intermediate cell mass) (Fig. 6.10); this will give rise to the nephrogenic cord (Chapter 14).

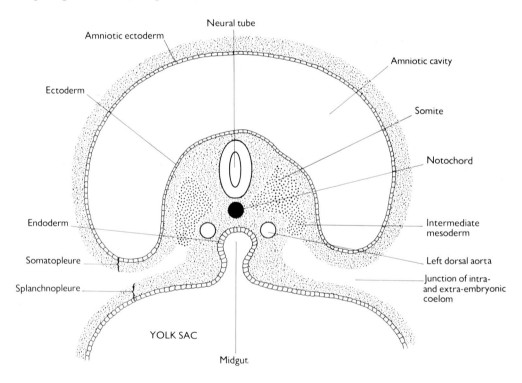

Fig. 6.10. The embryonic disc is beginning to bulge into the amniotic cavity to form the lateral folds. The intra-embryonic mesoderm has split to form the intra-embryonic coelom, which is continuous at the edges of the disc (in this region at least) with the extra-embryonic coelom (see Fig. 6.11 A—A).

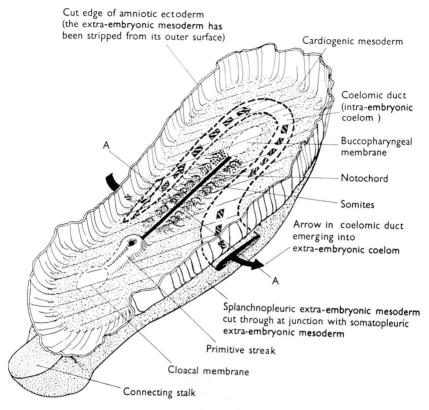

Cut edge of amniotic ectoderm
(the extra-embryonic mesoderm has
been stripped from its outer surface)

Cardiogenic mesoderm

Coelomic duct
(intra-embryonic
coelom)

A

Buccopharyngeal
membrane

Notochord

Somites

Arrow in coelomic duct
emerging into
extra-embryonic coelom

A

Splanchnopleuric extra-embryonic mesoderm
cut through at junction with somatopleuric
extra-embryonic mesoderm

Primitive streak

Cloacal membrane

Connecting stalk

Fig. 6.11. A diagram to show the extent of the intra-embryonic coelom. The amnion and extra-embryonic mesoderm (except for the connecting stalk) have been removed. A section through level A–A is seen in Fig. 6.10.

By the late primitive streak stage of development the connecting stalk has restricted the area of its attachment and now connects only a relatively small posteriorly situated region of the embryonic disc and the amnion to the chorion (Fig. 6.7). A posteriorly directed diverticulum from the caudal extremity of the yolk sac roof known as the *allantois* grows into the connecting stalk immediately behind the cloacal membrane (Fig. 6.7). This structure is well developed in some animals. It forms a large embryonic and fetal bladder in land-living, egg-laying vertebrates and has a similar function in some mammals especially among the ungulates (hoofed animals). It is essentially rudimentary in man though it forms a small portion of the endodermal lining of the urinary bladder and a fibrous cord connecting the apex of this organ to the umbilicus (Chapter 15).

The intra-embryonic coelom

Small fluid-filled spaces appear in the lateral plate mesoderm and eventually coalesce to form the *intra-embryonic coelom*. The latter at this stage is a horse-shoe

shaped cavity; its lateral arms are connected anteriorly across the midline in front
of the buccopharyngeal membrane (Fig. 6.11). It will be remembered that the layer
of mesodermal cells that migrates forward from the primitive streak on either side
of the notochordal process meets its counterpart of the opposite side in front of the
buccopharyngeal membrane (p.81); in this region it is known as the *cardiogenic
mesoderm* and the coelomic cavity within it will develop into the pericardial cavity.
At the extreme caudal ends of the 'horseshoe' constituting the embryonic coelom,
the cavity breaks through the mesoderm of the rim of the disc to communicate
with the extra-embryonic coelom on either side (Figs. 6.10 and 6.11) in the region
of the future midgut (p.88). The squamous epithelial lining of the coelomic cavity
is derived from flattened mesenchymal cells of the lateral plate mesoderm; it is
therefore a mesothelium (*vide supra*). As in the case of the extra-embryonic
membranes (p.79), mesoderm with a covering of ectoderm constitutes *somatopleure* while endoderm and mesoderm together form *splanchnopleure.* Fig. 6.10

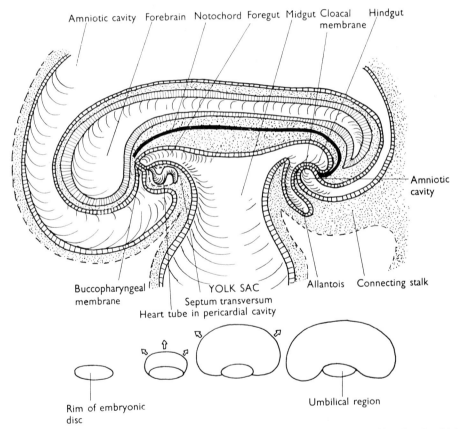

Fig. 6.12. A longitudinal section through the embryonic disc after the formation of head and tail folds
(compare with Fig. 6.7). These folds, together with the lateral folds result in the formation of fore-,
mid- and hindguts. The four lower diagrams are intended to show how the head, tail and lateral folds
result from the bulging upwards and outwards of the embryonic disc from its relatively fixed rim in
the manner of a soap bubble being blown.

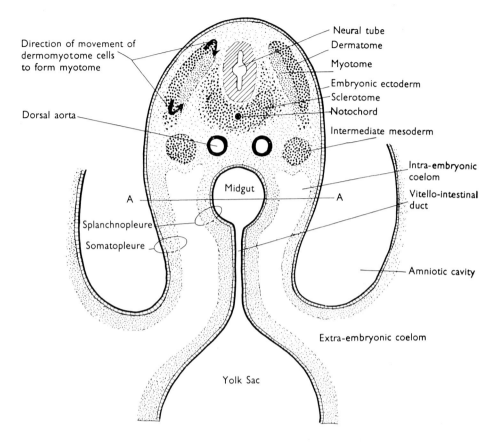

Neural tube
Dermatome
Myotome
Embryonic ectoderm
Sclerotome
Notochord
Intermediate mesoderm
Intra-embryonic coelom
Vitello-intestinal duct
Amniotic cavity
Extra-embryonic coelom

Direction of movement of dermomyotome cells to form myotome

Dorsal aorta

Midgut

A

A

Splanchnopleure
Somatopleure

Yolk Sac

Fig. 6.13. A transverse section through the embryo after the formation of the lateral folds. The midgut is now connected to the yolk sac remnant only by a narrow vitello-intestinal duct. The mesodermal somites are beginning to break up and the intermediate mesoderm forms a well defined longitudinal column of cells. Another view is seen in Fig. 6.14.

shows how the embryonic layers are continuous with their extra-embryonic counterparts at the lateral edge of the embryonic disc.

The formation of the head, tail and lateral body folds

During the fourth week after fertilization the trilaminar embryonic disc, which has always presented a convex surface to the amniotic cavity, bulges even further into the latter. Gradually a *head fold* and a *tail fold* are formed by a folding under of the cranial and caudal parts of the disc (Fig. 6.12). The process can be pictured by imagining that a probe in the yolk sac has pushed the anterior part of its roof forwards and the posterior part of its roof (just in front of the allantoic diverticulum) backwards. At the same time quite marked folding also takes place along the lateral margins of the embryo (Fig. 6.13). As a result of the folding of the

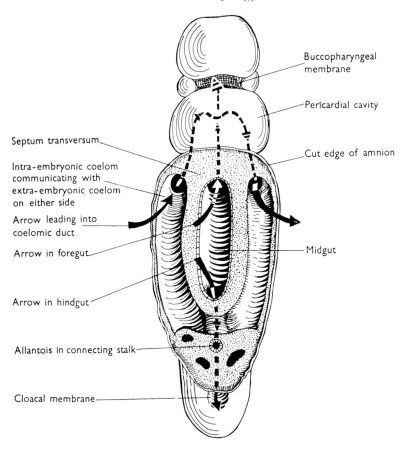

Buccopharyngeal membrane

Pericardial cavity

Septum transversum

Cut edge of amnion

Intra-embryonic coelom communicating with extra-embryonic coelom on either side

Arrow leading into coelomic duct

Arrow in foregut

Midgut

Arrow in hindgut

Allantois in connecting stalk

Cloacal membrane

Fig. 6.14. A diagrammatic ventral view of an embryo in which the ventral region has been removed along the line A–A in Fig. 6.13 (20 somites, 26 days).

embryo a primitive endodermally-lined *foregut* is formed within the head fold and a primitive *hindgut* with an allantoic diverticulum in the tail fold. Between them the roof of the yolk sac constitutes the roof of the *midgut*. The lateral folds serve to constrict the cavity of the midgut from the remainder of the yolk sac and the elongated *vitello-intestinal duct* thus produced (p.286) connects the midgut with a shrivelled yolk sac remnant until quite late in pregnancy (see Chapter 16).

As a result of the formation of the head fold, the pericardial cavity (i.e. the midline (anterior) portion of the intra-embryonic coelom) comes to lie below the foregut and behind the buccopharyngeal membrane (Fig. 6.12). The caudal wall of the pericardial cavity at this stage is formed by an extremely important landmark consisting of a mass of mesenchyme and known as the *septum transversum* (Fig. 6.12). It contributes to a broad ventral mesentery for the caudal portion of the foregut and the caudal margin of this mesentery marks the anterior extremity of the midgut. The septum transversum is also the anterior limit of the connection between the intra-embryonic and extra-embryonic coelom (Fig. 6.14) and is, therefore, a region in which vessels can pass from the somatopleure to the splanchnopleure (p.199).

The intra-embryonic coelom now consists of a midline pericardial cavity (Fig. 6.12) from which paired coelomic ducts pass dorsally and caudally on either side of the posterior portion of the foregut to become continuous with the extra-embryonic coelom caudal to the septum transversum and on either side of the midgut (Figs. 6.13 and 6.14).

The connection between the intra-embryonic and extra-embryonic coelom surrounds the junction of midgut and yolk sac (Fig. 6.14). The coelomic ducts will give rise to the pleural cavities, while the portion of the intra-embryonic coelom which surrounds the midgut (Fig. 6.13) gives rise to the peritoneal cavity.

In the tail fold region, the attachment of the connecting stalk is now on the ventral aspect of the embryo just behind the opening between the midgut and the yolk sac cavity (Figs. 6.12 and 6.13). The main part of the endodermal allantois has now been taken into the embryo but it also still extends into the connecting stalk for a short distance. Behind the embryonic attachment of the connecting stalk the cloacal membrane separates the hindgut from the amniotic cavity and immediately behind this the remains of the primitive streak overlie the extreme caudal extension of the hindgut. At the tail fold stage the hindgut is in the form of a single cavity the greater part of which will form the *cloaca* (p.277). Subdivision of this region by means of a septum will eventually give rise to an anterior portion (the *primitive urogenital sinus*) concerned in the formation of the bladder and urethra and a posterior portion which will give rise to the rectum and a part of the anal canal. These relationships are dealt with in detail in Chapters 14, 15 and 16.

Gastrulation

Gastrulation is a term used in all animals higher than the coelenterates to denote the early embryonic process whereby the single layer of cells comprising the blastoderm is transformed to thin germinal layers — the ectoderm, endoderm and mesoderm. The term is used in this way in the present chapter although human development has become slightly modified in this context. Thus the embryonic endoderm is delineated from the lower portion of the inner cell mass and no single layered blastoderm such as is seen for instance in the chick ever exists. The reader should consult a textbook of general embryology, such as Balinsky (1975) for comparative details. Some of the inductive processes manifested during gastrulation are discussed in Chapter 18.

Developmental stages

9—13 days : Bilaminar embryonic disc.

14—15 days : Beginning of primitive streak. Extra-embryonic coelom appears.

16 days : Beginning of notochordal process.

17—18 days : Neural plate appears.

19—20 days : Intra-embryonic coelom begins to develop.

24 days : Head, tail and lateral body folds have established basic embryonic shape.

Further reading

Balinsky, B.I. (1975) *An Introduction to Embryology*, 4th edn. W.B. Saunders & Co, Philadelphia, London, Toronto.

Boyd, J.D. & Hamilton, W.J. (1970) *The Human Placenta*. Heffer, Cambridge.

Bryce, T.H. & Teacher, T.H. (1908) *Contributions to the Study and Early Imbedding of the Human Ovum.* Jas. Maddox & Sons, Glasgow.

Hamilton, W.J., Boyd, J.D. & Mossman, H.W. (1972) *Human Embryology*, 3rd edn. Heffer, Cambridge.

Nishimura, H., Tanimura, T., Semba, R. & Uwabe C (1974) Normal development of early human embryos: observation of 90 specimens at Carnegie stages 7 to 13, *Teratology*, **10**, 1—8.

7

Implantation, the Fetal Membranes and Placenta Formation

Implantation

We have seen that on the fourth or fifth day after ovulation the ovum enters the uterine cavity in the form of a morula, or perhaps an early blastocyst (p.74). One or two days later the process of implantation begins with the swelling of the blastocyst and disappearance of the zona pellucida. At about the same time amniotic epithelium is formed from the inner layer of the polar trophoblast and becomes separated from the embryonic cell mass by the appearance of an amniotic cavity (Fig. 6.1). The polar trophoblast becomes attached to the uterine epithelium and begins to burrow into the endometrium. The cellular processes involved are ill understood and differ in various species. An insight into the mechanisms concerned with implantation would constitute a fundamental advance in the study of human reproduction but, at present, our knowledge is confined to data obtained from comparative embryology and we are able to say little more than that the process represents an *interaction* between the blastocyst and the endometrium which is to some extent hormonally dependent. The surface cells of the penetrating trophoblast fuse and their cell membranes disappear to form a layer of *syncytiotrophoblast* arising from the cellular *cytotrophoblast* on its embryonic aspect (Fig. 6.1). Invasion of the endometrium continues until at about 10 days the conceptus is completely buried (Fig. 6.2); its site of penetration on surface view is now marked by a slight swelling and, for a time, a small plug of fibrin. Even the latter eventually disappears with complete re-epithelialisation of the endometrial surface. Human implantation is, therefore, described as *interstitial*.

In the majority of cases implantation occurs high up on the posterior wall of the uterus. The endometrium is in the progestational state (p.51) and the cells of the pars functionalis (p.50) at the implantation site become laden with glycogen, closely packed and polyhedral in appearance; in this condition they are known as *decidual cells.* They degenerate in the region of the penetrating syncytiotrophoblast and no doubt together with maternal blood and uterine secretions provide a rich source of material for early embryonic (*histiotrophic*) nutrition. Gradually the area of decidualisation spreads from that immediately surrounding the implanted ovum to involve the greater part of the endometrium. Implantation of the blastocyst at an abnormal site may give rise to serious complications during pregnancy, a subject we discuss in a later section.

Formation of the chorionic villi

The formation of the *primary extra-embryonic (fetal)* membranes was described in Chapter 6. They constitute the yolk sac, the amnion, the chorion and the connecting stalk (Fig. 6.3). Quite early during implantation lacunae appear in the syncytiotrophoblast overlying the embryonic pole (Fig. 6.1); these are first filled with tissue fluid and uterine secretions but, as the penetrating trophoblast erodes small endometrial vessels, maternal blood begins to seep through (Fig. 6.2). When the conceptus (now called the chorionic vesicle — see Chapter 6) has buried itself in the endometrium its outer surface becomes completely clothed by radially orientated columns of syncytiotrophoblast lying on a *chorionic plate* of cytotrophoblast (Fig. 6.2). Deep to the latter lies the extra-embryonic mesoderm which later surrounds the extra-embryonic coelom (Fig. 6.3). Some 22–23 days after fertilization (two weeks after implantation) a fetal circulatory system (Fig. 7.1) begins to develop almost simultaneously in the mesoderm of the embryo (embryonic vessels), the yolk sac mesoderm (vitelline vessels) and the chorion and connecting stalk (umbilical vessels). The first heart beats, therefore, serve to carry material which has crossed the feto/maternal membrane, i.e. the composite membrane between the fetal and maternal blood, to reach the rapidly growing embryo, via the umbilical vessels. Embryonic nutrition of this type is termed *haemotrophic*. Its inception coincides with a time when embryonic nutrition is no longer adequately

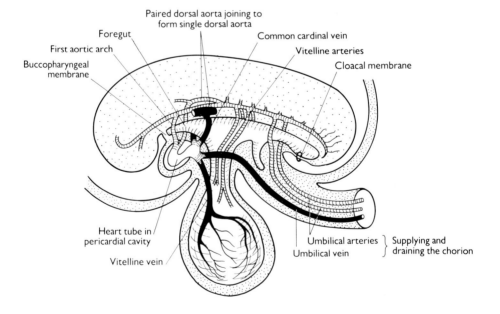

Fig. 7.1. The development of a primitive vascular system in the intra- and extra-embryonic mesoderm. Cardinal, umbilical and vitelline veins join the caudal end of the heart tube and a pair of (first) aortic arches leave its cranial end. See Chapter 12 for a more detailed description.

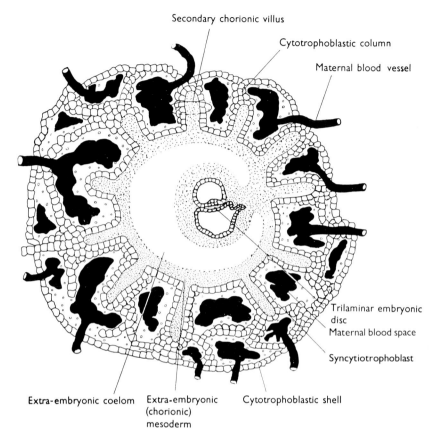

Secondary chorionic villus

Cytotrophoblastic column

Maternal blood vessel

Trilaminar embryonic disc

Maternal blood space

Syncytiotrophoblast

Extra-embryonic coelom

Extra-embryonic (chorionic) mesoderm

Cytotrophoblastic shell

Fig. 7.2. The extra-embryonic (chorionic) mesoderm penetrates the villi to form a core, thus forming secondary villi. The conceptus is totally enclosed by a cytotrophoblastic shell.

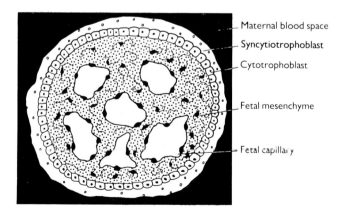

Maternal blood space

Syncytiotrophoblast

Cytotrophoblast

Fetal mesenchyme

Fetal capillary

Fig. 7.3. Transverse section of a tertiary chorionic villus. The fetal blood in the capillaries is separated from the maternal blood by fetal endothelium, fetal mesenchyme, cytotrophoblast and syncytiotrophoblast.

served by diffusion across the extra-embryonic coelom and yolk sac, which was
the method used at the primitive streak stage of development.

Short branching outgrowths of the cytotrophoblast all around the chorionic
vesicle now begin to extend into the syncytiotrophoblastic columns. These cytotrophoblastic structures together with their syncytiotrophoblastic covering constitute the primary *chorionic villi* (Fig. 6.3). Gradually the cytotrophoblast penetrates
through the syncytiotrophoblast that forms the outermost layer of the chorionic
vesicle and extending circumferentially at the junction of maternal and fetal
tissues forms a *cytotrophoblastic shell* around the conceptus (Fig. 7.2). Next,
chorionic mesoderm penetrates the primary chorionic villi converting them to
secondary villi (Fig. 7.2) which very soon become vascularised by fetal capillaries
and are then called *tertiary villi* (Figs. 7.3 and 7.4). The villous blood vessels, like
the mesenchyme in which they arise may differentiate *in situ* to some extent.
However, they soon join the vessels in the chorionic mesenchyme adjacent to the
extra-embryonic coelom and thus become continuous with the embryonic circulation through the connecting stalk (Fig. 7.1). At this stage of development *stem villi*
(anchoring villi) are seen to pass from the inner cytotrophoblastic wall of the
chorion (the *chorionic plate*) to the cytotrophoblastic shell (Fig. 7.4). Their tips are

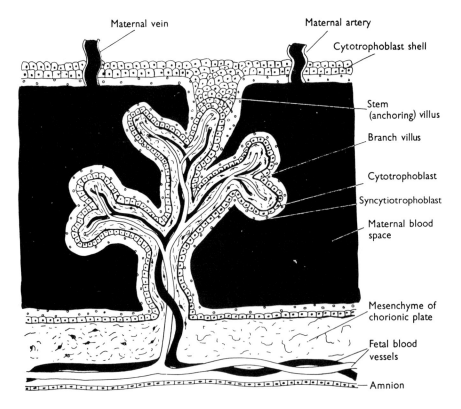

Fig. 7.4. A stem, or anchoring villus, with a number of branch villi.

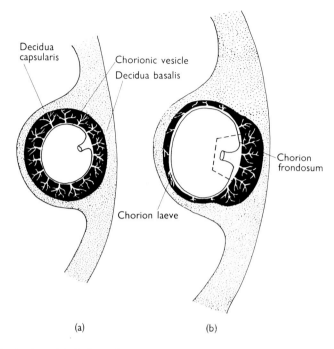

Fig. 7.5. (a) The chorionic vesicle in its early stages, surrounded by villi; (b) 3−4 months, the villi proliferate on the side facing the decidua basalis (chorion frondosum) but degenerate on the other side (chorion laeve). The dotted line indicates the area depicted in Fig. 7.10.

usually devoid of mesoderm and they should be distinguished from *branch villi* which grow from their sides into the maternal blood spaces lying between them (Fig. 7.4). It is through the branch villi that the main exchange of material between mother and embryo eventually takes place. Like the embryonic ends of their parent stem villi they consist at this stage of a vascular mesenchymal core surrounded by cytotrophoblast (usually only a single layer in branch villi) and covered by a layer of syncytiotrophoblast, i.e. they are tertiary villi. At first villi grow more or less uniformly over the whole surface of the chorionic vesicle but, during the third month of pregnancy, those facing the uterine lumen degenerate leaving a more or less smooth chorionic surface, the *chorion laeve*, on this aspect. On the other hand villi facing towards the uterine wall grow even more profusely to form the *chorion frondosum* (Fig. 7.5a and b). The stromal cells of the endometrium have by now been largely converted into decidual cells (p.91). Endometrium overlying the chorionic vesicle is called the *decidua capsularis* and the region deep to the vesicle is the *decidua basalis* (Fig. 7.7). The remainder of the uterine mucosa, i.e. that lying to the side of the implantation site and also on the opposite wall of the uterus is the *decidua parietalis* (or decidua vera). Gradually the chorion frondosum, together with the adjacent decidua basalis, forms the definitive flattened circular organ known clinically as the *placenta* (Fig. 7.6). Expansion of the cytotrophoblastic shell, particularly in the region of the decidua basalis, increases the extent of the

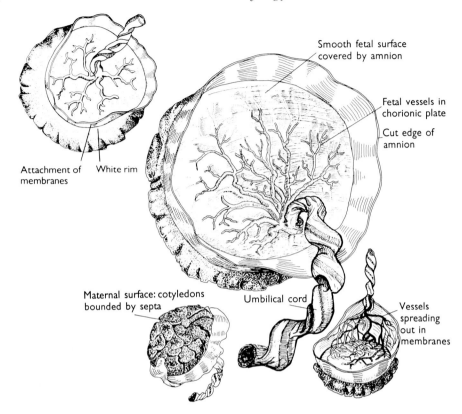

Smooth fetal surface
covered by amnion

Fetal vessels in
chorionic plate

Cut edge of
amnion

Attachment of   White rim
membranes

Maternal surface: cotyledons   Umbilical cord
bounded by septa

Vessels
spreading
out in
membranes

Fig. 7.6. A full-term placenta. The fetal surface is lined by amnion and is therefore smooth while the maternal surface (inset, bottom left) is ragged and split up into cotyledons. Inset (right) a placenta with a velamentous insertion of the cord. Inset (top left) A circumvallate placenta.

maternal blood space (i.e. the intervillous space filled with maternal blood) and new anchoring villi as well as branch villi are continually added by interstitial growth.

Expansion of the chorionic vesicle in the region of the decidua capsularis, on the other hand, causes a thinning of the cytotrophoblastic shell as well as a bulging into the uterine lumen (Fig. 7.7). The stretching of the endometrium over the surface of the chorionic vesicle leads to an attenuation of its blood supply and, as a result, most of the decidua capsularis covering the chorion laeve degenerates during the fourth month of pregnancy. Shortly thereafter what is left of the decidua capsularis fuses with the decidua parietalis covering the opposite uterine wall and thus the uterine lumen is obliterated (Fig. 7.7). The uterine epithelium in the region of fusion disappears and the cytotrophoblastic shell remains only a few cells thick.

Growth and maturation of the placenta

The growth of the chorionic vesicle is extremely rapid between the end of the first month and middle of the fourth month of pregnancy (corresponding to an

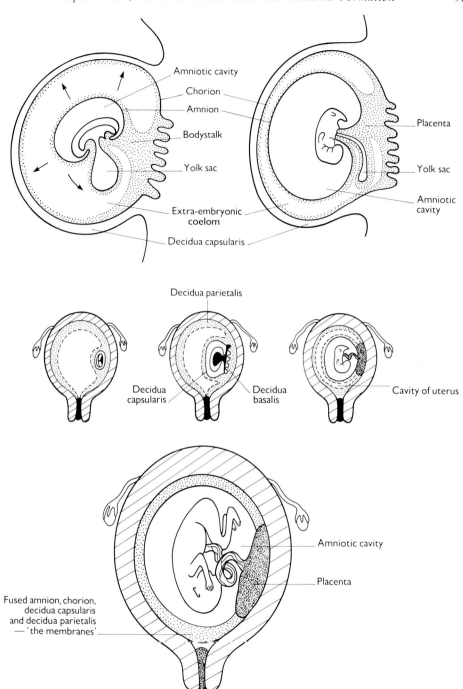

Fig. 7.7. The top two diagrams show how the increase in size of the amniotic cavity eventually causes the amnion and chorion to fuse, trapping the remains of the yolk sac between them. The central three diagrams show how the decidua capsularis and decidua parietalis fuse as the embryo increases in size, so that the cavity of the uterus is obliterated. In the lower diagram, all these layers have come together to form a composite layer termed 'the membranes'.

embryonic crown–rump length of between 5 and 65 mm). The cytotrophoblastic shell itself never acquires a mesenchymal core and, in general, consists of closely packed cells; nevertheless, maternal blood vessels, both arteries and veins pass freely through gaps in the shell and open into the maternal blood spaces through which there is now a good circulation. There is also evidence for accumulation and absorption of maternal cell detritus and glandular secretion by the cytotrophoblastic shell. This is particularly well marked in the early stages of development.

Towards the end of the fourth month the decidua basalis is almost entirely replaced by fetal placental tissue. At the same time, the cytotrophoblastic shell adds to its peripheral mass while its embryonic surface is 'scooped out' to extend the maternal intervillous space leaving a number of septa which therefore project from the cytotrophoblastic shell towards the chorionic plate. They consist of trophoblastic cells with a core of maternal tissue and they divide the maternal aspect of the mature placenta into about 20 *cotyledons* (Figs. 7.6 and 7.8). Between the fifth month and full term the placenta grows in diameter rather than in thickness, its expansion essentially keeping pace with that of the uterine wall.

Histological changes also take place in the villi beginning at the fourth month of pregnancy. At this time the cytotrophoblast in many of the branch villi becomes attenuated and eventually disappears over quite large areas leaving only thin plates of syncytiotrophoblast to separate the fetal mesenchyme with its peripherally situated blood vessels from the maternal blood in the intervillous spaces (Fig. 7.9). Some cytotrophoblast persists until term, however, and there is now no doubt that syncytiotrophoblastic nuclei in the human are non-mitotic. At all stages of pregnancy *syncytiotrophoblast is formed entirely from the underlying cytotrophoblast.* The tissues between the fetal and maternal blood streams (i.e. fetal endothelium, a small amount of fetal mesenchyme and the thinned out syncitiotrophoblast) constitute the so-called *placental membrane* and the changes in its morphology as the placenta matures suggest that its permeability increases during the second half of pregnancy. Coupled with an increase in the functional surface area of interchange this has important physiological implications which will be discussed later.

At the end of pregnancy the flattened placenta (Fig. 7.6) is over 15 cm (6 inches) in diameter and weights about 500 g. The attachment sites of the septa delineating the cotyledons usually enclose one stem villus together with its branches (Fig. 7.8). The fetal surface of the placenta is smooth since it is covered by amnion and here the main stems of the umbilical vessels diverge. The amnion is usually fused with the chorion during the later periods of gestation (*vide infra*).

The vascular arrangements within the placenta are of considerable physiological importance. It must be clearly understood that, although there is never any appreciable intermixture of maternal and fetal blood, placental function is concerned with extensive exchange of materials through the placental membrane. Fetal villi are supplied by branches of the umbilical arteries and eventually drain

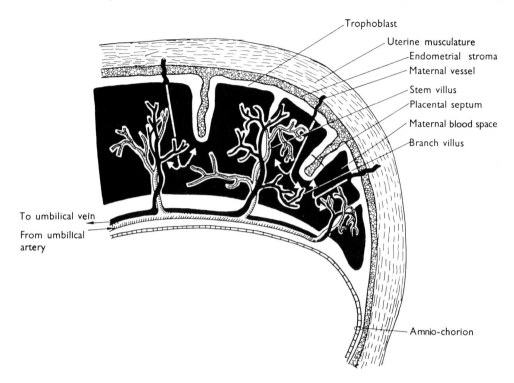

Fig. 7.8. The edge of the placenta. The maternal surface is split up into cotyledons by the placenta septa. No distinction between syncytio- and cytotrophoblast has been made in this diagram. The white arrows indicate the direction of maternal blood flow.

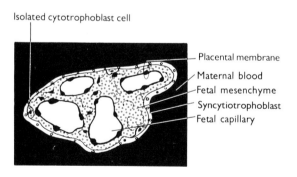

Fig. 7.9. The placental membrane after the fourth month of pregnancy becomes greatly thinned as a result of the almost complete loss of the cytotrophoblast and the thinning-out of the other components.

into the umbilical vein. On the maternal side, arteries discharge into the maternal blood spaces through gaps in the cytotrophoblastic shell. The head of pressure is sufficient to direct the stream towards the chorionic plate where it is deflected back towards the cytotrophoblastic shell. On the way it permeates between the branch villi before it leaves again through venous openings in the shell (Fig. 7.8). Inter-cotyledonary septa may serve to produce a 'baffle' effect and ensure an even flow of maternal blood through the placental bed. A good maternal circulation in the intervillous spaces is probably not established until the fifth week or so of pregnancy. In mid-pregnancy, cells of the cytotrophoblastic shell invade the lumina of the maternal arteries feeding the placenta and partly occlude them; this may be another important factor in the regulation of blood flow through the intervillous space.

The development of the umbilical cord

The early development of the amnion has been described in Chapter 6. We have seen that after the formation of the extra-embryonic coelom the mesodermal connecting stalk joins the amnion and the caudal end of the embryo to the wall of the chorionic vesicle (Figs. 6.3, 6.7 and 6.12) and that, after the formation of the tail fold, the attachment of the stalk to the amnion and embryo becomes ventrally situated (Figs. 6.12 and 6.14). Just cranial to it lies the junction of the midgut and the future vitello-intestinal duct surrounded on all sides by the connection between the intra- and extra-embryonic coelom (Fig. 6.14). With the growth of the embryo the enlarging amniotic cavity fills more and more of the extra-embryonic coelom until the remnant of the yolk sac and the elongated vitello-intestinal duct are pushed right up against the connecting stalk. The vitello-intestinal duct with a surrounding sleeve of the extra-embryonic coelom then gradually becomes embedded in the connecting stalk (Fig. 7.7 and 7.10). The latter is now called the *umbilical cord* and is surrounded on all sides by amnion. At its embryonic end, the enclosed extra-embryonic coelom containing the vitello-intestinal duct will be the site of herniation of the midgut loop into the umbilical cord later in development (Chapter 16). The umbilical cord consists chiefly of fetal mesenchyme known as *Wharton's jelly*. It contains the tip of the allantoic diverticulum as well as two muscular umbilical arteries and the left umbilical vein (also very muscular) which convey fetal blood to and from the placenta (the primitive right umbilical vein disappears early in pregnancy). The vessels differ from the majority by being devoid of a nerve supply. By mid-pregnancy the vitello-intestinal duct, yolk sac and surrounding extra-embryonic coelom have usually disappeared. In mammals the yolk sac never contains any yolk but Figs. 6.2, 6.3 and 7.2 show that early in development it is in a position to transmit nutrients directly from the trophoblast and, later, from the extra-embryonic coelom to the embryonic mass. In later pregnancy the mesodermal outer covering of the amnion usually fuses with the apposed inner surface of the chorion and the two layers are frequently inseparable at birth. Together they form the *chorio-amnion* (Figs. 7.7 and 7.8) across which some (probably unimportant) materno-fetal exchange mechanisms may operate.

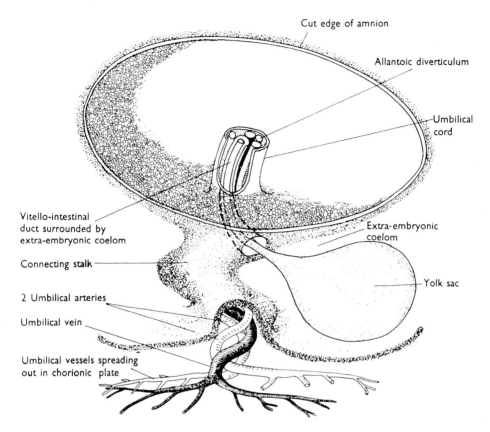

Cut edge of amnion

Allantoic diverticulum

Umbilical cord

Vitello-intestinal
duct surrounded by
extra-embryonic coelom

Extra-embryonic
coelom

Connecting stalk

Yolk sac

2 Umbilical arteries

Umbilical vein

Umbilical vessels spreading
out in chorionic plate

Fig. 7.10 A diagram corresponding to the dotted area in Fig. 7.5, showing the relations of the connecting (body) stalk before the complete formation of the true umbilical cord. The yolk sac remnant eventually becomes trapped between amnion and chorion (see Fig. 7.7). Note the extra-embryonic coelom around the neck of the yolk sac which is important in the development of the midgut (Chapter 16).

Classification of the placenta

A placental structure has been defined as 'any intimate apposition of fetal and maternal tissues for the purpose of physiological interchange' and, from a functional point of view, this unifying definition is very logical. Nevertheless, in man, the clinical usage of the term 'placenta' implies that region of the wall of the chorionic vesicle developed from the chorion frondosum and the adjacent decidua. The umbilical vessels are homologous with the allantoic vessels of other mammals and, for this reason, the human placenta is *chorio-allantoic*. Furthermore, since some of the decidual tissue is shed with the placenta at birth the term *deciduate* is often used to distinguish the human type of chorio-allantoic placenta from the indeciduate type found in many hoofed animals. Finally, a histological classification of chorio-allantoic placentae has been devised to take into account the different degrees to which the trophoblast penetrates the endometrium during placental formation in various species. Three major types are distinguished according to the maternal tissue in contact with the trophoblastic covering of the chorion. Firstly, the *epitheliochorial* form in which trophoblast has not penetrated the uterine epithelium but lies adjacent to it is characteristic of ungulates. Secondly, the *endotheliochorial* form, found in carnivores, is one in which penetration of the uterine epithelium and stroma has occurred and the trophoblast lies against maternal endothelium. Finally, the *haemochorial* form of rodents and of higher primates, including man, is one in which the trophoblast has penetrated through the vessel wall and lies in direct contact with maternal blood.

In summary, then, we may classify the *anatomical* 'placenta' in man as discoidal in shape, chorio-allantoic, haemochorial and deciduate. We should bear in mind, however, that other structures such as the chorio-amnion or the yolk sac may be placental in the functional sense defined at the beginning of this section.

Immunology of the placenta

The placenta (containing on average 50 per cent paternal genes) is, strictly speaking, a homograft in the uterus yet it is not rejected. The reasons after many years of research are still unclear but it is believed that one of the principal causes is that the syncytiotrophoblast lacks crucial antigens which allow it to act as an immunologically 'neutral' covering to the placental tissue. In support of this theory is the fact that there is no evidence of HLA antigens on trophoblast.

Additionally, pregnancy is associated with some degree of lymphopoenia and this is accompanied by some depression of the thymolymphatic system; pelvic lymph nodes in pregnant women often lack germinal centres so that there may well be some systemic immunosupression. Pregnancy plasma, possibly due to raised cortisol levels, exerts a *non-cytotoxic* immunosuppressive effect *in vitro* while high hormone concentration at the placental interface itself has been put forward as having a local influence on maternal *cellular* immunity. The hormone involved in the latter case is unknown but is no longer thought to be chorionic gonadotrophic which was originally postulated as the responsible factor.

Apart from these rather general factors, the possibility of specific immunological unresponsiveness has also been raised. It is suggested that the trophoblast, although forming a general barrier to fetal histocompatibility antigens, does allow a strictly limited access of antigens to the mother. This may have two results. Firstly, immunological tolerance may be established. This is a well documented phenomenon which occurs when an organism is subjected to multiple small doses of antigen (as in desensitization therapy practised in cases of pollen allergy). Repeated low doses of paternal antigen may produce just such an effect in pregnancy. Secondly, it is possible that weak antigenic sites on the trophoblast become coated by blocking antibodies. This low-grade antigen–antibody response has no cytotoxic effect but serves to protect cells from attack by sensitised lymphocytes. The response is known as immunological enhancement.

The fetus has a poor capacity to produce antibodies until well after birth. To compensate for this, maternal IgG can pass into the fetus (see p.216) to give it *passive* immunity. Only 7S antibodies can pass the placental membrane so that, for example, diphtheria antibodies can enter the fetus and give it immunity for about 4 months postnatally. It is noteworthy that during these 4 months the passive antibodies can interfere with active immunization.

Placental function

The fetal membranes must perform an enormous variety of complex functions in order to maintain the embryo and fetus within the maternal organism. Their activities are so comprehensive that only the most primitive attempts at the construction of an 'artificial placenta' have been made. We are nowhere near the point at which it is possible to foresee the design of a mechanism which will ensure the growth, differentiation and morphogenesis of a human ovum from fertilization to the point at which it is able to maintain an independent existence.

From a mechanical point of view the fetal membranes must ensure that the conceptus is firmly anchored to the uterine wall but that a natural site of cleavage is present at term so that easy shedding of the placenta can occur. In the human these conditions are provided by the decidua. The fetus must be able to grow free from local mechanical pressure, and this is possible because of the buoyant environment afforded by the amniotic fluid. The secretion of the latter is by no means clearly understood. Early in pregnancy it is largely produced from maternal extracellular fluids but later on it is in balance with the fetal circulation. The full term fetus excretes as much as 1 litre of hypotonic urine daily into the amniotic cavity and resorbs about a half of this by swallowing it. The rest is removed at sites which have not been fully determined but probably include transfer to the fetal circulation by diffusion across the amnion into the allantoic (umbilical) vessels of the chorion and into the maternal circulation by passage across the chorio-amnion. At full term there are about 700 ml of amniotic fluid. A great excess (*hydramnios*) or deficiency (*oligamnios*) in volume often indicates the presence of a malformed fetus.

Laboratory examination of the amniotic fluid obtained by amniotic puncture (*amniocentesis*) has recently become an important diagnostic criterion for determining the well-being of the fetus (see also Chapter 17). Although the procedure of puncturing the amnion in itself carries a certain risk this is within acceptable limits when specific abnormalities are suspected. A needle is inserted into the cavity avoiding the placenta, which is first located by ultrasound, and a small volume of fluid is withdrawn. Karyotyping of the contained fetal cells will establish a diagnosis of Down's syndrome so that amniocentesis is recommended for all pregnancies in women over the age of 35, after which age non-disjunction of chromosome 23 is very common. Biochemical examination can yield many important findings. For example, a raised α-fetoprotein (suspected by virtue of finding raised levels in the maternal blood) is indicative of an open lesion in the fetus such as spina bifida or, more rarely, omphalocoele. Later in pregnancy the lecithin/sphyngomyelin ratio indicates the degree of development of surfactant (p.240) and therefore the state of the lungs.

The paramount function of the placenta as an organ of transfer is beyond question; it must allow food materials and respiratory gases to reach the embryo and also provide a route for the excretion of fetal waste materials. At the same time it serves as a protective organ with respect to a variety of metabolites, toxins and hormones which, though present in the maternal circulation, are unable to reach the fetus in sufficient concentration to damage it. Physico-chemical factors will obviously influence placental transfer rate, among them being the molecular weight of the compound in question, its charge and its fat solubility as well as the permeability constant of the placental membrane. In addition physiological factors influence placental transfer. These include the functional area available for materno-fetal exchange (which depends in part upon the proximity of the maternal and the fetal circulation), the relative affinities of the two circulations for a substance (such as oxygen) and the proportion in which some substances are present in the free form as compared to the protein-bound form in the fetal circulation on the one hand, and the maternal on the other.

Placental function can conveniently be considered under five headings.

1: Biological characteristics of the placental membrane

In early placental development fetal and maternal circulations may be separated by many cell layers (p.91). At later stages the membrane between the two circula-tions is attenuated in areas to a single layered thin area of syncytiotrophoblast together with its basement membrane separated by a minimal distance from a fetal capillary cell resting upon its basement membrane. The capillaries are un-fenestrated but it is possible that some macromolecules (IgG perhaps) may pass between the cells at junctional complexes. The syncytiotrophoblast has a brush border and is actively pinocytic; in it can be seen mitochondria, granular and smooth endoplasmic reticulum, Golgi complexes and a comprehensive vacuolar system. Little wonder, therefore, that the placenta is metabolically active at a high level, compared by some with that of the kidney. Fetal capillaries, on the other hand, look relatively passive. There is little evidence of pinocytosis in their cells.

2: The placental transport mechanisms

Passive transport by simple diffusion is usually characteristic of substances passing from high concentration areas to areas of lower concentration. In the case of facilitated diffusion this seems to occur more rapidly than would be predicted physically. Unexpected results can follow when a Donnan equilibrium is established. For example, the chloride concentration in amniotic fluid is greater than in maternal blood while the protein concentration is lower. The barrier between blood and amniotic fluid is freely permeable to positively charged ions and an equal positive charge is therefore present on both its sides. An increased amount of negatively charged chloride ions must pass into the amniotic fluid in order to make up for the inability of large negatively charged protein ions to diffuse into it from maternal blood.

Many substances enter the embryonic circulation or are expelled from it by active transport. Such systems may involve the intervention of enzymes which temporarily combine with the materials in question. Besides many more complex substrates some inorganic ions (iron, calcium) fall into this category. Another method of transport usually reserved for larger molecules is that of pinocytosis.

Drugs use the same transport mechanisms as other metabolic chemicals and will pass the placental membrane to some degree. Fat-soluble materials as a rule gain entry to the embryo more easily than water-soluble ones and, as pregnancy proceeds, thinning of the placental membrane facilitates drug passage. For many compounds the rate of passage to the embryo has been well worked out. Only in the case of 'unphysiological' toxins and drugs does the old-fashioned term *placental barrier* seem relevant as a substitute for *placental membrane*.

3: Placental transport of specific substances

The vasculature of the placental villi forms an extensive network so that about half of the fetal cardiac output passes *directly* to the placenta. In the villi as well as in the maternal blood spaces the blood is moving slowly so that oxygen and carbon dioxide exchange is relatively efficient. The gases cross the membrane by direct diffusion and although the CO_2 levels are nearly equilibrated the oxygen levels differ greatly even after interchange between maternal and fetal blood. Towards the end of pregnancy the fetus is, in fact, at an oxygen level equivalent to that found in an unacclimatised person at over 25,000 ft and if fetal haemoglobin had a dissociation curve identical to that of adult haemoglobin this would, of course, lead to serious anoxia. For this reason fetal haemoglobin (HgbF) takes up oxygen at a lower partial pressure and also dissociates at a lower partial pressure than does adult haemoglobin (HgbA). The reason for the unsatisfactory level of fetal oxygenation is no doubt a result of the vascular arrangements of the maternal blood spaces in the placenta (p.98) where 'arterial' and 'venous' blood are mixed in a sluggish circulation.

The rate of transfer of nutritional substances is to some extent dependent upon their concentrations on either side of the membrane but many other factors play a part. Water, sodium, potassium and most monovalent cations as well as urea diffuse easily and rapidly. Indeed sodium diffusion increases in rate as pregnancy advances. Uric acid, amines and *some* amino acids also cross by simple diffusion.

On the other hand active transport appears to be involved in the passage of at least some amino acids from mother to fetus because the concentration is higher on the fetal side. Glucose, the principal energy source for the embryo, is probably actively transferred from the maternal to the fetal circulation but there is no evidence of a reversed concentration gradient. The situation is further complicated here by the presence of stores of glycogen in the placenta and later in the fetal liver. The enzymes also present in these tissues suggest that this polysaccharide may provide a ready source of glucose which would thus modify the amount required by transplacental passage. The divalent ions of calcium and iron are significantly more concentrated on the fetal side. In spite of complicating factors introduced by the fact that both iron and calcium are largely protein bound and that possibly there is a different proportion of free to bound element in the fetal and maternal blood, it is nevertheless highly likely that the placenta selectively concentrates both in the fetal tissues. Fatty acids cross the placenta fairly rapidly but the fetus probably requires very little lipid from the mother. Its own fat synthesising capacity is probably adequate to meet its demands.

Many substances are present in higher concentrations in maternal plasma but are nevertheless actively transported by complex enzyme systems. They are broken down into relatively simple compounds and then resynthesised in the placental syncytium. Proteins are degraded to amino acids, lipids to acetate and carbohydrates to glucose (but *vide supra*, glucose) and fructose. Some proteins (*vide supra*, IgG) pass directly across the placental membrane in small quantities by pinocytosis. Minerals are often transferred as conjugates with protein and vitamins are often reduced to simpler forms to be reconstituted again in the trophoblast.

4: Histiotrophic nutrition

Before the establishment of tertiary placental villi and of a reasonably rapid maternal circulation through the placental bed the embryo grows largely by virtue of its capacity to take up maternal protein molecules and break them down in its fetal membranes. Degenerating decidual cells, stagnant maternal blood and secretions of the uterine glands provide a rich *histiotroph* for this type of nutrition. Trophoblastic cells absorb maternal cell fragments by *phagocytosis* and soluble proteins by pinocytosis. The macromolecules are then broken down in vacuoles within the cells by catabolic enzymes. The breakdown products (amino acids, etc.) are able to escape from the vacuoles and eventually leave the trophoblast; they diffuse into the chorionic vesicle and thus reach the embryonic disc. Histiotrophic nutrition continues well into the fifth month of pregnancy although a functional chorio-allantoic placental mechanism is established during the somite stage with the formation of tertiary placental villi in the first month of development. Until mid-pregnancy decidual glands continue to be secretory and decidual erosion continues, albeit at a decreasing pace.

5: Endocrine functions of the placenta

These are referred to in detail in various parts of this book and will only be summarised here. As soon as the embryo is implanted the trophoblast secretes human chorionic gonadotrophin (HCG) which maintains the corpus luteum and therefore stops the onset of the next menstrual period. HCG continues to be secreted until just before parturition but maximal levels are found at about the end of the second month and much lower levels are produced from the middle of the third month to full term. The placenta also secretes oestrogens and progestogens but these are only produced in sufficient quantities to maintain pregnancy from the third month onwards. Before that time ovariectomy results in abortion. Placental secretion of oestrogens and progestogens rises throughout pregnancy and urinary oestriol levels are important to the obstetrician in monitoring the normal course of pregnancy. The placenta also secretes human placental lactogen (HPL) which probably has many functions. Besides being lactogenic it also has some of the properties of growth hormone. Its most important function, however, seems to be in changing the maternal metabolism in adaptation to pregnancy (see Chapter 8).

Abnormalities of implantation and placental structure

The commonest site of implantation and of subsequent placental formation is high up on the posterior wall of the uterus. Occasionally it takes place at the fundus or high on the anterior uterine wall. At all these sites pregnancy can proceed and placental function is unimpeded. For certain diagnostic procedures, such as obtaining a sample of amniotic fluid, it is necessary to know the position of the placenta so that it is not damaged during puncture of the amnion. A number of safe, accurate and ingenious methods for placental localisation have been devised but ultrasonic methods are the only ones now used.

The rare cases in which implantation of the ovum occurs at sites other than in the body of the uterus are known as *ectopic gestations*. For example, the ovum can implant in the ampulla of the uterine tube rather than in the body of the uterus. This dangerous condition may be caused by a delay in the passage of the fertilized ovum along the tube and usually leads to serious complications. The trophoblast erodes the tubal wall, which may lead to its rupture often between the fourth and eighth weeks of pregnancy. Sudden massive, and sometimes fatal, haemorrhage into the abdominal cavity can result; implantation in other portions of the uterine tube frequently lead to early, and often complicated, abortion. Ectopic sites on the surface of the ovary and in the peritoneal cavity are extremely rare and frequently secondary to a ruptured tubal pregnancy. Cases have been described in which such pregnancies may go to full term but such examples are really no more than medical curiosities.

Uterine implantation near the internal os rather than towards the fundus results in the formation of a *placenta praevia*, in which the placenta partially or completely occupies a position in the lower uterine segment. When labour begins the lower segment is 'taken up' and the placenta becomes prematurely detached.

The full term placenta may be abnormal in form. Usually the umbilical vessels enter its fetal surface towards the centre but occasionally they may be inserted at the edge (the *battledore* placenta) or even run for a distance in the chorion before entering the placental mass. This so-called *velamentous insertion* of the cord (Fig. 7.6) may give rise to complications at birth. Another aberrant placental form occasionally seen is one in which patches of placental tissue called *succenturiate lobes* are developed in the chorion at some distances from the main placental mass. These are sometimes retained in the uterus when the placenta is expelled at birth, they readily become infected and prevent normal post partum involution of the uterus.

Abnormal growth of trophoblast can complicate pregnancy. If the trophoblast penetrates too deeply, completely destroying the endometrium and reaching the uterine musculature then the natural cleavage plane of the placenta at parturition is destroyed. Under such circumstances the placenta is retained as a *placenta accreta* and this gives rise to serious obstetric problems. Occasionally benign (*hydatidiform mole*) or even malignant (*chorionepithelioma*) growths of the trophoblast occur during pregnancy; they are often detected by alterations in blood and urine gonadotrophin levels.

Occasionally the trophoblast invades not only directly into the decidua but also laterally underneath the decidual margin. As a result the area of the chorionic plate is less than that of the decidual plate. This is called a *circumvallate placenta* (Fig. 7.6). Its incidence is 18 per cent and it occasionally causes ante-partum haemorrhage.

Development stages

6−7 days after fertilization: Implantation of the blastocyst.

9−10 days after fertilization: Blastocyst fully implanted; Maternal blood spaces present in syncytiotrophoblast.

12 days after fertilization: Amniotic cavity formed.

12−13 days after fertilization: Sluggish blood flow through maternal blood spaces begins.

22−23 days after fertilization: Development of placental villi culminating with the inception of a rudimentary villous circulation of fetal blood.

3rd month: Chorionic vesicle differentiated into two areas, the chorion laeve and the chorion frondosum.

4th month: Obliteration of the uterine lumen by fusion of the decidua capsularis with decidua parietalis.

End of 4th month: Placenta has cotyledons and from now on grows in diameter rather than thickness.

Further reading

Beaconsfield, P., Birdwood, G. & Beaconsfield, R. (1980) The placenta. *Scientific American*, **243**, 2, pp.80−90.

Bernischke, K. (1972) Implantation, placental development, uteroplacental blood flow. In: *Principles and Management of Human Reproduction*. Reid, D.E., Ryan, K.J. & Bernischke, K. W.B. Saunders. Philadelphia.

Boyd, J.D. & Hamilton, W.J. (1970) *The Human Placenta*. Heffer, Cambridge.

Steven, D, (ed.) (1975) *Comparative Placentation*. Academic Press, London, New York.

8
Maternal Changes During Pregnancy and Lactation

A hormonally-induced change in metabolism occurs during pregnancy. It is typified by the rather placid disposition and flushed features characteristic of this period in a woman's life.

Endocrine changes in pregnancy

Almost immediately after implantation the trophoblast begins to secrete hormones vital for the continuation of pregnancy. The secretion unique to this tissue is human chorionic gonadotrophin (HCG). Serum levels of the hormone rise rapidly to the middle of the third month of gestation and then fall to a level which is maintained until full term. HCG maintains the life and secretory activity (oestrogen and progesterone) of the corpus luteum until such time as the secretion of these hormones by the placenta itself is sufficient to maintain pregnancy. The serum levels of HCG then fall and pregnancy can continue, even after ovariectomy, though there is some evidence that HCG controls the levels at which the placenta itself secretes oestrogens and progestogens.

The placenta also secretes human placental lactogen (HPL), otherwise called human chorionic somatotrophin, which to some extent acts synergistically with growth hormone. This affects the establishment of lactation (*vide infra*) but also seems to have a more generalised effect on metabolism. It may be that HPL is related to the diabetic diathesis of pregnancy because, like growth hormone, it has a diabetogenic action.

Progestogens, in the form of progesterone, are produced by the corpus luteum early in pregnancy but after about 60–70 days the syncytiotrophoblast secretes all that is required to maintain pregnancy. The hormone reduces excitability of the smooth muscle not only in the uterus but also, to a lesser degree, in the ureters and gut. The lesser understood actions of progesterone are a degree of regulation of the body fat and the stimulation of mild hyperthermia (1°F at maximum).

As already mentioned, the oestrogens are first produced by the corpus luteum but this function is quickly taken over by the placenta and, to some extent, by the suprarenal cortex. Oestrogenic functions are manifold. It is well known that they enhance protein synthesis but they also reduce the adhesion of collagen fibres in connective tissue (cervical softening is a sign of pregnancy). Oestrogens aid the growth of uterine muscle as well as the ducts and, to a lesser degree, the alveoli of

110

the breast and cause a certain amount of fluid retention to occur during pregnancy.

Other endocrine glands are also involved in pregnancy though less so. The pituitary secretes excess ACTH, melanocyte stimulating hormone and perhaps also thyrotrophin. The adrenal glands, besides producing some oestrogens, also increase their corticosteroid production and the thyroid gland is enlarged because a reduced level of circulating iodine results from an alteration in kidney function. More pituitary thyrotrophic hormone is probably released for this reason. In addition there is an increase of the basal metabolic rate.

Changes in the genital tract

The major changes are uterine. Blood flow increases some five-fold and operations in this area are, therefore, more hazardous. The blood vessels become coiled and hypertrophied in the first half of pregnancy and straighten out as uterine growth proceeds during the second half. Uterine muscle weight increases by a factor of 10, chiefly by hypertrophy of existing fibres. From the 20th week onwards muscle growth virtually ceases and increase in the size of the uterus is due to distention and thinning of its walls by the fetus which becomes greater in weight than the uterus from 28 weeks onwards. The thickest muscle layers (mainly those in the intermediate layer of the myometrium) lie at the fundus and in modern clinical practice Caesarian sections are, therefore, done in the region of the so-called lower segment of the uterus which is the junction between uterus and cervix anteriorly. Here the muscular disposition is ideal for the operation. As previously mentioned the cervix becomes soft during pregnancy due to a change in its collagen fibres and it is thus more easily dilatable during parturition.

Oestrogens cause the vagina to thicken and dilate in the later part of pregnancy. The mucosal cells are shed at an increased rate and the possibility of vaginal infection increases.

The level to which the uterus is palpable in pregnancy is an important clinical sign indicating the age of the embryo and the normality or otherwise of its rate of growth (p.301). Towards the end of gestation the level of the fundus falls slightly as the head of the fetus 'engages' in the true pelvis. Clinical measurements of uterine growth and details of the process of parturition are outside the remit of this book.

Cardiovascular changes during pregnancy

Total blood volume increases from about 4 litres to 5.5 litres by 32–33 weeks. The increase is mainly due to a rise in plasma volume which begins to fall again at 33 weeks or so. The red cells count on the other hand rises slowly but steadily throughout the pregnancy although its increase is to a lesser extent than that of the plasma. As a result, the haemoglobin concentration falls and this has misleadingly been called the physiological anaemia of pregnancy (about 12 g per cent at 32 weeks). There is also a leucocytosis of 10,500 cells/ml. Serum protein patterns alter — albumin and α-globulins fall while β-globulins and fibrinogen rise. The erythrocyte sedimentation rate cannot, therefore, be used as a diagnostic tool. Serum cholesterol, the precursor of the steroid hormones, is high. Most of these changes are thought to be related to circulating oestrogen levels.

Cardiac output rises by some 20 per cent but the peripheral resistance is reduced due to the high level of circulating steroids so that the blood pressure remains more or less constant in normal pregnancy. The blood vessels, due to previously mentioned changes in collagen, become more distensible and varicose veins are common in pregnancy, especially because of partial blockage of pelvic venous return by the enlarged uterus.

The uterus receives the greater part of the increased blood flow as arterial blood enters the maternal placental blood spaces (Fig. 7.8) under pressure from the endometrial arteries and streams through the otherwise slow-moving maternal blood to reach the chorionic plate. The stream then loses much of its force and swirls back over the branch villi, thus facilitating the exchange mechanisms. Blood eventually drains away through the veins of the endometrium which pierce the cytotrophoblastic shell interspersed with the maternal arteries to the placenta. Renal blood flow is also increased steadily up to the fifth month and remains at this level until full term. Smooth muscle in the renal pelvis and ureter relaxes and the system begins to dilate at about the 10th week; the middle portion of the ureter can often kink and dilate the renal pelvis even further (from 15 to perhaps 75 ml). Bladder muscle relaxation encourages urinary stasis and ascending urinary infection in pregnancy is, therefore, an ever present risk. Frequency of micturition early in pregnancy is normal and due to increased water excretion by the kidney. Gradually this subsides but frequency later in pregnancy may be due to pressure of the uterus on the bladder itself. The glomerular filtration rate rises by 60 per cent and since tubular resorption is effectively unchanged, clearance of urea, uric acid, glucose, amino acid and folic acid is increased.

The blood flow through the skin and mucous membranes also increases and peripheral vasodilatation is characteristic of the pregnant woman who also complains of sweating easily.

Changes in the respiratory and alimentary systems

Pregnant women overbreathe because raised progesterone 'resets' the respiratory centre. The result is a feeling of breathlessness at rest and a lowered pCO_2 level which is of advantage to the fetus but uncomfortable for the mother. Tidal volume may be increased by as much as 20 per cent. As a result of the changes in the pCO_2 Na^+ and HCO_3^- are excreted in excess and plasma osmolality falls by about 10 mosm/kg. Possibly the osmoreceptors are also 'reset' to accommodate this.

Changes in the alimentary system include 'sponginess' of the gums due perhaps to fluid retention. In common with other smooth muscle that of the alimentary tract is also relaxed so that oesophageal reflux, retention of food in the stomach, reduced peristalsis and constipation (aggravated by pressure from the fetal head) all contribute to the minor discomforts of pregnancy.

Breast changes in pregnancy

At puberty breast development in the female is stimulated chiefly by raised levels of circulating oestrogens. Progestogens, prolactin, corticoids and growth hormone also play a part. At this stage growth is largely due to duct proliferation. During pregnancy raised oestrogen levels again stimulate breast development but, at this time, the sustained increase in levels of progesterone also result in the full development of alveoli. The breasts increase in size from the second month of pregnancy onwards but subjective feelings of tenderness or tingling before this are sometimes the first symptoms of pregnancy experienced by the mother to be. The initiation of milk secretion is due to prolactin probably aided by corticosteroids and insulin. When oestrogen levels fall at the end of pregnancy the full effect of prolactin in the stimulation of milk production is released. This effect may be enhanced by co-incident falls in progesterone and placental lactogen levels. Oxytocin is essential for milk ejection by causing contraction of the myo-epithelium of the breast. A reflex release of oxytocin is induced by stimulation of the nipple as in suckling.

General metabolic changes

In spite of a raised metabolic rate, relative quiescence of general maternal metabolism as well as a decline of the rate of exchange between the maternal blood and tissues is an important adjunct to pregnancy. There is a general reduction in insulin sensitivity so that glucose remains longer in the blood even though there is a greater excretion rate and some glucose may be lost by this route. In addition, increased fat deposition, a larger cardiac output, greater tidal volume and reduction of muscle tone all aid the survival of the baby in periods of crisis.

Pregnancy and weight gain

In general, women who are of normal build may expect to gain some 12–13 kg during pregnancy. Excessive gain and fluid retention is often associated with a serious hypertensive complication of pregnancy known as toxaemia of pregnancy. Most, but not all, of the weight is put on during the second half of pregnancy and is due to both the products of conception and to a purely maternal component (*vide infra*).

The birth weight of babies is genetically related to the mother rather than to the father, paternal genes in this respect are chiefly expressed post-natally. Socio-economic standing still has some effect and the better-off tend to give birth to heavier babies. It is not clear, however, whether this is entirely due to available diet rather than to dietary habits and other features characterising different life styles. The fetus begins to grow rapidly at about 20 weeks (*vide supra*) while the weight gain of the placenta is maximal during the first 16 weeks at the end of which period the fetus overtakes it in weight and, at term, the placenta weighs about 20 per cent of the total conceptus.

The liquor amnii has already been mentioned (p.100); it increases from 300 ml at mid-term to 1000 ml at 38 weeks but then falls rapidly to 600 ml at term. Its circulation is of importance to the baby (p.314).

Maternal components of weight gain are multiple. The uterus increases in weight most rapidly in the first 20 weeks and, at term, weights about 1 kg more than in the non-pregnant state. Increments in breast weight, blood volume and fat deposition all add to maternal weight. The last is variable depending on the diet but usually is in the order of 4 kg, most of it being deposited in the first half of pregnancy. The fat is easily mobilised and liberates the excess calories used in the second half of pregnancy and in the *puerperium*, the period immediately following parturition. During pregnancy there is normally an increase of total extra-uterine body water of about 2.5 litres. Fluid retention is not considered pathological unless it exceeds 3.5 litres up to 30 weeks and 3.0 litres from then until full term. Excessive fluid retention is dangerous and can be detected by regular weighing even before the onset of tissue oedema. A gain of weight of 1 kg or more within a week should cause concern.

A great deal has been written about diet during pregnancy, much of it ill-informed and some positively harmful. We must accept that the developing child is susceptible to external influences and this includes the maternal diet. For this reason it would seem most important that the mother does not indulge in any dietary excesses in either direction and that, if her normal diet has been of good quality, she adheres to it throughout pregnancy. At the time of writing it seems quite possible that marginal vitamin deficiencies (as yet of unknown nature) are causally associated with the development of spina bifida and anencephaly (see Chapter 10). At present by far the best advice is that pregnant women eat a normal balanced diet with vitamin supplementation at physiological levels.

The diagnosis and maintenance of pregnancy: onset of parturition

The cardinal sign of pregnancy is amenorrhea (cessation of the menstrual periods) but there are other clinical reasons for this condition and specific pregnancy tests have been developed and used for a considerable time.

Recently, immunological tests have largely replaced biological tests for pregnancy. Anti-chorionic gonadotrophin serum is prepared by immunization of a suitable animal recipient with the hormone. The urine to be tested and serum containing anti-chorionic gonadotrophin are mixed in the first part of the test. Subsequently, red blood corpuscles or latex particles, both coated with chorionic gonadotrophin, are added. If the original urine contained significant amounts of chorionic gonadotrophin then this will have neutralized the serum antibodies and there will be no effect on the added corpuscles. On the other hand urine from a non-pregnant female will not affect the anti-chorionic gonadotrophin serum and, when the coated corpuscles are added, they will be agglutinated and lysed by the antibodies still present in the mixture. The production of human chorionic gonadotrophin is sufficient to give a positive pregnancy test ten days after a missed period and reaches a maximum around the 60th day of pregnancy. Thereafter serum levels fall progressively and remain quite low from the fifth month of pregnancy to full term. These observations, together with the result of culture experiments, suggest that the hormone is produced by cytotrophoblast and its serum level therefore falls as cytotrophoblastic cells become attenuated in the placental villi (p.98). Other techniques of localization, however, suggest that the syncytiotrophoblast is the true site of production and the question must therefore remain open. Human chorionic gonadotrophin is similar to, but not identical with, pituitary LH (p.55) both in chemical structure and in biological activity.

The corpus luteum of pregnancy begins to regress at the end of the fourth month of pregnancy (though it is still morphologically identifiable at term) and surgical removal of the ovaries after the second month does not interrupt pregnancy. Clearly, therefore, the human placenta produces increasing amounts of both progestogens and oestrogens, probably in the syncytiotrophoblast, as pregnancy proceeds. In addition, some of the oestriol found in maternal pregnancy urine is probably produced by the placenta as a metabolic breakdown product of fetal adrenal cortical hormones. The chief function of oestrogens during pregnancy seems to be connected with growth of the uterus and of the duct system, as well as the alveoli of the breasts. Progesterone is responsible, at least in part, for the establishment of the progestational endometrium into which the blastocyst implants (p.91). Thereafter uterine secretory activity is maintained for a considerable period and, more importantly, progesterone renders the uterine musculature quiescent throughout pregnancy. The hormone is also responsible for the further development of ducts as well as of alveoli in the breast in preparation for lactation. After the 12th week of gestation the syncytiotrophoblast produces placental prolactin in addition to oestrogens and progesterone. Like pituitary prolactin this hormone is probably concerned with breast growth and acts synergistically with the placental steroids in this respect (p.110).

Gestational length in the human is around a mean of just under 10 months (280 days) if counted from the first day of the last menstrual period. This calculation is, of course, about 10−14 days longer than actual fetal development because ovulation (p.43) occurs at mid-cycle. A rough, but effective, method of calculating the expected date of delivery which is widely used is to add seven days to the first day of the last menstrual period and then to count forward nine calendar months. The range of normal pregnancy length seems to be between 266 and 294 days. Very often calculations go astray because it is impossible to be sure of the time of the last menstrual period. Clinical estimations of the stage of pregnancy can then be made by palpation of the uterus but details of this are beyond the scope of this text.

The onset of parturition poses many unsolved physiological problems. Labour is almost certainly precipitated by the action of a number of factors principally, but not exclusively, hormonal in nature. Progesterone is known to inhibit the onset of parturition in many experimental animals and a rise in blood oestrogen levels just before the onset of labour has been reported in many species. There thus appears to be a definite partnership between oestrogen and progesterone levels in the blood which at certain relative concentrations work to maintain pregnancy and at others to terminate it.

Other important endocrine factors appear to be operative also. Progesterone appears to antagonise the smooth muscle-stimulating effect of oxytocin by preventing the propagation of muscular contraction but, as the uterus becomes increasingly distended later in pregnancy, its sensitivity to oxytocin increases. Increasing levels of oxytocin, secreted by the posterior pituitary gland late in pregnancy, might be an important factor in the onset of labour but unfortunately no fall in placental oxytocinase (a hormone antagonising the effects of oxytocin) level has been demonstrated until labour is already under way.

The maintainance of pregnancy and mechanisms of parturition vary greatly with species. For a more detailed treatment of these subjects the reader is referred to textbooks of reproductive physiology (see Johnson and Everitt, 1984).

Further reading

Ciba Foundation Symposium 47. (1977) *The Fetus and Birth* Elsevier.
Fuchs F. & Klopper, A. (1977) *Endocrinology of Pregnancy*, 2nd edn. Harper Row.
Hytten, F.E. & Leitch, I. (1971) *The Physiology of Human Pregnancy*. Blackwell Scientific Publications, Oxford.
Johnson, M.H. & Everitt, B.J. (1984) *Essential Reproduction*, (especially Chapters 10−13). Blackwell Scientific Publications, Oxford.

9
The Mesodermal Somites

In the youngest of the three embryos shown in Fig. 9.1 it will be noticed that immediately caudal to the developing face and the pharyngeal region lies the large bulging pericardial cavity and the shape of the developing heart may be seen within it. This embryo is at about 33 days of development. Later, the lung buds will enlarge and grow ventrally on either side of the heart and pericardium, which will therefore lie between them. The cranial end of the mesonephros (p.249) will extend up as far as the lung buds. At this stage, however, both sides of the heart as well as its ventral surface are visible through the very thin pericardium. A further reason why the heart is so clearly visible is that the body wall is semi-transparent, both in the region of the heart and in the abdomen, so that the abdominal contents, too, are visible through it. This is because the dermatomes (*vide infra*) have not yet invaded this area. A large part of the ventral abdominal wall is occupied by the relatively large umbilical cord.

A very noticeable feature of the embryo at this stage is the series of *mesodermal somites* which lie on either side of the midline down the dorsal aspect of the embryo (Fig. 9.1). From the surface they have the appearance of a number of square opacities within the rather transparent tissue of the embryo. It is by means of growth and migration of the cells of the somites that the body wall becomes thicker and develops bone and muscle. Somite-derived tissues will spread medially to form the vertebrae, dorsally to form the extensor musculature of the back and ventrally into the body wall to form the ribs, intercostals and the abdominal muscles. The deeper layers of the skin are also of somite origin. It must be stressed again that up to the end of the first month of development the body wall consists only of somatopleure, that is to say of ectoderm together with a thin layer of somatic or parietal mesoderm. It is, therefore, semi-transparent and it is not until it is invaded by the cells derived from the somites that it becomes thicker and more or less opaque. The somatopleure forms only a part of the connective tissue and blood vessels of the thoracic and abdominal wall, the most substantial part being made up of tissues derived from the dermatomal cells of the somites.

As has been seen (p.84), the mesoderm at the trilaminar disc stage of development may be subdivided into the paraxial portion that lies on either side of the midline, the intermediate cell mass and the lateral plate mesoderm that extends out to the edge of the embryonic disc where it becomes continuous with the extra-

117

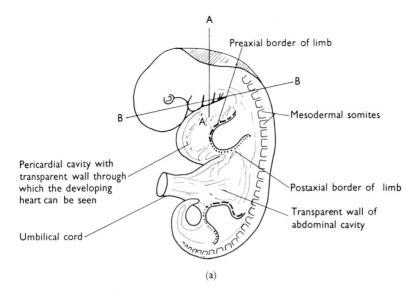

(a)

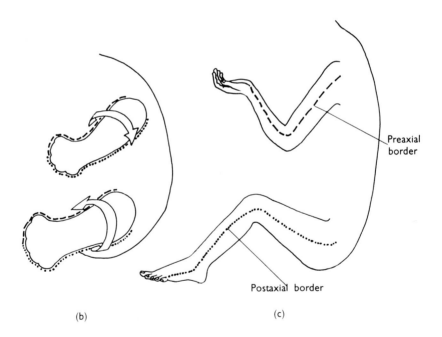

(b)   (c)

Fig. 9.1. (a) An embryo in the somite stage (approximately 33 days) before the invasion of the body wall by cells from the somites. The limb buds are just beginning. Preaxial borders are marked by a broken line, postaxial borders by a dotted line. A–A and B–B show the planes of section of Figs. 11.1 and 11.2.
(b) and (c) Later stages in the development of the limbs to show their change in position.

embryonic mesoderm. The intermediate cell mass is important in the development of the urogenital system and will not be further considered in this chapter. At the end of the third week the paraxial mesoderm, which is already heaped up on either side of the neural groove, begins to become divided up into mesodermal somites which are a prominent feature during the fourth and fifth weeks after fertilization. In transverse sections the somites are roughly triangular in shape and, for a short period, they contain a cavity but this soon becomes obliterated. One side of the triangle faces the neural tube and the opposite angle is continuous with the intermediate cell mass and the lateral plate mesoderm which will later split to contribute to the somatopleure and splanchnopleure (Fig. 6.10). Each somite consists of a densely aggregated mass of epitheloid cells which are, at first, clearly demarcated from the surrounding loose mesenchymal tissue but which soon become less well defined as the cells of which they are composed migrate in various directions.

It has already been observed that, during the development of the primitive streak and notochord, there is a cranio-caudal gradient of maturity and a similar gradient is seen in the development of the somites, as well as in numerous other embryonic structures that will be described later. The somites thus appear first in the future occipital region of the embryo although, of course, the region cannot be recognised as such at this stage. Further somites rapidly appear caudal to those that are first laid down until eventually about 44 pairs develop (Fig. 17.4). The most cranial somites begin to break up before the caudal ones are completed so that the whole number cannot be identified at any one time. It is important to stress that the paraxial mesoderm of the cranial end of the embryo (the future head region) remains unsegmented.

There are about 4 *occipital somites*, although the most cranial of these are difficult to recognise and the exact number is uncertain. These are followed by 8 *cervical somites*, 12 *thoracic*, 5 *lumbar*, 5 *sacral* and 8–10 *coccygeal somites*. On surface view the square appearance of the somites resembles a series of vertebral bodies but this appearance is misleading since the development of the vertebrae is more complicated than appears at first sight.

Subdivisions of the somites

Soon after its formation, each somite becomes differentiated into three parts (Fig. 6.13). The ventro-medial part first loses its well defined outline and the cells spread out and migrate medially towards the notochord and the neural tube. These cells are known collectively as the *sclerotome* and they will later take part in the development of the vertebrae and ribs. The remainder of the somite is known as the *dermo-myotome* and the cells of its dorsal and ventral edges proliferate and move medially to form the *myotome*. These cells also migrate widely (p.127) and become differentiated into myoblasts or primitive muscle cells. The thin layer of cells which finally remain are known as the *dermatome* and they spread out to form the dermis of the skin (p.128).

Reference to Fig. 6.13 will show that the myotomes are conveniently situated with regard to the neural tube so that it is easy for developing nerves, which are growing peripherally from the neural tube, to reach this region. In fact, the myotome of each somite receives a single spinal nerve which is destined to innervate its future muscle derivatives, no matter how far they eventually migrate from the position of their parent somites. For this reason, nerves in the adult often travel a long way before supplying a muscle and perhaps the best example of this phenomenon is the phrenic nerve which is described on p.240. The dorsal aortae (or single aorta in the more caudal region of the embryo) lie adjacent to the somite region and these large vessels give off a series of *intersegmental arteries* which, as their name implies, lie between the somites (Fig. 9.2a) and pass dorsally to supply the neural tube. Thus, the spinal nerves are segmental in position whereas the arteries are intersegmental. The significance of this will be appreciated when the development of the vertebrae is considered.

The sclerotomes and the development of the vertebrae

Although much of the final development of the vertebrae takes place fairly late in the fetal period and is not, in fact, wholly completed until a long time after birth, it will be convenient at this stage to deal with the whole period of their development from beginning to end.

As has been seen, the mesodermal cells of the ventral and medial part of each

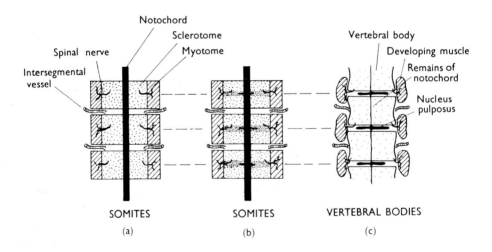

Fig. 9.2. Each vertebral body is formed from adjacent halves of two somites. One nerve supplies the myotome of each somite, and one intersegmental artery passes between each pair of somites. With the formation of the vertebral bodies, the nerves become intervertebral in position and the arteries run in relation to the vertebral bodies.

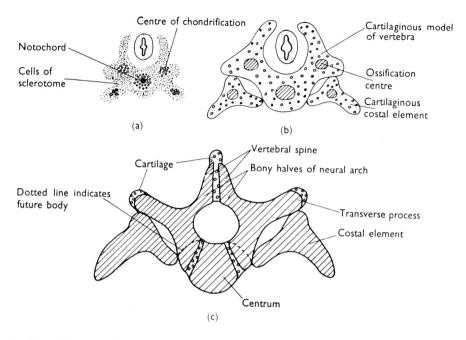

Fig. 9.3. (a) The cells of the sclerotome migrate towards the neural tube and form the rough shape of a vertebra. (b) Cartilaginous models of vertebrae and costal elements develop, with centres of ossification for the centrum, for each half of the neural arch and for each rib. (c) The vertebra and costal elements are almost completely ossified, but some cartilage remains so that, at birth, each bony vertebra is in 3 pieces.

somite which form the sclerotome lose their dense epitheloid arrangement and begin to stream medially to surround the neural tube (Fig. 6.13). The largest accumulation of these migrating cells lies ventral to the neural tube where they surround the notochord. In transverse sections of an embryo at this stage some idea of the outline of the vertebral body can soon be made out (Fig. 9.3). In longitudinal sections of the embryo, however, it can be seen that the condensations of cells around the notochord are not uniform in density but are packed closely together in one region of the sclerotome. This dense band of cells eventually comes to lie near the centre of the sclerotome (Fig. 9.2b); the caudal portion of each sclerotome unites with the cranial portion of the next to form a single vertebral body, the dense band of cells forming a primitive intervertebral disc (Fig. 9.2(c)). There is no great change, at this stage, at least in the position of the spinal nerves and intersegmental arteries, so that the nerves which originally innervated each of the somites now come to lie between the vertebrae, while the arteries which originally passed between the somites now lie close to the bodies of the vertebrae (Fig. 9.2). Spinal nerves, in the adult, therefore emerge through the intervertebral foramina and are closely related to the intervertebral discs. The fate of the intersegmental arteries will be described in Chapter 12.

The fate of the notochord

The notochord can, for some time, be recognised as it runs through the centre of the vertebral body but eventually it disappears. In the central part of the inter-vertebral disc, however, the notochordal cells spread out to form a major part of the nucleus pulposus (Fig. 9.2c). Cranially, the notochord is incorporated into the base of the skull, its anterior extremity lying in the region of the future hypo-physeal fossa. This part of the notochord normally disappears entirely. Occasion-ally tumours of persistent notochordal tissue occur (*chordomas*) and, since these are nearly always formed at one or other end of the notochord, they are found in the sphenoidal or the sacrococcygeal regions.

The formation of the vertebrae

As described above, the body of each vertebra develops from the caudal part of one somite together with the cranial portion of the next. Cells of the sclerotome also migrate dorsally around the neural tube to form a *neural arch* and a suggestion of a transverse process (Fig. 9.3). Chondrification (the conversion of mesodermal cells into cartilage) now begins from a number of centres in this mesodermal condensation and it soon spreads to form a cartilaginous model of the vertebra with a dorsally projecting spine and a pair of transverse processes which extend out laterally into the region of the myotomes (*vide infra*). Chondrification also begins in a pair of costal elements which are in close relation dorsally with the transverse process and more ventrally with the base of the neural arch (Fig. 9.3).

Ossification in the cartilage now commences from three centres, one in the region of the future vertebral body and one in each half of the neural arch. The centre for the body is at first paired but the two centres rapidly fuse. The ossification spreads from the first named centre to form a bony *centrum*; as will be seen later, the centrum does not coincide exactly with the adult body. The centres in each side of the neural arch also spread until the only cartilage remaining is that lying in the midline dorsally, and that lying between the bases of each side of the neural arch and the centrum ventrally (Fig. 9.3c). Further growth in size occurs, but this is essentially the state of the vertebra at birth. By three years of age the ossified portions of the neural arch have fused with each other and with the centrum so that the vertebra is now complete except for a number of secondary centres of ossification that appear after puberty and fuse still later. It can be seen from Fig. 9.3(c) that the adult vertebral body consists of the centrum together with the expanded lower end of the neural arch.

Atlas and axis

In the case of the atlas and axis (the first two adult cervical vertebrae) there is some modification of this pattern. Development here is somewhat complicated but

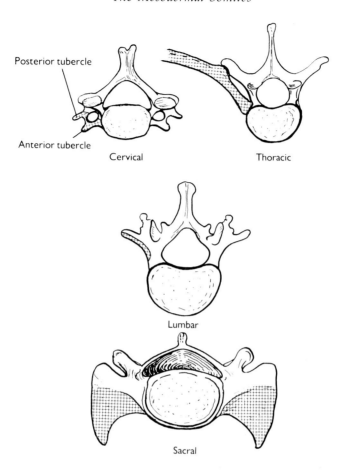

Fig. 9.4. Cervical, thoracic, lumbar and sacral vertebrae. In each case the costal element is shaded.

may be summed up by saying that the centrum belonging to the atlas becomes fused to that of the axis to form the dens.

Costal elements

The fate of the costal elements varies in different regions of the spine. As can be seen from Fig. 9.3, the dorsal end of the costal element develops in close relation to the transverse process and the base of the neural arch. In the thoracic region synovial joints develop at these areas of contact and, since the base of the neural arch is incorporated into the vertebral body, the heads of the adult ribs articulate with the sides of the bodies. The shaft of the costal elements grows into the body wall between adjacent myotomes so that the alternating sequence of ribs and intercostal muscles in the fully developed thorax is formed. The ventral ends of some of the costal elements become continuous with a longitudinal mesodermal condensation and these bilaterally placed 'sternal bars' become united in the midline to form the rudiments of the sternum in which chondrification, and later ossification, will occur.

In the cervical region the costal elements do not form synovial joints with the neural arches but fuse with them at two points and the whole mass becomes ossified. It can thus be seen (Fig. 9.4) that in the cervical region the true transverse processes are represented by part of the posterior tubercles of the adult transverse processes, while the costal elements form the rest of the posterior tubercles, the anterior tubercles and the bar of bone which connects them. The foramen transversarium in a cervical vertebra thus corresponds to the space between the neck of the rib and the transverse process of a vertebra in the thoracic region. In the lumbar regions of the spine the costal element forms part of the adult transverse process so that no distinction can be made between the two. In the sacral region

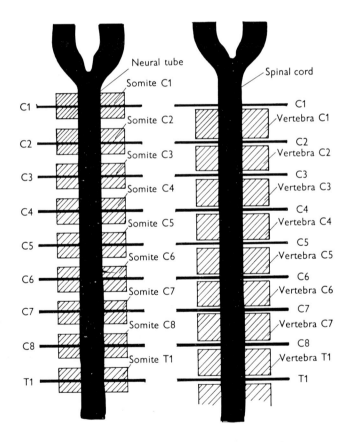

Fig. 9.5. A diagram to explain the relation of spinal nerves to vertebrae. One nerve supplies each of the eight cervical somites so that there are 8 cervical nerves. As a result of the formation of vertebrae from two adjacent somites, the 8th cervical nerve comes to lie *caudal* to the 7th cervical vertebrae.

similarly the costal element forms part of the lateral mass of the sacrum which is thus composed of both transverse and costal elements.

Development of the skull

The skull ossifies partly in membrane and partly in cartilage. The base of the skull, including the petrous part of the temporal bone and the greater and lesser wings of the sphenoid, ossify in cartilage. The main cartilaginous precursor in the midline consists of a base plate (*parachordal plate*), into which the occipital somites are incorporated and which is extended forwards to the nasal region by other centres of chondrification. To this are later fused the more laterally placed auditory and nasal capsules and cartilage masses which will later form the greater and lesser wings of the sphenoid. The whole is called the *chondrocranium* and, since the cranial nerves are already present before it develops, the various components leave gaps between them which become the foramina in the base of the skull (Fig. 9.6). Ossification commences in a number of centres for different bones and these spread until the whole base is ossified except for a cartilaginous plate between the basi-occiput and the body of the sphenoid. This is an important growth centre until it closes at about the age of 25. The vault of the skull (*membranous neurocranium*) ossifies in membrane to form the frontal, parietal, occipital and squamous temporal bones. There are, in the fetus, two frontal bones and the diamond shaped area between these and the parietals forms the anterior fontanelle, which closes at about 18 months of age. The bones of the face (including the mandible) are ossified partly in membrane and partly in cartilage. As will be described in Chapter 11, certain derivatives of the branchial arches are incorporated into the skull.

Development of the limbs

Although the limb musculature in mammals possibly develops *in situ* rather than from the somites as it does in the chick, this will nevertheless be a convenient place briefly to discuss the formation of the limbs. They make their appearance as flipper-like outgrowths, the *limb buds* (Fig. 9.1), the forelimb bud appearing first. Each bud consists of a mass of mesenchyme covered by ectoderm with a thickened ectodermal ridge at the tip. The ridge is part of a complicated system controlling the normal morphogenesis of the limb. Details of the mechanisms involved are beyond the scope of this book. They may be studied by reading the reference to Wolpert (1978) given in *Further Reading* at the end of this chapter. At the beginning of the second month the prominences of the future knee and elbow region can be recognised, both projecting laterally and backwards. The hand and foot plates appear at the same time as flattened expansions at the end of the limb buds and between 36 and 38 days, 5 radiating thickenings which develop into the fingers and toes can be distinguished. The webs between these thickenings then disappear, thus freeing the digits. The appropriate spinal nerves grow down into the

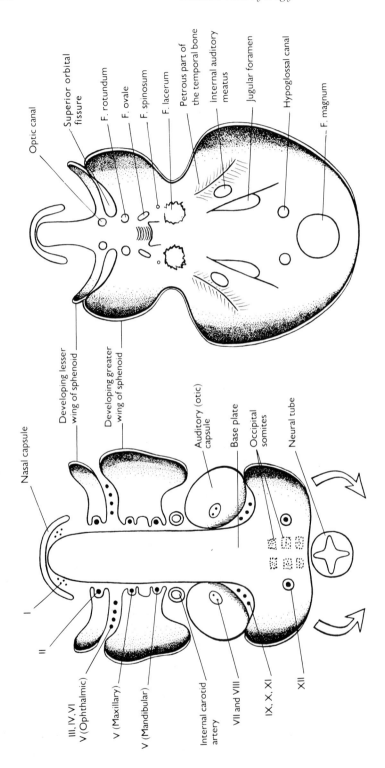

Fig. 9.6. Development of the chondrocranium. On the left are shown the cranial nerves (which are present before the chondrocranium develops) and on the right the foramina which are formed as a result of the fusion of the various components of the chondrocranium.

limbs (C5, 6, 7, 8, T1 for the upper limb; L2, 3, 4, 5, S1, 2, 3 for the lower limb) and the bones differentiate from the mesenchyme of the bud. At present, doubt exists concerning the origin of the musculature.

The limbs grow in such a way that they appear to rotate in opposite directions, the upper limb laterally and the lower limb medially (Fig. 9.1). Thus the thumb becomes the lateral (*preaxial*) digit of the hand and the big toe the medial (*preaxial*) digit of the foot. An understanding of the development of the limbs makes it easy to understand why true flexion at the ankle corresponds to plantar flexion while extension is obviously dorsiflexion.

The dermo-myotomes

As has been stated (p.119), the lateral part of each somite after the migration of the cells that form the sclerotome is known as the dermo-myotome. After a short time the dermo-myotome begins to break up, the cells moving both dorsally and ventrally.

The myotomes

The dorsal myotome cells move into a position between the transverse process and the spine of the vertebra while the cells of the ventral part of the myotome move into the body wall, or somatopleure, which thus becomes thicker and less transparent. The spinal nerves that originally supplied each myotome become divided into an anterior and a posterior *primary ramus*, the former supplying the ventral part of the myotome (*hypomere*) and the latter the dorsal part (*epimere*). The cells of the myotome become spindle-shaped, with large spherical nuclei and these primitive muscle cells (*myoblasts*) later become differentiated into skeletal muscle fibres. When the cells migrate, their nerves of supply follow them so that the site of origin of any of the trunk muscles in the adult can be deduced from its nerve supply. Thus the muscles of the abdominal wall in the adult are supplied by the lower six thoracic and first lumbar nerves so that it may be inferred that they developed originally from the corresponding somites and have migrated over a considerable distance to reach their adult position. This is why the lower thoracic anterior primary rami (intercostal nerves) enter the abdominal wall whereas the corresponding intercostal arteries remain in the intercostal spaces.

The epimeres form the extensor musculature (sacro-spinalis muscle) and the hypomeres form the prevertebral muscles such as the scalenes, quadratus lumborum, psoas major and pyriformis together with the muscles of the thoracic, abdominal and pelvic walls. Certain somites are somewhat atypical. Thus, it seems probable that the occipital myotomes whose nerves are represented by the rootlets of the hypoglossal nerve, migrate ventrally into the mass of mesoderm formed by the first and third branchial arches (p.186) to form the tongue musculature. Similarly, the skeletal muscle of the diaphragm is developed from the third, fourth and fifth cervical somites, the myotomic cells of which move into the septum transversum at the time when this lies in the immediate vicinity of these somites (p.240). Later, when the developing diaphragm undergoes a relative descent to its adult position, the nerves follow it down to produce the long and unbranching course of the adult phrenic nerve.

It must be appreciated that the above account is partly based upon obser-vations and experiments upon lower animals. The actual migration of myotomic cells in the human embryo can only be deduced by a study of numerous single embryos. In fact, there is some evidence that the human tongue musculature may develop *in situ*.

The relation of nerves to vertebrae

The first cervical vertebra (atlas) develops from the caudal part of the first cervical somite and the cranial part of the second; the cranial portion of the first somite together with the occipital somites lose their identity. The first cervical nerve originally supplied the first cervical somite so that, in the adult, the first nerve is related to the upper surface of the atlas. There are eight cervical somites and, therefore, eight cervical nerves. The seventh cervical vertebra is formed from the caudal part of the seventh somite and the cranial half of the eighth, so that the adult eighth cervical nerve lies caudal to the seventh vertebra and, from this level down, each nerve lies below the corresponding vertebra (Fig. 9.5).

Development of the skin

In the early stages of development the embryo is covered by ectoderm which consists only of a single layer of cuboidal cells. During the second month a more superficial layer of rather flattened cells appears, covering the original cuboidal cells (Fig. 9.7). This is the *periderm* and it persists as a surface layer while the remaining layers of the skin (and its derivatives, such as sweat glands and hair) develop beneath it. In the later stages of pregnancy the periderm is shed and this, together with cast-off cells derived from the stratum corneum and the secretions of the sebaceous glands, form a whitish slippery coating known as the *vernix caseosa* which may help to render the skin more waterproof (p.311) and, by virtue of its slippery nature, allows childbirth to take place without undue abrasion of the birth canal.

The dermatomes

The cells of the dermatomes (p.119) migrate in similar directions to those of the myotome. They spread out immediately deep to the ectoderm and form the major part of the dermis of the skin, although this is also partly formed from the mesenchyme which already lies deep to the ectoderm. Like the myotomes, the dermatomes take their nerve supply with them. Textbooks of topographical anatomy describe the distribution of dermatomes in the adult. These are of clinical importance in localizing lesions of the spinal cord and spinal nerves.

The skin appendages

Hairs begin to develop as solid ingrowths of epidermis called *hair buds*. Each grows down into the dermis and expands at the end to form a *hair bulb* (Fig. 9.7) which becomes invaginated by a core of mesoderm to form the papilla. The basal columnar cells of the hair bulb and of the sides of the hair bud proliferate and the central core of cells becomes keratinised to form the hair itself. Further cell division in the bulb causes the hair to elongate until it protrudes from the surface of the skin. The first hairs develop all over the body; they are very fine hairs and are known collectively as *lanugo*. The lanugo is normally shed before birth and is replaced by coarser hairs which develop from new follicles. The peripheral cells of the hair bud also proliferate laterally to form solid collections of

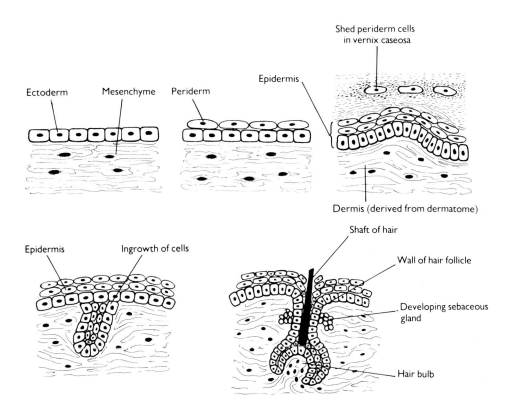

Fig. 9.7. The upper three figures show the development of the skin and the lower two the development of a hair.

cells, the forerunners of the sebaceous glands. The central cells of these clusters degenerate to form the sebum which is discharged into the hair follicle. Sweat glands develop as individual ingrowths of ectoderm which become canalized and tortuous.

The nails appear first as thickenings in the ectoderm at the tips of the digits — the *primary nail fields*. The nail fields grow dorsally and proximally to take up the normal position of the nails and the cells at the proximal end proliferate to form the nail itself. The nail then slowly grows towards the tip of the finger, which it reaches round about birth or a little later. Finger nails which stop short of the fingertips are an indication of prematurity.

The mammary glands

In the early stages of development (about 35 days) ectodermal thickenings appear along a pair of mammary ridges (*milk lines*) which run from the region of the future axilla to the inguinal region on each side. In the human embryo further development occurs only in the pectoral region although accessory nipples (or even mammary glands) are not uncommon in other situations along the mammary ridges. In some animals, such as pigs, mammary glands develop all along the milk line whereas in cows for example the glands are restricted to the lower end.

From the ectodermal thickening in the region of the future nipple about 20 solid cords of cells grow radially into the surrounding mesenchyme. These become canalized to form *lactiferous ducts* and then alveoli develop at their end. The region of the nipple is, at first, marked by a depression but this later becomes elevated to form a true nipple. Failure of this process to occur may give rise to the condition of *inverted nipple* which may cause difficulty in breast feeding in later life. Post-natal breast development is under hormonal control. Occasionally, in the neonate, some secretion may be seen, presumably as a result of stimulation by maternal prolactin.

Developmental anomalies of somite derivatives and the limbs

Vertebral column and skull

Spina bifida

The most important anomaly of the vertebral column and skull, *spina bifida*, is closely associated with anomalies of neural tube development and is, therefore, dealt with in Chapter 10.

Fusion of cervical vertebra (Klippel–Feil syndrome)

In this defect the bodies of the cervical vertebrae fuse together to cause a congenital short neck. The hair line is low, the head immobile and not uncommonly there is an associated cervical meningomyelocele. Neurological problems from cord and root compression often occur: the condition may sometimes be recognised by the extension of the scalp hair down the back.

Agenesis of sacrum

Vertebrae in the sacral region can fail to differentiate. This abnormality, for poorly understood reasons, occcurs more commonly in babies of diabetic mothers. Its major consequence is a tethering and maldevelopment of the lower part of the spinal cord with faulty innervation to the bladder leading to urinary retention, dribbling micturition and gluteal muscle wasting and weakness.

Hemi-vertebrae

These are due to failure of one of the paired ossification centres in the vertebral arch to develop. Any vertebrae can be involved, but those in the thoraco-cervical region are most commonly affected. Hemi-vertebrae commonly occur with anorectal anomalies and anomalies of the mesenteries such as mesenteric cysts. Hemi-vertebrae lead to lateral curvature of the spine (*scoliosis*) which, later in life, can cause serious problems not only for locomotion but also for breathing since the rib-cage development is also likely to be abnormal.

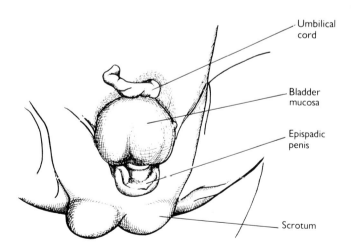

Fig. 9.8. Exstrophy (ectopia vesicae). The mucosa of the bladder is exposed above an epispadic penis. The ureteric orifices are not visible in this drawing but they could be found by inspection of the mucosa.

Rib abnormalities

Bifurcate xiphisternum

If the two halves of the sternal plate do not unite in the lower thoracic region a split sternum results. It is of cosmetic disadvantage only and is a relatively common anomaly, leading to a deep concavity in the chest at the lower end of the sternum.

Cervical rib

Sometimes the costal element of the transverse process of the seventh cervical vertebra will enlarge to form a cervical rib. Anteriorly this is joined to the first rib or costal cartilage directly or by a fibrous band. A cervical rib can be diagnosed during the course of a routine chest X-ray. Sometimes it is diagnosed following the investigation of vascular symptoms in the arm (due to compression of the subclavian artery by the rib) or neurological symptoms (tingling, weakness of palmar intrinsic muscles) of irritation of the lower trunk of the brachial plexus.

Anomalies of body wall musculature

Cells of the dermomyotome sometimes fail to migrate ventrally into the somatopleure in the region of the abdomen. The abdominal wall will, therefore, be very thin or even absent due to sloughing off of the thin epidermis and somatopleure. The following anomalies can result.

Exomphalos (Fig. 16.15)

This abnormality might be regarded as a persistent physiological hernia of the midgut into the extra-embryonic coelom, due to failure of the mesoderm to invade the somatopleure around the umbilicus. It will be dealt with in Chapter 16.

Exstrophy (ectopia vesicae) (Fig. 9.8)

Although principally an abnormality of the bladder this defect (much more common in boys) has its origins in somite dysmorphogenesis resulting in failure of the mesoderm to invade the somatopleure of the cloaca below the umbilicus. It will be discussed in Chapter 15.

Gastroschisis

Although similar at first sight in appearance to an exomphalos, gastroschisis is anatomically distinct and has a different aetiology. The abdominal contents

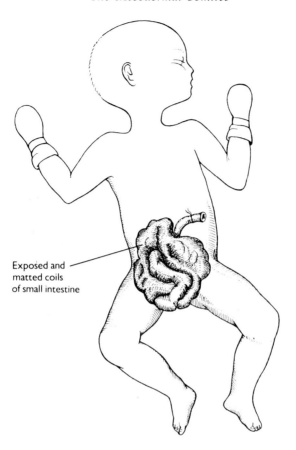

Exposed and
matted coils
of small intestine

Fig. 9.9. Gastroschisis (see text for description).

herniate through a defect in the abdominal wall musculature usually to the right of a normally inserted umbilical cord (Fig. 9.9). In contrast with exomphalos, organs other than stomach and small intestine rarely herniate and there is no covering sac. The prolapse is thought to occur in the last trimester of pregnancy. Because of the interaction of amniotic fluid and serosal secretions, loops of the prolapsed gut, often much shorter than normal, are frequently matted together. Management is by surgical reduction and patching up the defect in the abdominal wall. Unlike exomphalos, associated malformations are much less common and mainly involve the intestines, malrotation (p.293) being especially common.

Prune belly syndrome

This uncommon condition is almost always found in boys. The name describes the appearance of the abdominal wall which, because of an almost total absence of abdominal musculature, appears as lax and wrinkled as a prune skin. Abnormalities of the urinary tract are very common owing to defective muscularization and this causes dilatation and tortuosity of the ureters and bladder. Testes are always undescended. There is little to be done to make up the defect in abdominal wall musculature. Management is mainly directed towards the urinary tract problems. It has been suggested that the primary problem is not of defective musculature but instead a consequence of an obstruction in the penile urethra. The massive back pressure which results causes gross dilatation of the bladder and often of the ureters; the abdomen stretches. When the bladder is decompressed (usually by rupture) the abdomen is left lax with large redundant folds.

Abnormalities of the skin

Anomalies of ectodermal and mesodermal components of the skin can occur. The following are a few examples:

Ectodermal dysplasia

Partial or complete absence of sweat glands and other epidermal appendages including variable dental aplasia and sparse hair follicles constitutes an extremely rare condition. It occurs usually in males as a sex-linked recessive disorder. Major complications relate to hyperpyrexia due to inability to sweat.

Mesodermal anomalies

These are predominantly *naevi* (birth marks). They are growths of congenital origin involving the pigmented cells or vascular elements of the skin.

Pigmented naevi

Brown macules or papules of variable size resulting from overgrowth of melanin containing cells. Most are benign. Malignant changes can occur in those very deeply situated.

Vascular naevi

These are of two types. Superficial *cavernous haemangiomata* (strawberry naevus) are very common and are due to overgrowth of capillaries, usually on the face and trunk. They can increase rapidly in size over the first few months after birth and on the face they can be very disfiguring. They usually fade and grow smaller in time, but the whole process of resolution might, with large lesions, take many years. There is no available treatment to expedite resolution.

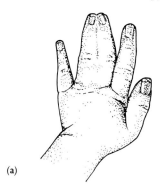
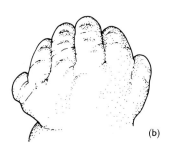

(a)

(b)

Fig. 9.10. (a) Syndactyly (b) Polydactyly.

Capillary angiomata (port wine stains)

These are wide, purple, flat lesions, usually on the face (where they are often very disfiguring) and limbs. They do not fade with age. On rare occasions they are associated with similar lesions on the course of the trigeminal nerve or in the brain (Sturge–Kalischer–Weber syndrome). Such lesions may rupture causing neurological damage.

Abnormalities of the limbs

A number of limb deformities appear relatively late in development as a result of mechanical factors, due to a deficiency in the volume of amniotic fluid or other constraints to growth. They will be dealt with in Chapter 17. Here three conditions of earlier onset are described.

1 *Phocomelia* is a condition in which there is a severe defect in limb development so that the limb is represented only by a short flipper-like appendage (phoca = a seal). This deformity may result from the action of a teratogen (thalidomide) taken during pregnancy (Chapter 18).

2 *Syndactyly* (Fig. 9.10a) is a condition in which one or more of the webs between the digits in the hand plate fail to break down, so that the digits are fused. They may be freed by a simple surgical operation. Many are inherited as autosomal dominants.

3 *Polydactyly* (Fig. 9.10b) is a condition in which more than five digits are present. It is unimportant; the extra digits may be amputated if they give rise to inconvenience. Some types of polydactyly are Mendelian dominant traits of variable expressivity.

Abnormalities involving the whole skeleton

Skeletal abnormalities which affect the relative proportions of the limbs and axial skeleton constitute very rare disorders, many being inherited in various Mendelian combinations. One example is provided.

Human Embryology

Achondroplasia (Fig. 9.11)

This condition, a defect in enchondral ossification, is characterised by short arms
and legs, stubby fingers and disproportionate growth of the base of the skull
(endochondral bone) and vault and face (membrane bone) and vertebral bodies. It
can be inherited as an autosomal dominant gene, but over 90 per cent are fresh
mutations. Life expectancy is usually excellent but two complications can seriously
affect well-being: (i) communicating hydrocephalus which might develop from
lack of space in the posterior fossa of the skull and (ii) peripheral nerve trauma
due to narrow intervertebral spaces.

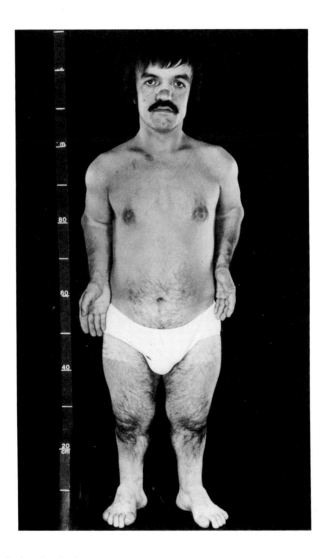

Fig. 9.11 A case of achondroplasia.

Developmental stages

20–30 days: Formation of somites

24–26 days: Limb buds appear

5 weeks: Hands and feet begin to develop

8 weeks: Primary centres of ossification appear in long bones

12 weeks: Formation of definitive body wall complete

3 months: Nails appear

4 months: Lanugo appears

5 months: Vernix caseosa begins to appear

7 months: Scalp and eyebrow hair develops

Birth: Vertebrae in 3 parts — centrum and 2 neural arches nails have grown to the
  end of fingers
  nipple everted
  anterior fontanelle easily palpable

Further reading

Breathnach, A.S. (1971) Embryology of human skin. A review of ultrastructural studies. *J. Invest. Dermatol.* **57**, 133.

Ebling, F.J.G. (1970) The embryology of skin. *In: An Introduction to the Biology of Skin*, eds. Champion, R.H., Gillman, T., Rook, A.J. & Sims, R.T. Blackwell Scientific Publications, Oxford.

Holbrook, K.A. (1979) Human Epidermal Embryogenesis. *Int. J. Dermatol.* **18**, 329.

Milaire, J. (1965) Aspects of limb morphogenesis in mammals, In: *Organogenesis*, eds. DeHann, R.L. & Ursprung, H. Holt, Rinehart & Winston, New York, Toronto & London.

Moffett, B.C. Jr. (1965) The morphogenesis of joints, In: *Organogenesis* eds. DeHann, R.L. & Ursprung, H. Holt, Rinehart & Winston, New York, Toronto & London.

Pinkus, H. (1958) Embryology of Hair. In: *The Biology of Hair Growth*, eds. Montagna, W. & Ellis, R.A. Academic Press, New York & London.

Prader, A. (1947) Die fruhembryonal Entwicklung der menschlichen Zwischenwirbelscheibe. *Acta Anat.* **3**, 68.

Prader, A. (1947) Die Entwicklung der Zwischenwirbelscheibe beim menschlichen Keimling. *Acta Anat.* **3**, 115.

O'Rahilly, R. & Gardner, E. (1972) The initial appearance of ossification in staged human embryos. *Am. J. Anat.* **134**, 291.

Sensenig, E.C. (1949) The Early Development of the Human Vertebral Column. *Contrib. Embryol. Carnegie Inst.* **33**, 23.

Wolpert, L. (1978) Pattern formation in biological development. *Sci. Am.* **239**(4), 154–164.

Zaias, N. (1963) Embryology of the Human Nail. *Archs Dermatol.* **87**, 37.

10
The Development of the Nervous System

As was explained in Chapter 6, the neural tube develops as a longitudinal infolding of a specialized region of columnar cell ectoderm along the dorsal aspect of the embryo. The edges of this infolding are raised above the level of the embryonic disc and are known as the *neural crests* (Fig. 10.1). Before the complete separation of the neural tube from the ectoderm, the neural crest cells themselves become segregated from the tube and arrange themselves on either side of it. Closure of the neural tube occurs first of all in the region corresponding to the future junction between brain and spinal cord and rapidly extends cranially and caudally until only small areas remain open at each end of the embryo. These are known as the *anterior* and *posterior neuropores* respectively. Before the anterior neuropore closes completely, certain changes occur which lead to the development of the eyes and optic nerves; these will be considered later.

The neuropores close soon after the formation of the head and tail folds and the neural tube, now complete, forms a prominent feature in transverse sections through the embryo (Fig. 10.1). The neural crest cells form a clump lying dorso-lateral to the neural tube and, from these, the posterior root ganglia and certain other structures will be formed (p.143). Immediately ventral to the neural tube, throughout the greater part of its length, lies the notochord but the cranial end of the tube (the future forebrain) projects beyond the cranial extremity of the notochord (Fig. 6.12), the latter only reaching as far forward as the region of the developing pituitary gland.

Histogenesis of the neural tube

The original neural ectoderm on the dorsal surface of the embryonic disc forms only a thickened layer of columnar epithelium but the cells soon begin to proliferate rapidly and, by the time the neural tube has become completely cut off from the surface, its wall consists of many layers of cells. These are destined to form the three types of cell that make up the nervous system, *ependymal cells, neuroglia (supporting) cells* and *nerve cells.*

In transverse sections through the neural tube at this stage it can be seen to have quite a complicated structure (Fig. 10.1) and three layers can be recognised. Nearest to the lumen can be seen a relatively thin pseudostratified layer containing a number of nuclei at various levels. This is now usually known as the

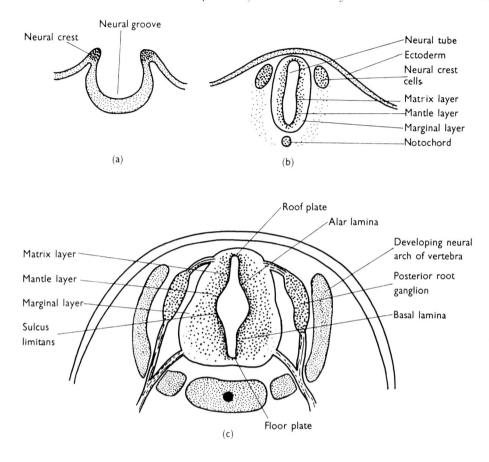

Fig. 10.1. (a) The neural groove and neural crest.
(b) & (c) The neural crest cells form *inter alia* the posterior root ganglia. The three layers of the neural tube can easily be distinguished.

matrix layer (also known as the ependymal or ventricular zone). External to this is a thick cellular layer called the *mantle layer* (or the intermediate zone) while on the outside is a layer of cell processes, the *marginal layer*. A continuous process of nuclear migration occurs in the neural tube during its development. Individual nuclei of the cells of the matrix layer immediately after DNA duplication move in turn towards the lumen, their cell bodies become spherical and the cells undergo mitosis in the innermost layer of the matrix. The nuclei of the daughter cells then either move back into the matrix layer where, in due course, they again move inwards to the zone of mitosis to repeat the process, or the cells lose connection with the luminal lining and enter the mantle layer as *neuroblasts*. The neuroblasts become nerve cells whose axons grow into the marginal layer in which they proceed to other levels of the nervous system. When all the required neuroblasts have been produced, the remaining matrix cells differentiate into neuroglia and ependymal cells, the latter forming the final lining of the cavity of the neural tube.

The derivatives of the three layers which have just been described are easily recognisable in the mature spinal cord (Fig. 10.2). Lining the central canal is a layer of ependymal cells. The grey matter of the cord consists of nerve cells derived from the mantle layer, while the peripheral white matter represents at least in part, the axons of nerve cells which originally grew cranially or caudally in the marginal layer. In certain regions of the brain this basic arrangement becomes modified by the migration through the marginal layer, of cells from the mantle layer which thus form an additional superficial layer of grey matter such as is seen, for instance, in the cerebral cortex. In the brain, too, the long columns of grey matter which are seen in the spinal cord become split up into separate discrete masses to form the nuclei of the cranial nerves. These may be motor or sensory and will be described in some detail later.

A further feature of the arrangement of cells in the neural tube may be seen in Fig. 10.1. The cells of the mantle zone are not uniformly distributed around the lumen of the neural tube. There are relatively few cells on the dorsal and ventral aspects of the tube (*roof* and *floor plates* respectively) but laterally there are two well marked accumulations of cells on each side, situated dorsally and ventrally and separated by a shallow groove, the *sulcus limitans*. The dorsal mass of cells is known as the *alar lamina* and is associated particularly with the sensory (afferent) part of the nervous system, while the ventral mass, the *basal lamina*, is associated with motor function. The alar and basal laminae project into the lumen of the

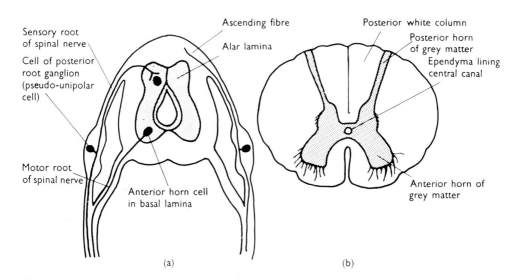

Fig. 10.2. (a) The axons of the basal lamina in the spinal cord grow out into the ventral nerve roots. The cells of the posterior root ganglion provide processes which grow out peripherally to form sensory nerve endings and others which grow into the spinal cord to synapse with cells of the alar lamina or to pass further up or down the spinal cord. (b) Mature spinal cord to show derivatives of the matrix, mantle and marginal zones of the alar and basal laminae.

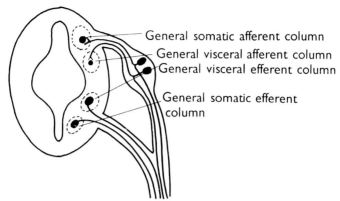

General somatic afferent column
General visceral afferent column
General visceral efferent column

General somatic efferent column

Fig. 10.3. Transverse section of the developing spinal cord to show the two types of efferent and two types of afferent columns of grey matter.

neural tube, narrowing it and giving it a characteristic shape (Fig. 10.1). These laminae can easily be recognised at least as far cranially as the lower part of the brain (hindbrain).

Cell groups within the spinal cord and the cranial nerve nuclei

The alar and basal laminae can be further subdivided according to the exact type of motor or sensory function involved (Fig. 10.3). In the spinal cord, motor fibres may be divided into two groups, those which supply skeletal muscle and those which supply the blood vessels and the glands and smooth muscle of the viscera. The particular group of cells whose axons are the motor fibres to skeletal muscle form a continuous column of cells throughout the length of the spinal cord. This is known as the *general somatic efferent column*, and will form the anterior horn of grey matter; the axons of these cells grow out to form the major part of the anterior (ventral) roots of the spinal nerves. More dorsally another column, which is restricted to the region of the sympathetic (thoraco-lumbar) and parasympathetic (sacral) outflows, is composed of cells whose efferents also travel in the anterior roots of the spinal nerves. They then leave the nerves to synapse in the sympathetic and parasympathetic ganglia, before travelling to their destination. This discontinuous column of cells is known as the *general visceral efferent column* and will form the lateral column of grey matter in the spinal cord.

Similarly, in the alar lamina, there are two main columns of cells. Ventrally, and, therefore, very close to the general visceral efferent column, lies a discontinuous column of cells that receives afferent nerve impulses from the viscera. This column is, therefore, known as the *general visceral afferent column* and lies in the ventral region of the future dorsal horn of grey matter of the spinal cord. Finally, a larger column of cells receives nerve impulses from the skin and deeper structures. These cells comprise the *general somatic afferent column* of cells and will form the remainder of the dorsal horn of grey matter. The fibres that reach the two afferent columns are the axons of pseudo-unipolar cells in the posterior root ganglia (p.143).

In the brain all four columns of cells are represented as discontinuous columns, and form the sensory and motor nuclei of various cranial nerves. There are in addition three extra columns; one motor, one sensory and one belonging to some of the special senses (the nuclei of the eighth nerve). These additional columns are shown in Fig. 10.4. Here, the four columns already mentioned can be recognised. Between the two efferent columns lies a third — the *branchial efferent column*, the axons of these cells supplying skeletal muscle derived from the branchial arch mesoderm (see Chapter 11). Between the two afferent columns is a third sensory column, the *gustatory column* which receives taste impulses chiefly from the tongue. The most dorsal and lateral column of all is the collection of sensory cells which form the vestibular and cochlear nuclei of the eighth (vestibulo-cochlear) nerve. This is sometimes called the *special somatic afferent column*.

Many of the cranial nerves are mixed and contain the axons from nerve cells that have developed from several of these columns of cells. Thus, for example, the facial nerve (VII) seen in Fig. 10.4, contains motor fibres which are derived from cells of the branchial efferent column and which supply muscles derived from the second branchial arch; secreto-motor fibres to the lachrymal, submandibular and sublingual glands, derived from cells of the general visceral efferent column; afferent (taste) fibres, from the anterior two thirds of the tongue, whose pseudo-unipolar cell bodies are found in the geniculate ganglion and which end in the gustatory column of cells. Textbooks of neuro-anatomy should be consulted for a complete account of the various components of the other cranial nerves.

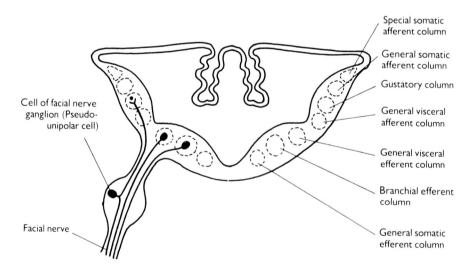

Fig. 10.4. Transverse section of hind brain to show the columns of grey matter. On the left, the facial nerve is illustrated as an example of the connections of a cranial nerve (see text for description).

The neural crest

The neural crest consists of those cells that lie along the prominent margins of the neural groove at the stage when it is still widely open (p.138). When the tube becomes closed off from the overlying ectoderm, some of the neural crest cells become isolated and form clumps of nerve cells on either side of the neural tube (Fig. 10.1). These cells are, at first, bipolar i.e., they have two processes. The parts of these processes nearest to the body of the nerve cell, however, fuse with each other to form a single process which thus appears to divide into two. Such cells are known as *pseudo-unipolar* cells (Fig. 10.2). In the spinal cord region, one of the processes grows peripherally to form a sensory fibre in a spinal nerve while the other grows centrally into the spinal cord, either to end in the grey matter of the alar lamina or to ascend or descend to other levels in the white matter (Fig. 10.2). In an exactly similar way, the neural crest cells form a collection of pseudo-unipolar neurones in relation to those of the cranial nerves which contain sensory fibres, such as the trigeminal nerve. Groups of nerve cells in the peripheral nervous system are called *ganglia* and these groups of pseudo-unipolar cells thus form the spinal and cranial nerve ganglia while their processes form the dorsal (sensory) roots of the spinal nerves (Fig. 10.2) and the sensory roots of the cranial nerves (Fig. 10.4).

Other cells of the neural crest migrate even further from their original position and they become differentiated into various types of cell. Our knowledge of their fate is largely derived from experiments with lower animals and it is not entirely certain how far this work is applicable to the human embryo. It seems fairly certain, however, that the neural crest cells develop into the sympathetic ganglion cells, the chromaffin cells of the medulla of the suprarenal gland (p.249) and the neurilemma cells of the whole of the peripheral nervous system. They probably also give rise to cells not associated with the nervous system, such as the calcitonin-secreting cells of the thyroid gland. Here only the first two groups need be discussed further. Having migrated ventrally from the neural crest, these cells form a long chain of *sympatho-chromaffin cells* on each side. These differentiate into neuroblasts destined to become multipolar *sympathetic ganglion cells* and *SIF (small intensely fluorescent) cells* and into *phaeochromocytes* which form collections of chromaffin cells. These are destined to form the para-aortic bodies and paraganglia. The former are related to the ganglia of the sympathetic trunk and the latter form two elongated brown bodies situated alongside the aorta in the region of the inferior mesenteric artery. They are prominent features at birth but almost disappear by the time of puberty.

The development of the spinal cord

Further development of the alar and basal laminae narrow the lumen still further until it is reduced first to a narrow slit and finally to a small central canal which is lined by ependyma. The mantle zone forms the grey matter of the cord. The anterior grey columns develop early as a bulky accumulation of cells in the basal lamina, while the cells of the alar lamina form the dorsal grey columns, into which the axons of many of the posterior root ganglion cells grow.

Since the neural tube is closely related to the notochord throughout its length (except at its cranial end), the spinal cord at first extends the whole length of the developing vertebral column and terminates in the coccygeal region. The spinal nerves leave the spinal cord at right angles. The vertebral column, however, grows more rapidly than the cord and since the latter is fixed at its cranial end by the development of the brain and skull, the caudal end gradually retreats up the vertebral canal, reaching the level of the third lumbar vertebra at birth and finally being situated at the level of the lower border of the first lumbar vertebra. This lag in the growth of the spinal cord accounts for the course of the nerve roots in the spinal canal of the adult. In the upper cervical region, the anterior and posterior nerve roots retain their earlier disposition and pass directly laterally to unite near the cord to form a spinal nerve. Below this level, however, the nerve roots become increasingly oblique until below the level of the first lumbar vertebra they descend vertically in a large bundle known as the *cauda equina*.

The development of the brain

Even before the closure of the anterior neuropore, modifications are beginning to appear at the cranial end of the neural tube and — by the time closure has been completed — it is possible to recognise three fairly well-defined subdivisions. These are the forebrain (*prosencephalon*), midbrain (*mesencephalon*) and hindbrain (*rhombencephalon*). The neural tube, however, is no longer straight. As well as the general curve, convex dorsally, of the spinal cord, two well marked flexures are present in the brain region (Fig. 10.5). In the region of the midbrain there is a very pronounced *midbrain flexure*, convex dorsally, while in the upper cervical region near the future junction between brain and spinal cord there is a rather less well

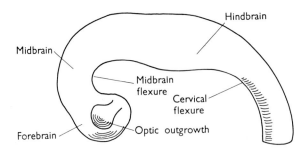

Fig. 10.5. The cranial end of the neural tube, subdivided into fore-, mid- and hindbrain. Two flexures, concave ventrally, have appeared (approximately 28 days).

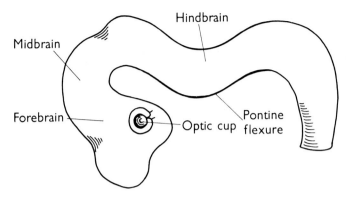

Fig. 10.6. A third flexure, the pontine flexure, has appeared and is responsible for the characteristic shape of the hindbrain (approximately 35 days).

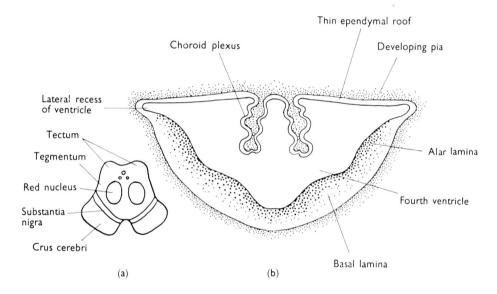

Fig. 10.7. (a) The crura cerebri have appeared along the ventral aspect of the midbrain and the central lumen has been narrowed to form the aqueduct, dorsal to which lies the tectum. (b) The pontine flexure causes the lateral walls of the hindbrain to spread out so that the roof plate becomes stretched and thin. The ependymal roof is invaginated by pia to form the choroid plexus of the future fourth ventricle.

marked *cervical flexure* which also has a dorsal convexity.

With further development, the forebrain and hindbrain dilatations become more pronounced and a new flexure, the *pontine flexure*, develops (Fig. 10.6). This flexure is convex ventrally and, because of this, the roof of the hindbrain becomes relatively thin and transparent, while the side walls, the alar and basal laminae, become opened out (Figs. 10.4, 10.7 and 10.8). The effect may be appreciated by rolling a sheet of paper into a U-section and then bending it to produce a ventral convexity.

When viewed from the dorsal aspect, the thin roof of the hindbrain takes on a rhomboid shape from which the term rhombencephalon is derived. At this stage there are few changes in the midbrain, which can be recognised mainly by the very marked midbrain flexure. This is so pronounced that the ventral aspects of the forebrain and the hindbrain are almost in contact (Fig. 10.8). A slight narrowing between midbrain and hindbrain is known as the *isthmus*. The *otocyst*, which is seen in Fig. 11.5, is derived from the ectoderm on either side of the hindbrain region. An area of ectoderm sinks below the surface and forms a hollow vesicle, the surface ectoderm closing up again over it. The otocyst will later form the membraneous labyrinth of the inner ear.

Meanwhile, the forebrain is also showing signs of increasing complexity. In addition to the developing eye and optic stalk, which will be described later, the original single forebrain vesicle (*prosencephalon*) now has a pair of lateral outgrowths, the future cerebral hemispheres. These are known as the *telencephalic vesicles*, the two vesicles and the intervening part of the forebrain (*telencephalon medium*) together forming the *telencephalon*. The posterior part of the forebrain forms the *diencephalon* (the 'between-brain'), so called because with the further development of the cerebral hemispheres it will come to lie between them (Fig. 10.9).

The telencephalic vesicles increase rapidly in size and soon hide the diencephalon completely. In addition to the changes in the form of the brain that have been described, the cranial nerves have also begun to appear. The motor fibres of these nerves have grown out from the cells of the various motor nuclei in the

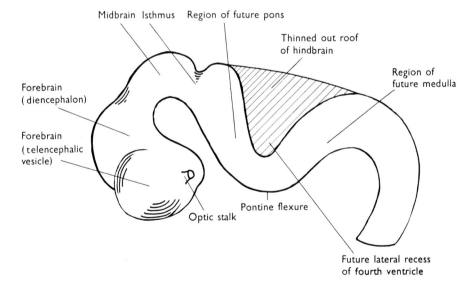

Fig. 10.8. Further development of the pontine flexure forms an acute bend in the hindbrain. The telencephalic vesicle is an outgrowth from the midline portion of the forebrain (approximately 37 days).

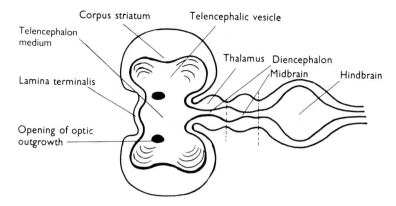

Fig. 10.9. A horizontal section through the brain (diagrammatic).

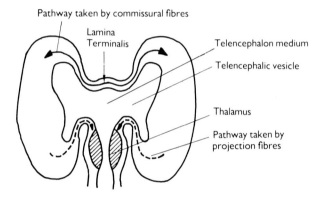

Fig. 10.10. A diagram of a horizontal section through the forebrain to show how the commissural fibres use the lamina terminalis as a pathway while the projection fibres have to bend sharply round into the diencephalon.

brain, while the sensory fibres with the exception of the mesencephalic nucleus of the fifth nerve and the special senses are the axons of the pseudo-unipolar cells of the ganglia of the cranial nerves. The nerves associated with the special senses will be described later.

The forebrain

The telencephalic vesicles, which appear soon after the formation of the brain flexures (p.145), grow rapidly in all directions but the wall remains relatively thin except in the floor and lateral wall of each vesicle, where a considerable thickening indicates the developing *corpus striatum* (Figs. 10.9 and 10.11) from which the adult basal ganglia will develop. A further thickening, the *thalamus*, appears in the lateral wall of the diencephalon. It will be seen from Fig. 10.10 that, owing to the growth of the telencephalic vesicles, the anterior extremity of the neural tube no

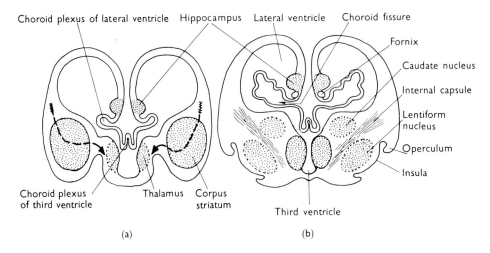

Choroid plexus of lateral ventricle   Hippocampus   Lateral ventricle   Choroid fissure

Fornix

Caudate nucleus

Internal capsule

Lentiform
nucleus

Operculum

Insula

Choroid plexus   Thalamus   Corpus
of third ventricle   striatum

Third ventricle

(a)   (b)

Fig. 10.11. A frontal section through the forebrain. (a) The arrows show the pathway taken by projection fibres through the corpus striatum and into the diencephalon. (b) Fusion has taken place between the lateral side of the diencephalon and the medial side of the telencephalon lateral to the thalamus. The corpus striatum has become divided into lentiform and caudate nuclei. Note also the choroidal fissue which is *below* the hippocampus and fornix.

longer forms the anterior pole of the brain. The original cranial end of the neural tube is called the *lamina terminalis*. As is indicated by an arrow in Fig. 10.10, it is a suitable region for nerve fibres passing from one side of the brain to the other (*commissural fibres*) to cross the midline. It is, therefore, in the region of the upper part of the laminal terminalis that commissural fibres, in particular the *corpus callosum*, will later develop. The other (dotted) arrow in Fig. 10.10 indicates the pathway taken by nerve fibres which leave the forebrain to pass down to the more caudal regions of the neural tube. As more and more of these *projection fibres* develop they will fill up the space between the telencephalon and the diencephalon until eventually these two parts of the forebrain fuse so that the mass of projection fibres and the developing corpus striatum lie immediately lateral to the thalamus.

This relationship can be seen more clearly in Fig. 10.11 which is a vertical section through the forebrain. The corpus striatum and thalamus can be seen on each side and projection fibres from the future cerebral hemispheres can be seen to be passing through the corpus striatum, dividing it into its two parts, the *caudate nucleus* and the *lentiform nucleus*. In Fig. 10.11(b) the increasing number of projection fibres has produced fusion between the telencephalon and dien-cephalon, so that something approaching the adult configuration can now be recognised. The cavities of the telencephalic vesicles form the *lateral ventricles* and that of the diencephalon and the telencephalon medium form the *third ventricle*. In the lateral wall of the latter is the *thalamus* and *hypothalamus*. Above and lateral to the thalamus and, therefore, in the lateral ventricle is the *caudate nucleus*. These two masses of grey matter are separated from the lentiform nucleus by the great mass of projection fibres now known as the *internal capsule*. When, at a later stage, the cerebral cortex becomes thrown into folds, the surface of the hemisphere overlying the lentiform nucleus develops only minor sulci and forms the *insula* over which the adjacent cortex grows to form the opercula (Fig. 10.11b).

Around the developing brain a condensation of vascular mesenchyme, known as the *meninx primitiva*, forms the membranous neurocranium (p.125) and three layers of the meninges (the *dura mater, arachnoid mater* and *pia mater*). The further development of the meninges need not be described in detail except for the formation of the choroid plexuses (Fig. 10.11). The medial wall of the telencephalic vesicles remains very thin in one region and no mantle or marginal layers develop, the wall consisting only of ependyma. The pia mater of this region, together with ependyma, forms the *tela choroidea*. The tela choroidea is invaginated laterally into the lateral ventricle and ventrally into the third ventricle to form the choroid plexuses. A slight longitudinal swelling above the thin part of the medial wall of the telencephalon develops into the *hippocampus*. The extent of this region can be appreciated from Fig. 10.12 which shows the medial wall of the cerebral hemisphere, the hippocampus and a bundle of partially decussating (commissural) fibres derived from the cells of the hippocampus which form the *fornix*. The linear invagination of the medial wall of the hemisphere which forms the choroid plexus is known as the *choroid fissure*. Immediately dorsal to it is the fornix and above this again is the hippocampus. The hemisphere continues to grow, particularly caudally, its caudal pole folding over to form the temporal lobe and the caudal part of its cavity forming the inferior horn of the lateral ventricle (Fig. 10.12b). As a result of this the choroid fissure, the fornix and the hippocampus become reversed in position in the temporal lobe, the hippocampus and the fornix (known as the *fimbria* in this region) lying below the choroid fissure. At a later stage the corpus callosum, which consists of commissural fibres developing first in the upper part of the lamina terminalis, grows backwards over the choroid fissue and the fornix; beneath it a large portion of the lamina terminalis becomes thinned out to form the *septum pellucidum*; the hippocampus almost disappears except for that portion which lies in the floor of the inferior horn of the lateral ventricle and a thin layer, the *induseum griseum*, on the upper surface of the corpus callosum.

The pituitary gland

The pituitary gland (*hypophysis*) develops in two parts. Soon after the formation of the head fold and just in front of the buccopharyngeal membrane, the stomatodaeum develops a midline upgrowth which meets a corresponding downward growing diverticulum from the forebrain (Fig. 10.13). The upgrowth is known as *Rathke's pouch*; it soon loses its connection with the stomatodaeum while its anterior and, to some extent, its posterior walls become thicker. A similar proliferation of cells occurs in the forebrain derivative which loses its internal cavity (Fig. 10.13c). The thickening in the anterior wall of Rathke's pouch becomes the *pars anterior* of the adult pituitary gland and a backward prolongation of this forms the *pars tuberalis*. The posterior wall of the pouch becoming attached to the

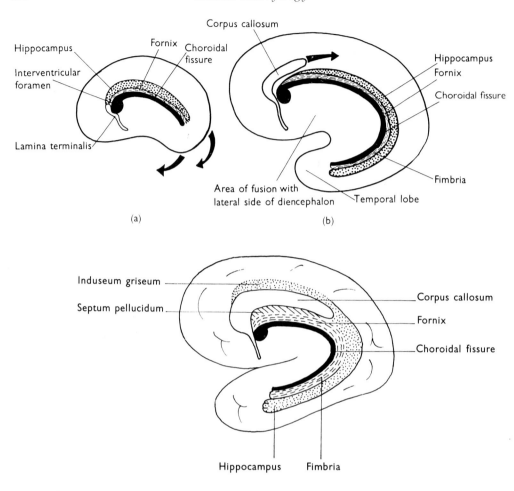

Fig. 10.12. (a) The medial side of the telencephalic vesicle which has been detached from the diencephalon. The arrows show the main direction of growth. (b) Growth of the caudal part of the telencephalic vesicle has now formed the temporal lobe. The fornix lies *above* the choroid fissure but its continuation, the fimbria, lies *below* the choroid fissue in the temporal lobe. (c) The corpus callosum has grown caudally and the upper part of the hippocampus is represented only by the induseum griseum.

downgrowth from the forebrain forms the poorly developed *pars intermedia*. The *pars nervosa* is developed from the forebrain downgrowth and therefore has, in the adult, a completely different structure from the other parts of the gland. Note that the pars anterior has no connection with the brain except for its blood vessels which form the hypophyseal portal system.

The midbrain

No very extensive changes occur in the midbrain during the course of development except for an enormous thickening of the walls. The growth of large tracts of

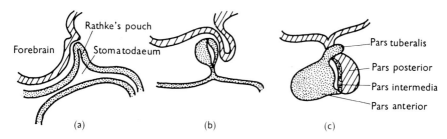

Fig. 10.13. The development of the pituitary. (a) An upgrowth (Rathke's pouch) form the stomatodaeum meets a downgrowth from the forebrain. (b) The walls of Rathke's pouch become thicker, particularly the anterior wall, and the pouch separates from the stomatodaeum. (c) The mature pituitary.

nerve fibre through the midbrain from higher and lower centres in the nervous system has the effect of narrowing the central lumen of the neural tube until it becomes relatively greatly reduced in size to the form the *aqueduct*. Cells of the basal laminae form the nuclei of two motor cranial nerves, the oculomotor and trochlear, and large masses of cells, probably derived from the alar laminae, migrate ventrally and cranially to form the *red nucleus* and the *substantia nigra*. The alar laminae also form the grey matter of the tectum which lies dorsal to the aqueduct. Cortico-pontine and cortico-spinal fibres are grouped together to form a large mass on each side of the ventral surface of the midbrain. This is the *crus cerebri* or basis pedunculi (Fig. 10.7a).

The hindbrain

When the pontine flexure is fully developed, the hindbrain is acutely flexed ventrally and its roof is composed entirely of ependyma, since the mantle and marginal zones do not develop in this region. As can be seen from Fig. 10.7, the alar and basal laminae come to lie dorso-laterally and ventro-medially respectively and the cavity within the hindbrain is now known as the *fourth ventricle*. Just as happens in the forebrain, the thin ependymal roof, together with a layer of pia mater, forms the tela choroidea and part of this becomes infolded into the ventricle to form the choroid plexus. The most lateral part of the cavity becomes the lateral recess of the fourth ventricle (Fig. 10.8). The thin roof of the lateral recess becomes perforated, as does the roof of the ventricle in the midline, thus forming the lateral and medial openings through which cerebro-spinal fluid is able to escape from the ventricular system of the brain to the subarachnoid space. The cranial limb of the pontine flexure becomes the *pons*, while the caudal limb becomes the *medulla* (Fig. 10.14). Cells from the alar lamina migrate ventrally and forwards to form the *pontine nuclei* and the *olivary complex*. The remainder of these cells and those of the basal lamina group themselves to form various cranial nerve nuclei which have already been referred to.

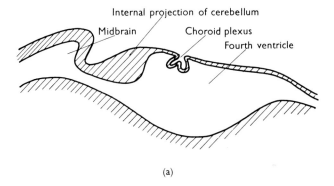

(a)

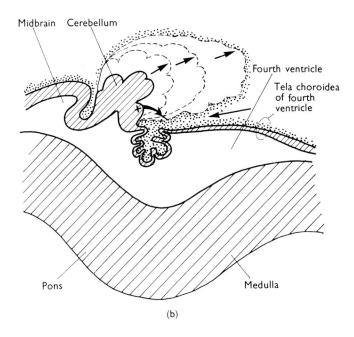

(b)

Fig. 10.14. (a) The cerebellum begins to grow into the 4th ventricle. (b) It then becomes everted to overhang the thin roof of the fourth ventricle. The small arrows indicate the enormous backward growth of the neocerebellum. The original posterior lobe (X) thus comes to lie on the inferior surface of the cerebellum (dotted X). The long arrow indicates the cerebello-medullary subarachnoid cistern of the adult.

The cerebellum

The cerebellum develops relatively late (i.e. at about 6 weeks). It begins as a bilobed thickening of the alar laminae at the cranial end of the hindbrain. The thickening is, at first, inside the cavity of the ventricle but it soon becomes everted so that the main mass of the cerebellum is extra-ventricular (Fig. 10.14). The cerebellum then grows rapidly backwards, the main growth forming the middle

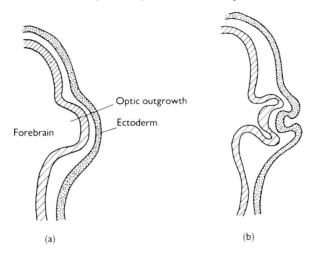

Forebrain

Optic outgrowth

Ectoderm

(a)   (b)

Fig. 10.15. (a) The optic outgrowth from the forebrain. (b) The surface ectoderm sinks in to form, eventually, a lens vesicle. The optic outgrowth becomes invaginated to form an optic cup.

lobe or *neo-cerebellum* which eventually conceals the roof of the fourth ventricle. As a result of this, in the adult, the pia mater appears to be invaginated forwards between the cerebellum and the dorsal part of the medulla (arrow in Fig. 10.14b), to form the tela choroidea of the fourth ventricle. The original posterior region of the cerebellum marked with an X' on Fig. 10.14b, comes to form a very inconspicuous region of the inferior aspect of the adult cerebellum (*flocculo-nodular lobe*).

The large overgrowth of the neo-cerebellum is a human characteristic and, together with its connections, it develops *pari passu* with the prominent pontine nuclei, and the extensive and folded cerebral cortex.

The eye and optic nerve

The first indication of the development of the eye occurs at a very early stage, even before the closure of the anterior neuropore, as a ventro-lateral outgrowth from the forebrain (Fig. 10.5). The outgrowth is hollow, its cavity being continuous with the lumen of the forebrain and it soon shows a dilatation at its distal end which is known as the *optic vesicle* (Fig. 10.15a). This reaches the surface and the area facing the ectoderm soon begins to become invaginated. As it does so, a thickening of ectoderm occurs opposite the invaginated region (Fig. 10.15b) and sinks below the surface to form a circular depression. The invagination of the optic vesicle finally becomes complete and the ectodermal invagination overlying it breaks away from the surface to form a closed vesicle, the *lens vesicle* (Fig. 10.16). The formation of the lens vesicle is a good example of induction (p.356). The presence of the optic vesicle induces the lens to form, probably through the

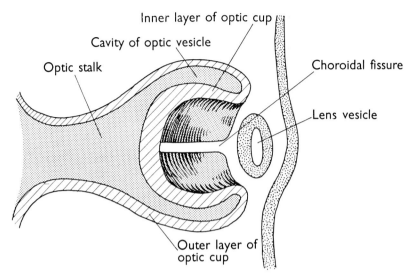

Fig. 10.16. A *horizontal* section through the optic cup, viewed from above. The original cavity of the optic vesicle is reduced to a narrow slit. The lens vesicle has detached itself from the ectoderm.

medium of a chemical mediator. Early classical experiments performed on lower animals showed that in many, if the optic outgrowth is removed no lens will form in the normal position, while if the outgrowth is transplanted to another situation

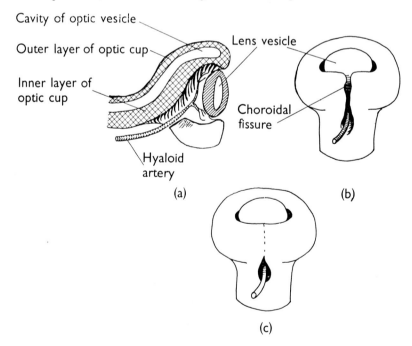

Fig. 10.17. (a) A midline vertical section through the developing eye. The section has passed through the choroidal fissure. (b) The optic vesicle seen from below. The hyaloid artery enters through the choroidal fissure. (c) Closure of the choroidal fissure.

at the appropriate developmental stage a lens will form from the ectoderm at the new site.

The invagination of the optic vesicle takes place not only from the surface which faces the ectoderm but also, to some extent, from the inferior aspect so that when the process is complete the result is a two-layered *optic cup* with a ventral fissure, the *choroidal fissure* (Figs. 10.16 and 10.17). This soon closes except for its most posterior part (Fig. 10.17c). The lens lies within the opening of the optic cup. The cup itself contains loose mesenchyme, through which runs a *hyaloid artery* which enters the cup through the still open posterior end of the choroidal fissure.

The final stages of the development of the eye and its adnexae can be seen in Fig. 10.18. In the optic cup, it will be seen that the inner (invaginated) layer has become much thicker and is now forming the *nervous layer* of the retina, the outer layer remaining relatively thin and forming the *pigmented layer*. The original cavity of the optic vesicle becomes obliterated by the fusion of the two layers of the optic cup but this is never very firm and, if an adult eyeball is dissected, it will often be found that the nervous layer floats away from the pigmented layer. A similar appearance is often seen in histological sections unless special precautions are

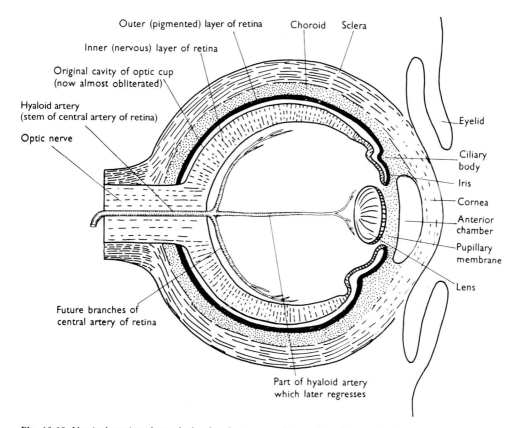

Fig. 10.18. Vertical section through the developing eye. For explanation, see text.

taken. Under certain conditions a similar separation of the nervous layer from the pigmented layer may take place during life and although this important condition is known clinically as *detached retina*, it will be appreciated that it is not a detachment of the whole retina from the underlying choroid, since the pigmented layer remains behind.

The cells of the nervous layer differentiate into the various layers of cells of the adult retina. The axons of the nerve cells in the innermost (most superficial) layer grow proximally, down the optic stalk (which until this time has not contained any nerve fibres), to the brain and as a result the cavity of the stalk becomes obliterated, the great mass of nerve fibres which have grown proximally along the stalk forming the *optic nerve*.

The anterior part of the optic cup in Fig. 10.18 has grown down in front of the lens to form the epithelium of the *ciliary body* and of the *iris* as well as the musculature of the latter. In this region, therefore, the two layers of the optic cup have remained thin and form the non-visual part (*pars caeca*) of the retina. The lens vesicle becomes transformed into the definitive lens by a series of changes which are shown in Fig. 10.19. As can be seen in Fig. 10.18, the hyaloid artery together with its retinal branches will form the central artery of the retina proximally, while the distal part of the artery normally disappears.

Just as mesenchyme condenses around the brain to form the dura, arachnoid and pia, so a similar condensation occurs around the eye which, it will be remembered, is in fact an outgrowth of the brain. Around the optic nerve the condensation forms meninges which are continuous with those of the brain. Around the developing eyeball, the inner part of the condensation forms the vascular coat of the eye which is known in the adult as the *uveal tract* and comprises the choroid, and the mesodermal parts of the ciliary body and of the iris (i.e. the non-epithelial muscular parts). This layer therefore corresponds to the vascular pia-arachnoid. The tougher outer layer of mesenchymal condensation forms the sclera.

Between the lens and the surface a cavity, the *anterior chamber*, appears and the

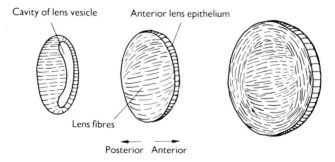

Cavity of lens vesicle   Anterior lens epithelium

Lens fibres

Posterior Anterior

Fig. 10.19. Three stages in the development of the lens. The primary lens fibres are elongated cells formed from the posterior lens epithelium. Secondary lens fibres are added to the outer sides of the primary fibres by proliferation from the equatorial region.

tissue forming the outer wall of this cavity becomes the *cornea* which is continuous posteriorly with the *sclera*. The lens is separated from the anterior chamber by a layer of mesenchyme which thus occludes the pupil and is known as the *pupillary membrane*. This will eventually disappear.

The ectoderm above and below the cornea grows in the form of two folds to form the eyelids. These meet and fuse, superficial to the cornea, to form a *conjunctival sac*. Many animals are born with their eyelids fused in this way but, in the human fetus, the lids separate during the seventh month so that the new-born baby is able to open its eyes quite readily.

Congenital anomalies of the central nervous system

The incidence in Britain of major anomalies of the nervous system (one of the largest single groups of congenital malformations) is about 3 per 1,000 births. Of these, *anencephaly* and *meningomyelocele* (anomalies resulting from abnormal development of the neural tube) contribute about 85 per cent. The remaining 15 per cent are made up of rather rare defects, such as *hydrocephalus, hydrencephaly* and *microcephaly*. There are interesting geographical variations in the incidence of neural tube defects. In Japan, for example, the incidence is only about 0.3/1,000: in Wales and Northern Ireland the incidence is about 4 per 1,000 whilst in South East England it is only 2/1,000. Within social classes there is also a marked gradient, ranging from 1/1,000 in social classes 1 and 2 to 5/1,000 in social class 5. As well as geographical and social variations, incidence differences also exist in the distribution of specific malformations. In Hong Kong, for example, anencephaly outnumbers meningomyelocele by a factor of 6:1; in the United Kingdom the ratio is nearer 1:1. Fronto-ethmoidal anomalies are far more common in South East Asia than the occipital encephalocele which predominates in Western European populations.

The aetiology of central nervous system malformations is unknown, although some helpful pointers are beginning to emerge. That there is a polygenic genetic predisposition is beyond doubt since the risk of recurrence in a mother with one affected child is in the order of 1 in 20, increasing to 1 in 10 if there has been more than one malformed child. Precipitating environmental insults must also exist but these have yet to be defined. At the present time a nutritional clue is being followed, namely the possibility that certain vitamin deficiencies — especially folic acid — interfere with normal neural tube closure.

There are three categories of developmental abnormalities of the nervous system.

1 *Structural anomalies* — due mainly to errors in organogenesis. These exist in two principal groups — those which result from abnormal development of the neural tube and those representing brain anomalies resulting from abnormal development of a brain which has passed normally through the stage of neural tube formation.

2 *Disturbances in the organisation* — of cellular elements in a structurally normal brain. These are caused by adverse influences, such as malnutrition, upon cell division (especially of glial cells). Later during development myelin formation and neuronal connections during the period of maximum brain growth are affected.

3 *Errors of metabolism* — many inherited, which can lead to severe and irreversible mental subnormality due either to the accumulation of toxic substances (e.g. *phenylketonuria* (p.24) or to deficiency of essential substances (e.g. *congenital hypothyroidism*). For many disorders in this category there is no effective treatment (e.g. *Tay−Sach's Disease* in which G_{m-2}-ganglioside accumulates in neurones because an enzymatic defect prevents its degradation.

In this chapter only structural anomalies of the brain and spinal cord will be considered.

Neural tube abnormalities

To understand the pathology of neural tube abnormalities it needs to be re-

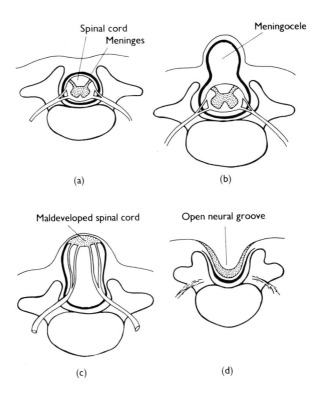

Fig. 10.20. Congenital anomalies of the spine. (a) Spina bifida occulta. (b) Meningocele. (c) Meningomyelocele. (d) Rachischisis.

membered that the central nervous system develops initially as an invagination of the mid-line ectoderm (Fig. 10.1). As the folding becomes progressively deeper the outer parts migrate towards each other until, with eventual fusion, a neural tube forms which becomes submerged within mesodermal structures (p.138). Fusion begins in the upper cervical region and extends in cranial and caudal directions, being complete by three weeks. It is failure of fusion which brings about the various neural tube defects, together with anomalous development of the bones (skull and vertebrae) which protect the brain and spinal cord.

A wide range of neural tube abnormalities results from abnormal fusion processes (Fig. 10.20). At one end of the spectrum is a *spina bifida occulta* which rarely causes problems: at the other there is a total failure of most of the brain to develop *anencephaly* which is incompatible with life. Between these extremes are the various types of *spina bifida cystica* in which there is herniation of the spinal cord and/or its coverings through posterior defects in the vertebral arches.

Anencephaly

This grotesque abnormality results from failure of the anterior portion of the neural tube to fuse (Fig. 10.21). There is total absence of cerebral hemispheres and basal ganglia together with absence or gross abnormality of the hypothalamus and pituitary gland. Frontal and parietal bones and squamous parts of the occipital bone are absent. Anencephaly is often associated with other congenital anomalies, especially of the cardiovascular system. Of physiological interest is an associated hypoplasia of the adrenal glands reflecting the lack of the trophic influence of ACTH which is produced in sub-optimal amounts from the malformed hypothalamus and pituitary gland. In view of the probable role of the fetal adrenal

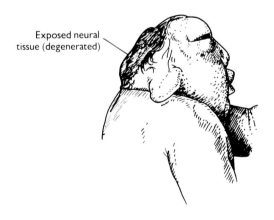

Exposed neural tissue (degenerated)

Fig. 10.21. A case of anencephaly.

gland in helping to initiate labour, gestation is often prolonged in anencephalic pregnancies.

Anencephaly usually results in a baby being stillborn. If the baby happens to be born alive, death will take place in the first day or so.

In this anomaly one or more neural arches, usually in the lumbo-sacral region, fail to develop dorsally (p.122), leaving an incomplete protective bony ring for the spinal cord. There is no protrusion of the meninges or spinal cord (Fig. 10.20a) so that neurological symptoms rarely occur. This not uncommon anomaly is usually incidentally diagnosed during the course of an X-ray taken for some unrelated purpose. On rare occasions the diagnosis may be suspected because of the presence on the skin of the back of a tuft of hair, pigmented naevus or, in very exceptional circumstances, a sinus which may communicate through the neural arch defect with the spinal theca. Surgical treatment is required only in the rare instance of there being neurological symptoms caused by accompanying neural tube abnormality or a risk of meningitis (as might exist with a sinus).

Spina bifida cystica

There are two principal anomalies in this category of neural tube defect — *meningomyelocele* and *meningocele*.

Meningomyelocele

In this abnormality the spinal cord and its coverings protrude through a large posterior defect in the neural arches (Fig. 10.20c). The lumbo-sacral region is most commonly affected. The sac contains part of the spinal cord, or cauda equina, which is exposed on the surface of the skin. The affected spinal cord is structurally and functionally grossly abnormal. In some instances there is no evidence of any neural tube folding — the spinal cord appearing like a large anchovy fillet on the surface of the back — rachischisis (Fig. 10.20d). Various other malformations are associated with this condition.

Examination of the ventricles at birth by ultrasound examination will reveal enlargement (*hydrocephalus*) in about 90 per cent of cases. This will sometimes be present clinically at birth with a large, tense anterior fontanelle, splayed sutures and a large occipito-frontal head circumference. Hydrocephalus associated with meningomyelocele is due to herniation through the foramen magnum of the cerebellar tonsils and medulla (*Arnold-Chiari malformation*) which causes obstruction to the flow of cerebro-spinal fluid. The herniation may be due to the fact that the spinal cord is tethered at the site of the spina bifida so that it cannot ride upwards when differential growth of the spinal cord and vertebral column occurs during normal development (p.144).

The clinical consequences of a meningomyelocele are best considered under two headings — (i) due to the spinal defect itself and (ii) to associated malformations (*hydrocephalus*). The spinal defect causes motor, sensory and autonomic dysfunction in the lower trunk, lower limbs, bladder and anus. Since it is really an open wound, the meningomyelocele is extremely vulnerable to infections which, untreated, can lead to meningitis and ventriculitis.

There is always some degree of muscle paralysis below the level of the lesion, the muscle groups most frequently involved being in the buttocks, thighs, legs and feet. Paralysis is usually flaccid (lower motor neurone type) but there is often a spastic (upper motor neurone) component. Muscle imbalance around various joints often causes severe contracture deformities (*arthrogryposes*), deformed hip joints (congenital dislocation) and ankles (*talipes*) as well as flexion deformities of hips and knees (Fig. 10.22). Along with the bony spinal defect, weakness of spinal column musculature can only lead to severe curvature of the spine (*kyphoscoliosis*). Sensory loss over the buttocks, perineum and lower limbs is common, though often difficult to assess in the newborn baby. These sensory disturbances do not usually cause problems at birth but, in older infants and children, lack of trophic influences will render the skin in these areas extremely vulnerable to trauma, causing pressure sores, ulcerated feet and poor circulation of the legs.

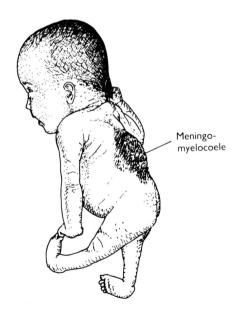

Meningo-
myelocoele

Fig. 10.22. Thoraco-lumbar meningomyelocoele. Note particularly the gross deformities of the lower limbs due to interference with their motor innervation.

Various combinations of functional disorders of the bladder can exist. A lower motor neurone lesion involving S2−4 (calf, foot and anus weakness) leads to a paralysed bladder with dribbling incontinence. An S2−4 upper motor neurone lesion (spastic calf and toe flexors with brisk reflexes) causes inco-ordination between the detrusor muscle and external sphincter leading to incomplete emptying, dribbling with overflow and later vesico-ureteric reflux with hydro-ureter and hydronephrosis causing urinary infection and pyelonephritis.

Weakness of the anal sphincter is indicated by a lax, pouting anus with an absent anal reflex and, on occasions, prolapse of rectal mucosa. This indicates a lesion involving S2−4. If the baby survives, progressive rectal and bowel inertia develops which, together with sensory loss in the rectum and anal canal, causes large amounts of stool to be accommodated in a hypotonic, floppy bowel. Constipation and diarrhoea with overflow will later occur. Problems of associated hydrocephalus are discussed on page 164.

Babies born with a meningomyelocele should be seen as soon as possible after birth by a paediatrician, a surgeon and a specialist in neuro-developmental paediatrics. This initial assessment has the prime object of determining the full extent of abnormality, including (i) an accurate description of the defect (its site and maximal diameter), (ii) whether there is leakage of cerebro-spinal fluid, (iii) presence of associated spinal abnormalities, such as kyphoscoliosis (confirmed by X-ray), (iv) motor and sensory function in the legs, (v) joint deformities, (vi) anal tone, (vii) the possible existence of hydrocephalus, aided by ultrasound examination of the head or computed axial tomography (CAT scan). From charts of myotomes and dermatomes the level at which useful spinal cord function terminates can be assessed.

At one time this initial assessment was a prelude to the early surgical closure of the spinal defect. However it gradually became evident that, although this aggressive approach increased survival rates with about 40 per cent of children still being alive at 11 years of age, the cost of this survival was immense; 80−90 per cent were severely handicapped at 5 years. So great was the suffering and handicap of many of these children who survived early surgery, with their need for multiple surgical procedures for hydrocephalus, limb deformities, bladder and bowel incontinence often leading to severely incapacitating mental and physical handicap, difficulties in social integration and disastrous effects on the lives of their families that a policy of *selective surgery* gradually evolved. This approach was pioneered by Lorber in Sheffield in 1971. From meticulous follow-up studies on about 400 children with meningomyelocele who had been operated on soon after birth, he arrived at the conclusion that certain features at birth were very accurate indices of a poor prognosis and that they could be used as a basis for a selective policy for early surgery. Included in these were (i) thoraco-lumbar meningomyelocele, (ii) flaccid paraplegia of the legs, (iii) hydrocephalus, (iv) lax anus, (v) kyphoscoliosis and (vi) other gross congenital malformations, such as heart defects.

This approach to the newborn baby with a meningomyelocele has been adopted by many doctors and parents alike, although there is still an opinion held by some that life must be preserved at all costs, whatever its ultimate quality for both child and family. Recent follow-up studies have confirmed the improvement in the quality of survival that has emerged when a policy of selective surgery as previously outlined is implemented. Those babies who are not operated upon are given nursing care, food and warmth and any pain or distress is relieved by appropriate drug therapy. Antibiotics are not given, nor any investigations carried out. The baby's parents must be kept fully informed throughout and indeed, where possible, should be encouraged to spend as much time as they can with their baby.

For those babies in whom surgery is undertaken (between 5 and 10 per cent) the defect in the spine is closed soon after birth by covering the lesion with dura and skin. Most babies who survive this procedure will develop hydrocephalus which will require therapy (see below). Long-term management is concerned with the disturbances in function which might be associated with the initial spinal defect: fortunately, with a selective surgical policy, these are now less frequent. Early closure of the back unfortunately makes little difference to later lower limb, bowel and bladder problems. Several operations to correct main joint deformities of hip, knee and ankle will be needed in childhood and calipers required to help walking in the powerless joints. For the urinary tract the long term aims of management are to prevent renal damage from vesico-ureteric reflex and to maintain continence as much as possible: surgery is often needed to treat bladder neck obstruction from external sphincter imbalance and urinary diversion in a bladder fashioned from ileum will sometimes be indicated for severe hydronephrosis. Neurodevelopmental handicap will often require education in special schools although it is essential for these children to be integrated as much as possible into the life of the community in which they live. In adolescence, pyscho-sexual problems will often emerge as the children develop insight into the restrictions to their sexual life due to their handicapped state.

Meningocele

In this abnormality the spinal cord and roots are not usually involved. The spinal protrusion is only a sac of meninges and fluid usually without any neural tissue (Fig. 10.20b). The covering is intact skin. It is a rare abnormality. It is unusual for there to be any neurological complications but, if these do exist, surgical repair will at some stage be indicated but there is not the urgency that might exist with meningomyelocele. Hydrocephalus is associated in only about 10 per cent of cases.

Encephalocele

This often grotesque abnormality results from anomalous development of the cranial part of the neural tube causing the brain to herniate through a defect in the skull bones. The size of the encephalocele varies considerably from a small meningeal sac, to one containing a large amount of brain tissue (Fig. 10.23). In Western European populations the site of an encephalocele is commonly in the occipital region: in South Eastern Asia fronto-ethmoidal encephaloceles emerging from the base of the nose predominate.

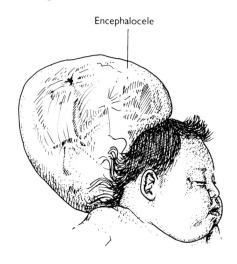

Fig. 10.23. A large occipital encephalocele.

The future of babies with these abnormalities is usually extremely poor. Even if surgery is undertaken to excise the sac there is a high incidence of later neuro-developmental handicap and limited life expectancy.

Other developmental anomalies of the brain

Hydrocephalus

The term *hydrocephalus* refers to an excessive accumulation of cerebro-spinal fluid (CSF) within the ventricles of the brain. It is usually due to an obstruction to the flow of CSF at some stage in its course from its production by the choroid plexuses in the ventricles to its absorption in the arachnoid granulations. In most instances congenital hydrocephalus (acquired forms are not considered here) is associated with meningomyelocele as in the Arnold-Chiari malformation (p.160). Other less common causes of congenital hydrocephalus include stenosis of the aqueduct of

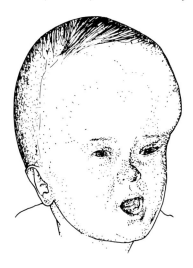

Fig. 10.24. Hydrocephalus.

the midbrain which is sometimes caused by intra-uterine infection (e.g. from toxoplasmosis, rubella, herpes, cytomegalovirus). Rarely aqueductal stenosis is inherited as an X-linked abnormality.

Clinical features

Hydrocephalus associated with meningomyelocele may be suspected at birth from clinical examination and confirmed by visualisation of the ventricular system by ultrasound examination or CAT scan. Hydrocephalus from aqueductal stenosis is rarely diagnosed at birth; instead it presents in the first few months after birth with a rapidly growing head, a large tense bulging anterior fontanelle, distended scalp veins, sutural splaying with the eyes partially downward and displaced showing the white sclera above the cornea (sun-setting) (Fig. 10.24). The head circumference growth will confirm hydrocephalus.

Treatment of congenital hydrocephalus aims at controlling the accumulation of cerebro-spinal fluid by a shunt procedure. The first method which evolved in the 1950's was the Holter ventriculo-caval shunt in which cerebro-spinal fluid is drained from one or other of the ventricles by silastic tubing carried subcutaneously to the neck at which point it is passed into the internal jugular vein and fed into the right atrium. Over the last decade the method of ventriculo-peritoneal diversion has become more widely used in which the catheter carrying CSF enters the peritoneal cavity. In about 5–10 per cent of children the shunts can be removed at about the age of 10 when a new level of equilibrium between CSF production and drainage is spontaneously achieved.

Miscellaneous abnormalities

Numerous other structural abnormalities of the brain exist but, as these are so rare, they will be only briefly mentioned.

Agenesis and *hypoplasia* of the corpus callosum and cavum septum pellucidi are often associated with severe mental subnormality and intractable epilepsy. *Microcephaly* is a term given to a very small head with prematurely fused sutures containing a grossly under-developed and abnormal brain, a condition which is frequently incompatible with life beyond a few months of birth. Microcephaly is sometimes associated with abnormalities of other organs (producing syndromes — for example Edwards' syndrome (Trisomy 18) and Cornelia de Lange syndrome). *Hydrencephaly* is an extreme degree of hydrocephalus in which the cerebral cortex is parchment thin. One aetiological explanation for this abnormality is that the condition is acquired, perhaps from extensive vascular occlusions, causing early damage to the cerebral cortex, rather than a true error of organogenesis. Diagnosis is made by transillumination of the skull, and later confirmed by ultrasound examination. The prognosis is appalling, death occurring within a few months of birth.

Developmental anomalies of the eye are uncommon but two are worth mentioning. *Coloboma* is the result of partial or complete failure of the choroidal fissure to close with the result that a defect occurs in the ventral part of the retina and of the choroid and iris. Remnants of the pupillary membrane (p.157) are commonly seen in the adult eye but, rarely, it may persist in part as a vascular membrane across the pupil.

Prevention of neural tube defects

Knowledge that a mother, previously having given birth to a baby with a neural tube defect, was at considerable risk of having another similarly affected baby, provided a vital stimulus in the 1960s to research methods into preventing a recurrence of the malformation in a later pregnancy. Two principles have emerged, those of primary and secondary prevention. Historically, methods for secondary prevention were the first to be developed.

Secondary prevention

This concerns identifying in the first half of pregnancy a fetus with an 'open' neural tube abnormality in order that termination of pregnancy might be offered to the mother. Anencephaly and about 80 per cent of meningomyeloceles constitute these 'open' lesions which cause fetal serum and lymph to leak directly through a thin or even absent membrane of neural tissue into the amniotic fluid and thereby into maternal serum. Using a biochemical marker for this fetal fluid it is, therefore, possible to diagnose major open neural tube defects in prenatal life. The fetal protein α-*fetoprotein* (AFP) (an α-globulin synthesised initially in the fetal yolk sac and later in the liver and which at 16–18 weeks of gestation has a concentration in fetal serum approximately 30 thousand times greater than that of maternal serum), provides such a biochemical marker.

In the late 1960s attempts were made to diagnose neural tube abnormalities in mothers at risk by measuring the AFP level in a small volume of amniotic fluid removed by amniocentesis at about 16 weeks of gestation. A level greater than an accepted upper limit of normality (for example, 2.5 times the median value) pointed to an affected fetus which could be removed by termination of pregnancy. This practice has now changed. In view of the fact that high levels of AFP exist in the serum of mothers carrying an affected baby and, with a spontaneous miscarriage rate of 1–2 per cent following amniocentesis, screening is now initially undertaken by determining at 16–18 weeks the level of maternal serum AFP. A significantly high level is followed by definitive investigations using both ultrasound scanning and amniocentesis.

In most areas of Britain, antenatal AFP screening is now offered not only to 'at risk mothers' but to all women who become pregnant. This is called the concept of *population screening*. Whilst few would doubt the need to offer women who had previously given birth to babies with neural tube defects, or other significant family history, the amenity of antenatal diagnosis, the value of routinely screening large populations of pregnant women has yet to be established. The incidence of neural tube defects in Britain has shown a very marked decline over the past 10–15 years. High maternal serum levels of AFP are associated with only 80 per cent of neural tube defects (those not detectable being closed lesions and encephalocoeles). A high AFP in serum or amniotic fluid is by no means specific to open neural tube defects (although measurement of acetyl cholinesterase in amniotic fluid, another marker of fetal fluid leak, might make screening more sensitive): high levels can also be found with other congenital abnormalities such as congenital nephrosis (extremely rare) and some anomalies of the gastro-intestinal tract (e.g. exomphalos (p.292), gastroschisis (p.293) and high gut atresia which are in most instances surgically correctable defects (Chapter 16). Add to these sources of concern a fetal mortality of about 1–2 per cent from abortion caused by amniocentesis and the considerable maternal anxiety which can result from the false positive initial AFP screen and the idea of population screening becomes less appealing. There is a further difficulty. The selective policy for early surgery now being widely used in babies born alive with neural tube defects is resulting in a survival rate beyond the first couple of months of only 5–10 per cent. In this situation, an already imperfect screening procedure perhaps cannot be justified to detect a condition which, in about 90 per cent of cases, is incompatible with life.

For all these reasons the idea that neural tube malformations might be primarily prevented is becoming increasingly attractive.

Primary prevention

This relates to the prevention of the abnormal closure of the neural tube early in embryogenesis. It is possible that, in genetically vulnerable embryos, a deficiency or unavailability of certain vitamins in the mother (in particular ascorbic acid, riboflavin and especially folic acid) might prevent the neural tube from developing normally. Preliminary studies give some hint of optimism that others who are especially at risk of having children with neural tube defects can have this risk considerably reduced if folic acid and/or other vitamins are taken in the periconceptional period up to about the 12th week of gestation. At the time of writing, the Medical Research Council has agreed to a large multi-centre prospective study to evaluate the efficacy of primary prevention of neural tube defects by the periconceptional administration of vitamins and folate. The results will be awaited with very great interest.

Developmental stages

21 days: Neural groove present and neural tube beginning to form.

25 days: Neural groove closed except for anterior and posterior ends.

30 days: Neuropores closed. Fore-, mid- and hindbrain recognisable. Three layers of neural tube differentiated.

5 weeks: Brain flexures beginning to form. Optic vesicle invaginated and lens formed. Cranial and spinal nerves and their ganglia present. Cerebral hemispheres well marked.

6 weeks: Cerebellum begins to develop. Sympathetic ganglia forming.

7 weeks: Large corpus striatum and thalamus. Components of pituitary gland meet.

8 weeks: Meninges formed. Cerebral cortex differentiating.

3−4 months: Brain beginning to resemble adult brain. Cerebral hemispheres covering much of brain. Large cerebellum. Corpus callosum and other commissures formed.

4 months to term: Cerebral gyri and sulci appear. Insula sinks below surface. Myelinization takes place (but not complete until well after birth).

Further reading

Fujita, S. (1963) The matrix cell and cytogenesis in the developing central nervous system. *J. comp. Neurol.* **120**, 37.

Gaze, R.M. & Keating (1974) Development and regeneration in the nervous system. *Brit. Med. Bull.* **30**, No. 2

Lemire, R.J., Loeser, J.D., Leech, R.W. & Alvord, E.C. (1975) *Normal and Abnormal Development of the Human Nervous System.* Harper & Row, Hagerstown.

Mann, I.C. (1964) *The Development of the Human Eye,* 3rd edn. Cambridge University Press.

O'Rahilly, R. & Gardner, E. (1971) The timing and sequence of events in the development of the human nervous system during the embryonic period proper. *Z. Anat. Entwickl.-Gesch.* **134**, 1.

11

The Branchial Region, Mouth, Palate, Nose and Face

During the first two months of its development, the human embryo bears little resemblance to a fully formed fetus and it is very difficult to identify the different regions at the cranial end of the embryo in terms of structures present in the adult. It can be seen from Fig. 9.1 that there is no recognisable thorax, the whole 'thoracic' region being represented by the relatively enormous pericardium which is visible externally because the lungs are still in a very early stage of development. Similarly, it is not possible to recognise a neck, although the cervical somites indicate the position of the future vertebrae and, therefore, of the spinal nerves of this region. The eyes of the embryo are directed laterally so that, even if there were anything to see *in utero*, the embryo could not use binocular vision. The face cannot be recognised at all, since the large bulging forebrain region is almost in contact with the pericardium. The developing face is, therefore, pressed against the pericardium as though the embryo were 'eating its heart out'. A little more caudally, the lateral surface of the embryo shows a characteristic series of elevations on the surface; these are the *branchial* (or *pharyngeal*) arches. The two most cranial of these are clearly marked but behind these the arches are progressively smaller and less noticeable and, at a later stage, are completely overgrown by the large second arch. It will be seen from Fig. 9.1 that the floor of the branchial part of the pharynx is formed by the cranial wall of the pericardium, while the immediate relation of the roof is the forebrain. It is thus very easy for nerves to grow down into the arches from the brain and for arteries to reach the arches from the cranial end of the heart (see Fig. 11.1).

It has already been seen (p.81) that, at the cranial end of the embryo, a slight invagination of ectoderm (the *stomatodaeum*) comes into close contact with the endoderm of the foregut with no mesoderm in between the two layers. This double layer is the *buccopharyngeal membrane* (Fig. 6.12). It is only a temporary structure and by the time the branchial arches have developed it has disappeared. The pattern of growth in this region is such that it is extremely difficult to relate the original site of the buccopharyngeal membrane to adult anatomy, so that it may be difficult to decide whether certain adult structures, for instance, the parotid glands, are ectodermal or endodermal in origin.

The branchial arches lie in the lateral wall of the future pharyngeal region. The funnel-shaped embryonic pharynx, anteriorly quite wide, tapers rapidly down to the beginning of the future oesophagus. The roof of the pharynx is separated from

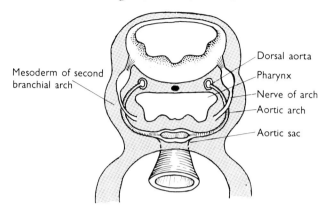

Fig. 11.1. A section through the pharynx and a pair of branchial arches (A−A in Fig. 9.1) seen from the front. Each arch contains a nerve and an artery.

the floor of the brain by only a thin layer of mesoderm. A diverticulum of the pharynx grows up in the midline just anterior to the original site of the bucco-pharyngeal membrane. This outgrowth is known as *Rathke's pouch* and it comes into contact with a downgrowth from the forebrain. The two components will later form the pituitary gland, which has been described in Chapter 10.

The branchial arches

The relation of the branchial arches to the forebrain and the pericardium may best be appreciated in a section, such as is shown in Fig. 11.1, that passes through the second branchial arch on each side. It will be seen that the branchial arch consists of a marked thickening in the mesoderm on each side of the pharynx; this is responsible for the ectodermal elevation that can be seen on the external surface. The mesoderm of each arch blends with the mesoderm lying in the roof and floor of the pharynx. In the mesoderm of the floor lies the *aortic sac*, the cranial end of the heart tube (p.196) which has just passed out of the pericardial cavity into the mesoderm. From the aortic sac an artery passes dorsally through the substance of the arch and joins one of the paired dorsal aortae; further caudally the two dorsal aortae fuse to form a single midline vessel. From the brain one of the cranial nerves (in the case of the second arch this is the seventh or facial nerve) passes ventrally into the arch, the nerve lying cranial to the artery. The other branchial arches are very similar; each thus contains a cranial nerve (or a branch thereof) and an artery, the latter being known as an *aortic arch* (not to be confused with the adult *arch of the aorta*). Later, some of the mesoderm of each arch will also differentiate into skeletal tissue (cartilage or bone) and into muscle.

A study of comparative embryology suggests that there are essentially six branchial arches on each side but, in most mammals including man, the fifth arch does not develop to any appreciable extent and may be ignored. The first (or mandibular) and the second (hyoid) arches are large; the third and fourth arches are much less conspicuous and the sixth cannot be recognized at all on the surface. The first arch sends, from its dorsal end, a process which grows forward below the developing eye. This is the *maxillary process*; it plays an important part in the development of the face (Fig. 11.13).

The large swellings produced by the thickened mesoderm of the arches are separated both internally and externally by shallow grooves. On the outside the ectoderm dips in between adjacent arches to form *ectodermal clefts* while, on the inside, the endoderm bulges outwards between adjacent arches to form *endodermal* or *pharyngeal pouches*. The endoderm and ectoderm thus approach each other very closely in between the arches, to form a *closing membrane*. In fishes the closing membrane breaks down between each pair of arches, so leaving a series of free communications between the cavity of the pharynx and the exterior. A series of gill slits is thus formed through which water may be passed, gaseous exchange taking place between the water and the plexus of vessels derived from the aortic arches. In the human embryo, however, this does not occur.

The ectodermal clefts and pharyngeal pouches can be seen in Fig. 11.2, which also shows the general shape of the pharynx and the structures that can be found in its floor. The ventral ends of the mesodermal thickenings that form the mass of the branchial arches extend into the floor to produce a series of transverse elevations. As might be expected, these are large cranially where the first two arches lie, but are progressively smaller and more oblique in the more caudal part of the pharynx. Between the first two arches, in the midline, lies a single elevation of the lining endoderm produced by a thickening in the underlying mesoderm. This is the *tuberculum impar*, the 'unpaired tubercle', and it is important only insofar as its caudal margin marks the site of a small midline outgrowth from the

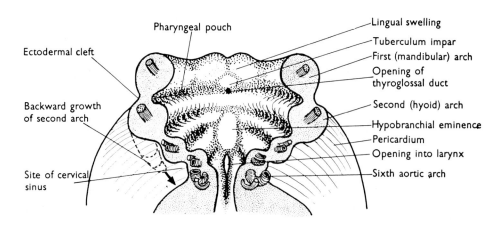

Fig. 11.2. A horizontal section through the pharyngeal region (B—B in Fig. 9.1) viewed from above. The first and second aortic arches have regressed. The third and fourth aortic arches lie *caudal* to the corresponding nerves but the sixth arch is *cranial* to the nerve.

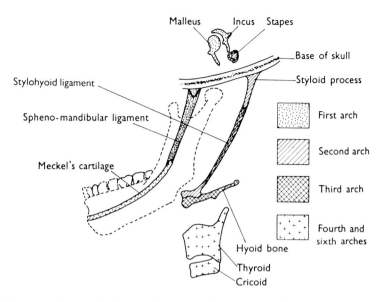

Fig. 11.3. The derivatives of the skeletal elements of the branchial arches.

pharyngeal floor. This is the *thyroglossal duct*, the caudal free end of which will form all or part of the thyroid gland (p.179). The elevations produced by the third and fourth arches do not reach the midline since they blend with another, larger, midline swelling known as the *hypobranchial eminence*. Just behind this is another opening, the site of the future glottis (the opening into the larynx and trachea).

The components of the branchial arches

The branchial arches make only a temporary appearance and their mesoderm later develops into various structures that may migrate a long way from their parent arch. It will, therefore, be convenient at this stage to consider each of the components of the arches in turn, i.e. the skeletal elements, the nerves, the muscles and the vessels.

The skeletal elements

In each arch some of the mesodermal cells form a longitudinal condensation which then becomes transformed into cartilage. The ultimate fate of these bars of cartilage varies in different arches (Fig. 11.3). In the first arch the cartilage forms a long rod that meets its fellow in the midline below the anterior part of the future mouth. This is *Meckel's cartilage* which marks the position of the future mandible. From its dorsal end, which projects above the level of the pharynx, the malleus and the incus develop. This part of the arch is cut off from the rest when the base of the skull develops and just below this level the cartilage disappears, leaving a fibrous band that forms the spheno-mandibular ligament. The remainder of Meckel's cartilage is incorporated into the mandible; the latter develops mainly by intra-membranous ossification around Meckel's cartilage, which subsequently disappears almost completely (Fig. 11.3).

The second arch cartilage is sometimes known as *Reichert's cartilage*. Its dorsal end lies near the dorsal end of the first arch and develops into the stapes. This is separated by the base of the skull from the remainder of the cartilage which forms the styloid process, the stylohyoid ligament and the lesser cornu and upper part of the body of the hyoid bone. The greater part of the skeletal element of the remaining arches disappears but small parts of their ventral ends remain. The ventral end of the third arch forms the remainder of the body and the greater cornu of the hyoid bone, while the fourth and sixth arches form the cartilages of the larynx, with the exception of the epiglottis which is derived from the hypo-branchial eminence (p.173).

The nerves

As can be seen from Fig. 11.1, the cranial nerves have only a short distance to travel from the brain to the branchial arches. The fifth (trigeminal) nerve supplies the first arch, mainly via its mandibular division although its maxillary division is involved in the innervation of the maxillary process. The seventh (facial) nerve runs caudally from its ganglion and then turns down to enter the second arch. A small branch of the seventh nerve runs forwards, until it becomes cranial to the first endodermal pharyngeal pouch and supplements the fifth nerve in the supply of the first arch. This is the *chorda tympani* and it is the only remaining representative of a whole series of nerves that, in lower animals, pass from each branchial arch into the preceding arch (*pretrematic branches*). The nerve of the third arch is the ninth (glossopharyngeal) nerve, while two branches of the vagus account for the remaining arches, the superior laryngeal nerve to the fourth and the recurrent laryngeal to the sixth. In each arch, except the sixth, the nerve lies cranial to the corresponding artery but it is important to note that in the sixth arch the nerve is caudal (p.213). The motor divisions of the nerve supply the muscles that are derived from the mesoderm of the corresponding arches.

The muscles

The mesoderm of the arches forms, among other things, all the skeletal muscles other than those derived from paraxial mesoderm; the motor nerves establish contact with the muscle fibres. Thereafter the developing muscle cells migrate to various parts of the head and neck, but they retain their original nerve supply so that the cranial nerves concerned have a very widespread distribution. Thus the motor division of the trigeminal nerve supplies the muscles of mastication and the mylohyoid as well as the tensor tympani and the tensor palati, all of which are therefore derivatives of the first arch mesoderm. The facial nerve supplies the muscles of facial expression, including the scalp muscles, the stapedius, the posterior belly of the digastric and the stylohyoid muscle, all second arch derivatives. The third arch gives rise to only one small muscle, the stylopharyngeus, which is therefore supplied by the ninth (glosso-pharyngeal) nerve. Finally, the superior laryngeal (via its external laryngeal branch) and the recurrent laryngeal nerves supply the muscles of the larynx and pharynx. These muscles are thus derivatives of the fourth and sixth arches. The axons of the cranial nerves that supply the branchial musculature are, of course, derived from the branchial efferent column of nerve cells (p.142).

The arteries

Each branchial arch contains an artery that links up ventrally with the aortic sac and dorsally with the left or right dorsal aorta (Fig. 11.1). These aortic arches are not, however, all present at the same time. As happens in so many regions there is a cranio-caudal growth gradient so that the first and second aortic arches appear in quick succession but, by the time the third aortic arch has developed, the first aortic arch has begun to regress and the second aortic arch soon follows suit as the more caudal aortic arches appear. Finally, the only aortic arches that remain are the third, fourth and sixth; these will be discussed in Chapter 12.

The formation of the neck

As can be seen in Fig. 9.1, the first and second arches are a great deal larger than those that follow and this disproportion becomes emphasized as the first arch makes its contribution to the lower part of the face and as the second arch becomes larger and grows caudally (Figs. 11.2 and 11.4). The third and fourth arches

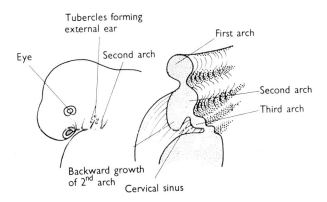

Fig. 11.4. Diagrams to show how backward growth of the second arch forms the cervical sinus (cp. Fig. 11.2).

soon disappear from view, when seen from the exterior, as the second arch grows back over them, and eventually they come to lie in the floor of a cavity the roof of which is formed by the large second arch and which is, for a time, open to the exterior at the caudal margin of that arch. This ectoderm-lined cavity is the *cervical sinus* and it normally disappears completely so that the external surface of the neck becomes smooth.

By the time the branchial arches have differentiated fully, the embryo is beginning to acquire a recognisable neck and thorax. This is due to several factors: the growth of the lungs which enclose the heart and hide it from view (p.239), the development of the ribs and the musculature of the body wall from the somites (p.127) and, less obtrusive but equally important, the so-called 'descent of the heart' (p.213). It must be stressed that this is only a relative descent; in the embryo at this stage of development growth is occurring throughout the body and many organs are rapidly changing their relations. In the absence of any fixed points of reference, it is impossible to describe the movements of viscera with any accuracy and the 'descent' of the heart and other associated structures is due more to the cranial end of the embryo growing away from the region of the septum transversum than to any true descent of the heart. The embryo, therefore, should really be imagined as 'sticking its neck out' but the relative descent of the heart thus produced is a useful descriptive term and will be referred to frequently in the next chapter.

The endodermal derivatives

The endodermal pouches lie between the branchial arches, the first pouch lying between the first and second arches. Fig. 11.5 is a transverse section through the pharynx similar to Fig. 11.1 but passing through a pair of pharyngeal pouches instead of through the arches. It can be seen that each pouch has a dorsal and

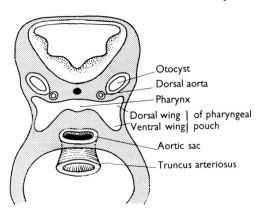

Fig. 11.5. A vertical section through the pharyngeal region (just posterior to Fig. 11.1) passing through the pharyngeal pouch on each side.

ventral prolongation or 'wing'. The first pouch becomes very large and retains its close relation to the ectoderm. It is known as the *tubo-tympanic recess* and will form the middle ear cavity and the pharyngo-tympanic (auditory) tube (Figs. 11.7, 11.8 and 11.9). The dorsal wing of the second pouch is probably incorporated into the tubo-tympanic recess, but the endoderm of the ventral wing proliferates to form a large mass that, during later development, becomes infiltrated with lymphocytes to form the tonsil, lying in the lateral wall of the pharynx (Figs. 11.6 and 11.7). Endodermal proliferations also occur in the dorsal and ventral wings of the third and fourth pouches (*vide infra*); these pouches ultimately lose their

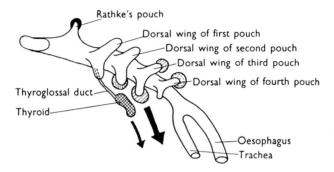

Fig. 11.6. A side view of the pharynx to show the endodermal proliferations of the pharyngeal pouches and the thyroid outgrowth from the pharyngeal floor.

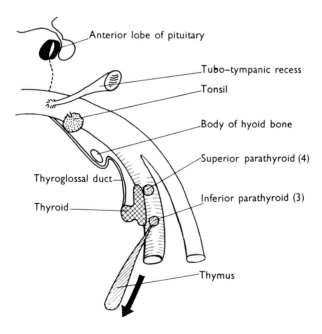

Fig. 11.7. A side view of the pharynx to show the fate of the structures in Fig. 11.6.

connections with the pharynx as they undergo a relative descent from their original positions. The ventral wing of the fourth pouch is small; it is sometimes known, together with a rudimentary derivative of a fifth pouch, as the *ultimo-branchial body* or the *caudal pharyngeal complex*.

The thymus gland

The endoderm of the ventral wing of the third pharyngeal pouch proliferates to form a large mass on each side. This is the rudiment of the thymus and it becomes invaded by cells from the surrounding mesenchyme that split the developing gland into lobules. The mass of cells on each side fuse ventral to the developing great vessels to form a single midline structure (Fig. 11.7). Together with the aortic sac and the heart, to which the gland is closely related, the thymus undergoes a relative descent. The original connection to the pharynx becomes stretched out and soon disappears. The endodermal tissue becomes infiltrated with special cells of the lymphocyte series (*thymocytes*) and their subsequent fate and function is described in Chapter 12. The thymus plays an important part in the development of the immune response and, in some experimental animals, removal of the thymus at birth interferes with the subsequent production of antibodies. Development of the thymus is not complete at birth. Although the gland is relatively largest at this time, in that it occupies a considerable part of the upper thorax, it continues to grow and reaches its greatest size at puberty. Thereafter it becomes smaller though it is an exaggeration to say that only an atrophied remnant remains in adult life.

Parathyroid glands

The parathyroids develop from the dorsal wings of the third and fourth pouches (Figs. 11.6 and 11.7). As with the thymus, the proliferating endodermal cells form the epithelial cells of the gland, while invading mesenchyme forms the supporting tissue and blood vessels. During embryonic life these glands are best named parathyroid III and parathyroid IV (denoting the pouch from which each is derived) but the position of the two glands later becomes reversed. As the thymus (derived from the ventral wing of the third pouch) descends, it carries with it the corresponding parathyroid gland (derived from the dorsal wing of the third pouch) so that parathyroid III comes to lie at a lower level than parathyroid IV. Both glands lost their connection with the pharynx at an early stage and they come to lie in relation to the posterior surface of the thyroid gland. Parathyroid III thus forms the inferior parathyroid and parathyroid IV the superior. Occasionally parathyroid III may retain its association with the thymus and may thus be found in the superior mediastinum.

The thyroid gland

This is a single midline structure, the greater part and possibly the whole of which is derived from the outgrowth that develops just caudal to the tuberculum impar (p.172). The outgrowth forms a bilobed mass of cells that descend to lie in relation to the ventral surface of the aortic sac, drawing out during its descent a long cord of cells known as the *thyroglossal duct* (Figs. 11.7 and 11.11). When the heart descends, it leaves the thyroid behind so that the two lobes lie on either side of the developing larynx, in close relation to the ultimo-branchial body, with which they fuse. Whether or not the latter contributes to the thyroid tissue proper is a subject for dispute, but animal experiments suggest that the ultimo-branchial body is responsible for the formation of the 'clear' or parafollicular cells of the thyroid which produce calcitonin, an important hormone that, to some extent, opposes the action of parathyroid hormone by inhibiting the transfer of calcium from bone to blood and thus lowering the plasma calcium level.

Reference to Fig. 11.2 shows that the site of the original thyroid outgrowth corresponds to the foramen caecum of the adult tongue. The thyroglossal duct, if it persists, will therefore extend from this point down to the isthmus of the thyroid, passing ventral to the body of the hyoid bone. The lower end of the duct contributes to the pyramidal lobe of the thyroid.

The development of the ear

Although the membranous labyrinth develops from the otocyst, which is closely associated with the hindbrain (p.146), it will be convenient here to deal with the development of the ear as a whole. The middle ear and the pharyngo-tympanic tube develop from the tubo-tympanic recess. This is formed from the large first

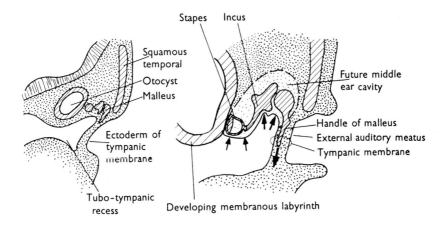

Fig. 11.8. The development of the middle ear. The ossicles develop in mesoderm and are not included in the middle ear cavity until it grows up in the direction of the arrows. The handle of the malleus develops in the mesoderm of the tympanic membrane.

endodermal pouch together with the dorsal part of the second. The lateral extremity of the recess lies very close to the ectoderm between the first and second branchial arches, with only a small amount of mesoderm between (Fig. 11.8). In the roof of the recess is the otocyst and in front and behind are the skeletal elements of the first and second arches, the dorsal ends of which extend up above the level of the roof of the recess and are themselves closely related to the otocyst (Fig. 11.9).

The flattened end of the tubo-tympanic recess, together with the mesoderm and ectoderm in relation to it, forms the tympanic membrane. The dorsal end of the first arch skeletal element forms the malleus and incus, and that of the second arch, the stapes. As can be seen in Fig. 11.8 the handle of the malleus grows down into the mesoderm of the tympanic membrane. The ectoderm and endoderm form respectively the outer and inner epithelial layers of the membrane while the mesoderm forms the fibrous central layer. The chorda tympani which, as has been seen, passes from the second to the first branchial arch (p.174), naturally passes through the central layer of the tympanic membrane, medial to the handle of the malleus.

The tubo-tympanic recess becomes constricted between its distal expansion and the pharynx to form the pharyngo-tympanic (auditory) tube. The dilated outer end gradually enlarges at the expense of the surrounding mesoderm and, in so doing, it engulfs the ossicles that originally lay in the mesoderm of the roof of the recess. Even in adult life the ossicles are still covered with an epithelial layer so that they are, strictly speaking, still outside the middle ear cavity. The otocyst becomes converted into the very irregular shape of the membranous labyrinth, and the mesoderm around it becomes condensed, chondrified and finally ossified, to form the petrous portion of the temporal bone. The squamous part of the temporal bone develops in membrane lateral to the petrous part (Figs. 11.8 and 11.9). Externally, a series of small hillocks at the dorsal ends of the first and second arches and around the first ectodermal cleft (Fig. 11.4) form the auricle of the ear and the cartilaginous part of the external auditory meatus.

Developmental anomalies of the branchial region

There are many developmental anomalies in which derivatives of the branchial arches are either missing or malformed. Most of these are so uncommon as to be of little clinical importance. Only two types will be described here — anomalies of the *first arch* and of the *cervical sinus*.

First arch syndrome

This usually refers to abnormalities which result from disappearance or anomalous development of the structures derived from the first pharyngeal arch.

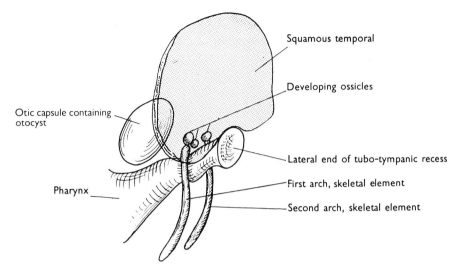

Fig. 11.9. The ossicles develop from the dorsal ends of the first and second arch skeletal elements. The squamous temporal ossifies in membrane on the surface of the temporal region. The contribution of the end of the tubo-tympanic recess to the tympanic membrane is shown in Fig 11.8.

Micrognathia

In this condition the mandible is hypoplastic (under-developed) giving rise to a shrew-like face. The tongue is inserted into the mandible very far back (*glossoptosis*). Sometimes a small mandible is associated with a midline cleft palate (with an intact lip) a combination recognized as the *Pierre Robin syndrome*. Aetiology of micrognathia is poorly understood. Impaired blood supply might be sometimes responsible and occasionally external pressure *in utero* (as can occur with a prolonged transversely lying fetus in relation to the uterus) will cause micrognathia — representing, therefore, more a deformity than a true malformation (see also p.315).

Babies with mandibular hypoplasia will often have difficulty in sucking so that feeding milk directly into the stomach through a naso-gastric tube might be initially required. Respiratory obstruction can even occur if the poorly anchored tongue falls backwards obstructing the oropharynx. The long term prognosis is usually excellent, the chin in time regaining its correct shape. Any associated palatal cleft will require surgical management.

Mandibular-facial dysostosis (Treacher Collins syndrome)

This is a rare hereditary condition transmitted as a dominant trait. In the complete form it constitutes mandibular and maxillary hypoplasia, high arched or cleft palate, antimongoloid (i.e. downward sloping) palpebral fissures, coloboma (cleft) of outer part of lower lid, deformed ear pinnae, absent external auditory meatus and middle ear abnormalities leading to deafness.

Oculo-auriculovertebral syndrome (Goldenhar's syndrome)

This is another rare syndrome of multiple congenital abnormalities not hereditary, characterised by deformed pinnae, ear tags, absent external auditory canal and deafness, small mandible, facial clefts, hemi-vertebrae and sometimes a congenital heart defect.

Cervical sinus anomalies

If the cervical sinus, made up of the remnants of the second, third and fourth ectodermal clefts, is not completely obliterated by proliferation of the mesoderm of the second arch an epithelial-lined cyst may remain in the neck, sited usually along the anterior border of the sterno-mastoid muscle. This is known as a *branchial* or *cervical cyst*. It sometimes connects with the surface through a narrow canal, a *branchial fistula*, which will often become infected and require surgical removal. Reference to Fig. 11.4 will show that the upper end of such a fistula passes immediately anterior to the third arch and, therefore, to the internal carotid. If treated surgically it thus has to be dissected out from between the internal and external carotids. It should be mentioned that there are a number of other theories of the pathogenesis of these cysts and there is insufficient evidence to choose between them.

Developmental anomalies of the pharyngeal pouches and the thyroid

Thyroid gland

Five principal types of developmental anomaly can affect the thyroid gland.

Aberrant thyroid tissue

If the normal descent of the thyroid is interfered with, an aberrant thyroid gland will result; this may be situated anywhere along the course of the thyroglossal duct from the foramen caecum on the tongue to the isthmus of the thyroid gland. This ectopic endocrine tissue frequently fails to function adequately thereby causing, through negative feedback via the hypothalamic-pituitary axis, a compensatory output of thyroid-stimulating hormone(TSH) from the anterior pituitary gland which stimulates thyroid tissue to increase in size (in the neck this is called a *goitre*). The accompanying increase in the output of thyroid hormones usually prevents the development of hypothyroidism.

Thyroglossal cysts

These are fluid filled swellings located close to, or in the midline, occurring along the migratory course followed by the thyroglossal duct. The thyroid gland is usually normally situated and functions normally. Both aberrant thyroid tissue and thyroglossal cysts share the common feature of presenting as a lump in the midline anywhere between the foramen caecum ('lingual thyroid') and the isthmus of the thyroid gland itself (Fig. 11.11). They usually move upwards on protrusion of the tongue. Surgical excision is usually needed, but this should not be undertaken without a preliminary thyroid scan with, for example, [132]I to establish whether the lump is aberrant thyroid tissue or a non-functioning thyroglossal cyst. Replacement thyroid therapy will be needed if aberrant thyroid tissue has to be removed.

Thyroid dysgenesis

The spectrum of thyroid dysgenesis (abnormal development) extends from complete failure of the thyroid gland to develop (*agenesis*) to the presence of a small thyroid remnant situated above the hyoid bone. Agenesis will usually present with congenital hypothyroidism from birth: partial dysgenesis is more likely to present with hypothyroidism later in childhood.

Thyroid dyshormonogenesis

These conditions represent a group of metabolic thyroid disorders, many genetically determined as autosomal recessives in which there are blocks at various stages in the synthesis of thyroid hormone (clinical textbooks should be consulted for a detailed account of these). The gross structure and position of the gland are normal. The hypothalamic-pituitary axis responds by increasing synthesis of TSH which in time causes diffuse thyroid hyperplasia. This might appear at birth as a swelling of the thyroid gland. If the metabolic block is incomplete this compensatory response will sometimes succeed in allowing sufficient thyroid hormone to be secreted. If the block is total, hypothyroidism will present from birth.

Congenital hypothyroidism

This condition describes the consequences to physical growth and development of inadequate levels of circulating thyroid hormones whose origins (dyshormonogenesis in 10–15 per cent of cases or, more commonly, various degrees of thyroid gland dysgenesis) are determined before birth. In exceedingly rare instances thyroid dysfunction is due to reduced secretion of TSH by the pituitary or TSH-releasing factor by the hypothalamus. In some instances congenital hypothyroidism can be diagnosed at birth, or very soon afterwards, by the presence of dysmorphic facial features (eyes set far apart, depressed nasal bridge), umbilical hernia, dry thickened skin and clinical features of aberrant physiological function including prolonged neonatal jaundice, slow pulse rate, constipation and a tendency towards hypothermia. Infants with some, or all, of these features have probably been hypothyroid for some time *in utero* — maternal thyroid hormones do not cross the placenta. In clinical practice, however, most infants with congenital hypothyroidism have more often been diagnosed at the age of a few months with various combinations of the features described above, yet were passed as normal at birth. Delay in diagnosis, largely on account of the often very protean clinical features of congenital hypothyroidism early in post-natal life, and in instituting treatment is of serious consequence since it can lead to irrecoverable neuro-developmental damage and physical growth retardation. Thyroid hormones play an essential role in brain maturation (myelination, synaptic and dendrite formation, timing of switches in the phases of brain devel-opment) and skeletal growth and osseous maturation. The sooner replacement therapy with thyroxine is instituted the less will be the likelihood of any per-manent deficit in growth and neuro-psychological function. It is for this reason that laboratory screening programmes have been set up in most economically developed countries to detect, in the first week of life, sub-clinical congenital hypothyroidism. The most widely used methods are the measurement of thyroxine and TSH (which, other than in the very rare hypothalamic hypothyroidism, is invariably raised) on dried blood spots on filter paper. The test is usually per-formed at the same time as the Guthrie filter paper test for phenylketonuria (p.24). between the 6th and 14th days of life. Indeed, the principle underlying biochemical screening for both these conditions is the same — the detection in an asymptoma-tic stage of a metabolic abnormality which, unless diagnosed early and appro-priately treated, will lead inevitably to irreparable mental subnormality and growth retardation. Screening programmes indicate an incidence of congenital hypothyroidism of about 1 in 3,500. The results to date on the neuro-developmental outcome of infants detected and treated from birth are very encouraging.

Thymus and parathyroid glands

Abnormalities in the development of the thymus gland are extremely rare. They occur as isolated anomalies or are associated with deviant development of structures derived from other pharyngeal pouches especially parathyroid glands: they generate a disproportionate amount of interest (at least in relation to their frequency in practice) because they provide an important model for the study of the development of the immune response. Thymic dysplasia is usually diagnosed in the investigation of severe chronic infections in the first few months of life. Symptoms particularly include failure to thrive, diarrhoea, chest and skin infections. Circulating immunoglobulins are normal but there is a very low lymphocyte count (*lymphopenia*) and impaired cell-mediated immunity due to deficiency of T cells which are normally processed in the thymus.

Hypocalcaemia is sometimes associated with thymic dysplasia due to failure of the development of the parathyroid glands from the third and fourth pharyngeal

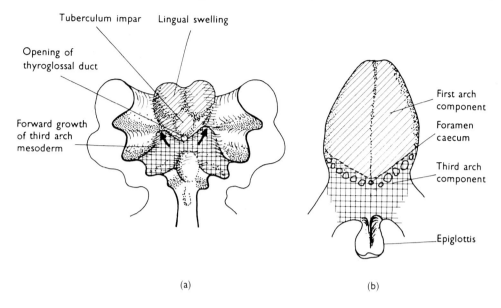

Fig. 11.10. (a) The tongue with the exception of its muscles develops from the first and third arches in the floor of the embryonic pharyngeal region. (b) Adult tongue, showing the first and third arch components.

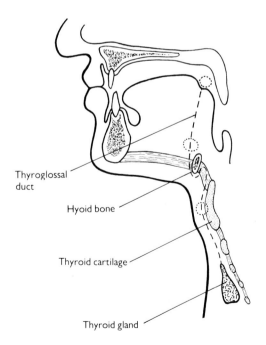

Fig. 11.11. Diagram to show the path of the thyroglossal duct, which indicates the possible sites of aberrant thyroid tissue or thyroglossal cysts.

pouches — the *Di George syndrome*. T cell deficiency is incompatible with normal life. The only treatment available is to maintain the child in a germ-free environment and attempt a bone marrow transplantation.

The tongue and mouth cavity

It will be seen from Fig. 11.2 that, at the ventral extremity of the first arch, the mesoderm has formed a pair of lingual swellings. These enlarge further and incorporate the tuberculum impar to form a large swelling on the pharyngeal floor in the region of the first arch (Fig. 11.10). The second arch plays no part in forming the tongue, but the mesoderm from the third arch grows forwards, deep to the epithelial covering but superficial to the mesoderm of the second arch, eventually to join the first arch swelling. The junction between these two components of the tongue is marked by the position of the upper end of the thyroglossal duct which, when the duct has disappeared, forms only a small pit known as the *foramen caecum* (Fig. 11.11). Thus the anterior two thirds of the tongue is of first arch origin so that it is supplied by a branch (lingual) of the mandibular division of the trigeminal nerve subserving ordinary sensation. Additionally, the chorda tympani, which is the pretrematic branch of the second arch nerve (facial), passes into the first arch (p.174) and subserves taste. The posterior third of the tongue including the circumvallate papillae is of third arch origin and is therefore supplied by the glossopharyngeal nerve for both taste and general sensation. The nerves just mentioned do not supply the muscle, since the arch mesoderm forms only the connective tissue basis of the tongue, together with the blood vessels. The muscle is probably derived from the occipital somites which migrate into the tongue, bringing with them their nerve supply, the hypoglossal nerve (p.127).

The tongue, at this stage, (later part of second month) is a squat, cushion-like structure, but its tip becomes progessively freed and this process is continued by the formation of two concentric horseshoe-shaped grooves that surround the tongue anteriorly. These form the sulci between tongue and gums and between gums and cheek respectively (Fig. 11.12a). The teeth develop in the gums, partly from mesoderm and partly from the ectodermal *dental lamina*, which grows from the surface epithelium into the underlying mesoderm and then breaks up to form a series of tooth germs, one for each of the ten deciduous teeth in the lower jaw. Each tooth germ consists of an invaginated sac derived from the dental lamina. together with the mesoderm that is enclosed within the invagination (Fig. 11.12b). The invaginated layer of ectodermal cells forms the *enamel organ* and its lower layer of cells become *ameloblasts*. The mesodermal cells in contact with the enamel organ form a layer of *odontoblasts*. The ameloblasts lay down enamel on their deep aspect and the odontoblasts lay down dentine on their superficial aspect (Fig. 11.12c). The loose mesoderm inside the layer of odontoblasts forms the pulp and is well supplied by free nerve endings subserving the sensation of pain. A further series of tooth germs from the dental lamina forms the primordia of the permanent

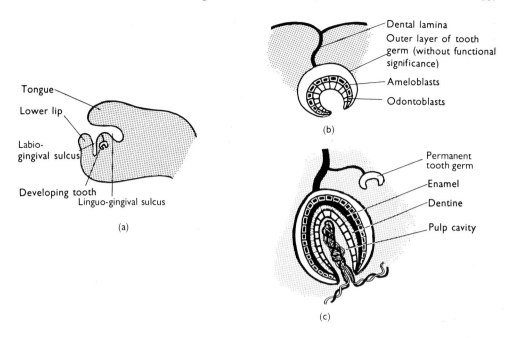

Fig. 11.12. (a) A midline sagittal section through the lower jaw to show the freeing of the tongue, gums and lips by two sulci. (b) and (c) Developing tooth, showing the laying down of dentine and enamel by odontoblasts and ameloblasts respectively at approximately seven months.

teeth. Similar development, of course, occurs in the upper jaw.

The salivary glands develop as invaginations from the surface epithelium of the stomatodeum which branch to form alveoli at their extremities.

The development of the face and palate

At the stage of development shown in Fig. 9.1 the stomatodaeum is bounded by the forebrain above, the first (mandibular) arch below (separating it from the pericardium) and the maxillary processes at the side (Fig. 11.13). In spite of their names, the maxillary and other processes to be mentioned later are not true processes that can reach out and bridge gaps (as is so often described) but are simply accumulations of mesoderm that cause bulges in the overlying ectoderm. When two such processes 'fuse', their mesodermal components become continuous and the slight groove in the ectoderm, which marked the junction between the two processes, becomes obliterated.

Bilateral thickenings in the ectoderm, the *olfactory placodes*, sink beneath the surface so that each comes to lie at the deepest part of a *nasal sac* to form the olfactory epithelium (Fig. 11.14a). The opening of the sac, the external nares, has mesodermal thickenings on each side of it which form the *medial* and *lateral nasal processes* (Fig. 11.13), the mesoderm of the latter soon becoming continuous with

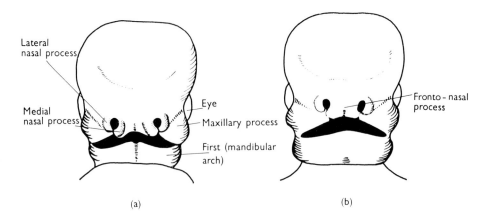

Lateral nasal process

Medial nasal process

Eye

Maxillary process

First (mandibular arch)

Fronto-nasal process

(a)

(b)

Fig. 11.13. The development of the face.

that of the maxillary process. The two medial nasal processes, together with the area between them, form the *fronto-nasal process* (Fig. 11.13).

The mesoderm of the maxillary process 'fuses' with the lateral part of the frontonasal process and the line of junction between them runs up to the eye (Fig. 11.13). Note that the eyes, at this stage of development, are directed laterally. There is a good deal of evidence that the maxillary process mesoderm overgrows the fronto-nasal process to meet its fellow of the opposite side to form the philtrum of the upper lip. The nasal sac soon establishes continuity with the stomatodaeum posteriorly to form the *primitive posterior nares* (Fig. 11.13) and the mesoderm of the maxillary process becomes continuous with that of the fronto-nasal process to complete the upper lip (Fig. 11.13). There are now both anterior and posterior nares and a *primitive nasal cavity* that is separated from the future mouth by a *primitive palate* (Fig. 11.14). The major part of the definitive palate,

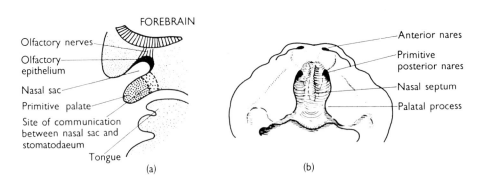

FOREBRAIN

Olfactory nerves

Olfactory epithelium

Nasal sac

Primitive palate

Site of communication between nasal sac and stomatodaeum

Tongue

Anterior nares

Primitive posterior nares

Nasal septum

Palatal process

(a)

(b)

Fig. 11.14. (a) Parasaggital section through the nasal sac. The sparsely dotted area will later break down to form a communication between nasal sac and stomatodaeum (primitive posterior nares). (b) A drawing of the palatal region of the human embryo seen from below to show the primitive posterior nares.

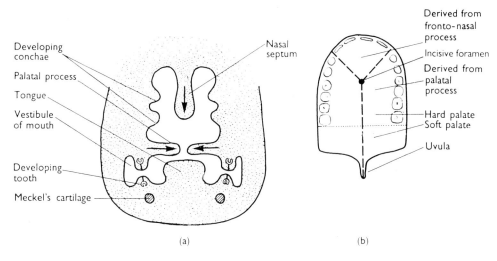

Fig. 11.15. (a) A coronal section through the mouth and nose of a human embryo to show the formation of the palate and nasal septum. This diagram is simplified — in a real embryo the tongue lies at first between the palatal processes so that its dorsum is in contact with the free border of the nasal septum. (b) The derivation of the adult palate.

however, develops behind this, when two *palatal processes* grow medially from the inner surfaces of the two maxillary processes (Fig. 11.15). At first, the palatal processes hang down on either side of the tongue, the dorsum of which is in contact with the nasal septum (this is not shown in Fig 11.15a). The septum has grown down from the roof of the nasal cavity. Later, as a result of the extension of the head and perhaps of muscular movement of the tongue, the palatal processes are freed and 'flip up' to meet and fuse with each other and with the lower edge of the nasal septum. The 'flip up' is partly due to the increasing turgor of the processes as a result of water imbibition by the glycosaminoglycans in their mesenchymal cores. The very small primitive nasal cavity thus becomes much larger and is separated from the mouth by a mesenchymal palate. Later, muscle and bone will differentiate here to form the hard and soft palates. The paranasal sinuses develop as outgrowths from the nasal cavity. Most are absent or only shallow depressions at birth and do not become fully developed until puberty.

Developmental anomalies of the face and palate

There are many forms of anomalous development of the face and palate but most are so rare as not to merit mention here. The commonest and most important anomalies are the various types of *cleft (hare) lip* and *palate*, which occur either separately or in combination with an incidence of about 1 per 1,000 live births. They result from failure of growth mechanism(s) which cause the various facial and palatal processes and the nasal septum to become continuous with each other in the 5th–10th week of development. For the majority of cases a specific

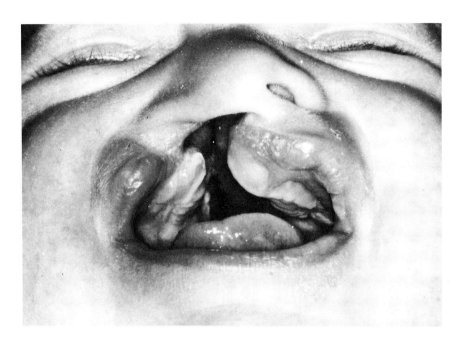

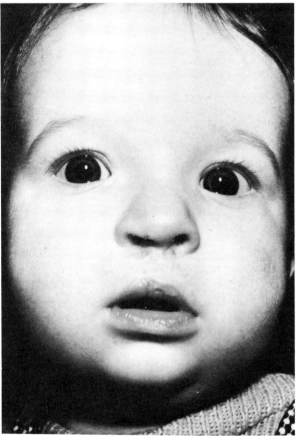

Fig. 11.16. Unilateral cleft lip and palate, before (at birth) and after treatment (aged 2 years).

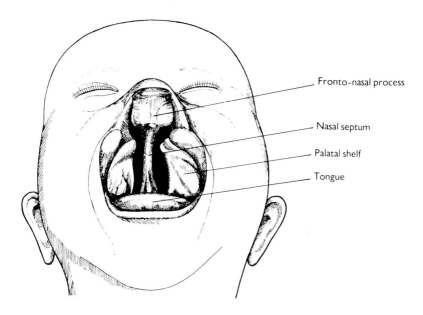

Fronto-nasal process

Nasal septum

Palatal shelf

Tongue

Fig. 11.17 Bilateral cleft lip and palate. The free edge of the nasal septum is clearly visible.

aetiology is unknown, and a multifactorial basis is assumed. In animals palatal anomalies can result from the administration of certain drugs to the pregnant mother or by rendering her deficient in certain nutrients. In the human, the role of environmental factors is unclear although anti-convulsants taken by the mother are believed to increase the risk of palatal anomalies threefold. Genetic factors play an important, though complex, role. In isolated cleft lip, for example, the risk of recurrence if parents are normal is about 1 in 20. If two siblings are affected the subsequent risk is 1 in 10. If either parent has a cleft lip as well, the risks to subsequent offspring are in the order of 1 in 5. Inheritance of cleft palate follows a similar pattern but with half the levels at birth. Cleft lip, with or without cleft palate, also occurs with other syndromes of congenital malformations, particularly those associated with chromosome abnormalities.

Deformities of the lip and palate can be divided into anterior and posterior cleft varieties, according to their relationship to the incisive foramen — the point at which the palatal shelves join the primitive palate (Fig. 11.15). Anterior defects include either *unilateral* or *bilateral cleft lip* and *cleft upper jaw* (Fig. 11.16). Posterior defects result from failure of one or both of the palatal shelves to grow normally across to the midline. A posterior cleft is often continuous with a cleft in the upper lip of the same side, due to failure of the maxillary process to fuse with the fronto-nasal process: this cleft joins the lip to the external nasal opening. If both palatal processes fail to grow towards the midline a large central cleft results with the nasal septum free margin being visible through the cleft and the isolated fronto-nasal process appearing as a distorted lump (Fig. 11.17). On rare occasions the palatal processes may just fail to join in the midline, and are separated by a thin midline cleft. If the palatal processes fuse in all but their most posterior part, simple cleavage of the uvula and soft palate will result.

The many permutations of palatal anomalies are most likely explained by the extent of the embryonic error and the timing in relation to the stage of development reached by the various parts. For example, in the 7th week the palatal process fuses with the primitive palate but it is only in the 10th week that each palatal process fuses with its partner on the other side.

Clinical features

An isolated cleft lip, other than being a cosmetic embarrassment which is readily corrected by surgery, will rarely cause problems. In contrast the baby with a cleft palate anomaly can cause major anxieties in both the short and long term.

Early problems

The prime purpose of the palate is to separate the nasal from the oral cavities and so allow feeding and breathing to take place concurrently. It is understandable, therefore, that in the baby with a cleft palate feeding is likely to cause problems. In the first place it will be difficult for sufficient negative intra-oral pressure to be created in order to draw milk into the mouth. Secondly, abnormalities in the soft palate will make it difficult for the oral cavity to be closed off. Milk will, therefore, easily be regurgitated through the nose. Skilled nursing management is needed if the baby is to be fed satisfactorily. Breast feeding should be possible in all but the largest clefts. Sometimes special devices will be needed to help feeding such as an obturator (a dental plate which occludes the cleft providing an 'artificial' palatal area) and special long teats (lambs teats) to allow milk to immediately enter the pharynx. Sometimes the only satisfactory method of feeding if suction is inadequate is to use a cup and spoon. Because of swallowing difficulties aspiration of milk into the lungs is not uncommon, with subsequent infection.

Late problems

The principal later problem, occurring in as many as 25 per cent of children, concerns speech disorders. An intact hard palate is essential for normal articulation: a normally functioning soft palate is required, through its various muscles, to perform fine co-ordinated movements for good speech and to create an air tight seal with the posterior pharyngeal wall to prevent nasal speech. The child with a cleft palate may have speech difficulties from three main sources: (a) from the defect itself, involving both hard and soft palates; (b) following plastic surgery for the palatal defect which might damage the pharyngeal muscles; (c) catarrhal conditions of the middle ear (*glue ear*) often leading to otitis media. The last is a very common problem as the muscles of the palate are inserted around the auditory tube as well as the base of the skull. Conductive deafness (often in the order of 10−15 decibels) is, therefore, a frequent occurrence, in as many as 50 per cent of children.

Management

The objective of surgery is to provide as normal a facial appearance as possible and the potential for competent speech. Cleft lip is repaired normally at about 6 months, although some authorities recommend repair as early as 48 hours to lessen the cosmetic problem. The palatal defect is closed later, usually between 9 and 12 months, together with correction of the nasal deformity. With modern surgical techniques the transition from what is often a very ugly malformation to a face which is almost normal is truly remarkable. To help parents understand and cope with the often unsightly appearance parent self-help groups are extremely valuable. One such example in Britain is CLAPA (Cleft Lip and Palate Association). Photographs showing the excellent results of treatment are invaluable (Fig. 11.16). In the long term there must be careful supervision of speech and hearing. Surgical management of middle ear effusions by myringotomy, i.e. controlled incision into the ear drum, and aspiration may be needed to reduce risks of permanent damage to hearing. Successful outcome depends as with so many congenital defects on multidisciplinary teamwork, in this case involving plastic and otorhinological (ENT) surgeons, speech therapists, orthodontists and paediatricians.

Developmental stages

4 weeks: Pharyngeal (branchial) arches, maxillary processes appear. Thyroid outgrowth recognisable. Buccopharyngeal membrane ruptures.
5 weeks: Tongue recognisable. Processes that will form face have appeared. Pharyngeal pouch derivatives appearing. Nasal cavities appear.
6 weeks: Primary palate developed.
8 weeks: Upper lip and nostrils formed and face recognisably human. Palatal processes and nasal septum begin to fuse (former first). Tongue fully developed.
11 weeks: Palatal fusion complete.

Further reading

Bertelli, A.P. & Freitas, J.P.A. (1971) Thyroglossal cysts and fistulae. *Eye, Ear, Nose and Throat Monthly*, **50**, 88.

Ferguson, M.W.J. (1977) The mechanism of palatal shelf elevation and the pathogenesis of cleft palate. *Virchows Arch. A.*, **375**, 97.

Gorlin, R.J. & Pindborg, J.J. (1964) *Syndromes of the Head and Neck*. McGraw Hill, New York.

Luke, D.A. (1976) Development of the secondary palate in man. *Acta Anat.*, **94**, 596.

Moseley, J.M., Matthews, E.W., Breed, R.H., Galante, L., Tse, A. & Macintyre, I. (1968) The ultimo-branchial origin of calcitonin. *Lancet* **1**, 108.

Paley, W.G. & Keddie, W.C. (1970) The aetiology and management of branchial cysts. *Brit. J. Surg.*, **57**, 822.

Poswillo, D. (1975) Causal mechanisms of craniofacial deformity. *Brit. Med. Bull.*, **31**, 101.

Shepard, T.H. (1965) The Thyroid. In: *Morphogenesis*, eds DeHaan, R.L. & Ursprung, H. Holt, Rinehart & Winston, New York, Toronto & London.

Slavkin, H.C. (1979) *Developmental Craniofacial Biology*. Lea & Febiger, Philadelphia.

Sperber, G.H. (1973) *Craniofacial Embryology*. John Wright, Bristol.

Tamarin, S. & Boyde, A. (1977) Facial and visceral arch development in the mouse embryo: a study by scanning electron microscopy. *J. Anat.*, **124**, 563.

Warbrick, J.G. (1960) The early development of the nasal cavity and upper lip in the human embryo. *J. Anat.* **94**, 351.

Weller, G.L. (1933) Development of the thyroid, parathyroid and thymus glands in man. *Contr. Embryol. Carnegie Inst.* **24**, 93.

12
The Heart and the Vascular System

In the early stages of development the embryo can obtain sufficient nourishment by diffusion from the surrounding tissues. As the size of the embryo increases, however, this becomes impossible and the early development of a transport system becomes necessary.

The blood vascular system, including the heart, is formed initially from endothelial tubes which develop in the mesenchyme both within the embryo and in the extra-embryonic tissues. Some of the mesenchymal cells develop into flattened endothelial cells which form thin-walled tubes while others, trapped within the tubes, develop into primitive blood cells. These endothelial tubes and developing blood cells form *blood islets* which appear first in the wall of the yolk sac but are soon found throughout the mesenchyme. The endothelial tubes rapidly become linked up with one another, to form a primitive circulatory system. There is, of course, no structural differentiation between arteries and veins at this stage but, later, condensations of cells surround the endothelial tubes to form the tunica media and adventitia of the vessels and the myocardium and the epicardium of the heart.

Early development of the heart and the primitive circulation

The earliest sign of the developing heart is the appearance of paired endothelial tubes in the floor of the future pericardial cavity when the embryo is still in the form of a trilaminar disc. These fuse to form a single tube which comes to lie in the dorsal wall of the pericardium when the head fold appears (Chapter 6). The heart tube then invaginates itself, with its surrounding mesenchyme, into the pericardial cavity (Fig. 12.1) so that it acquires a *dorsal mesocardium*. This soon becomes perforated and disappears so that the heart tube runs through the pericardial cavity, being attached only at its cranial and caudal ends. The mesenchyme adjacent to the tube becomes condensed and forms the *myocardium* and *epicardium*, the latter being equivalent to the visceral layer of pericardium in the adult. At the same time, a series of constrictions and dilations appears along the heart tube so that it is now possible to recognise a *sinus venosus*, an *atrium*, a *ventricle* and a *bulbus cordis* (Fig. 12.2). The caudal end of the tube, the sinus venosus, is partly embedded in the septum transversum, while the cranial end leaves the pericardium to lie in the floor of the pharynx (Fig. 11.1).

195

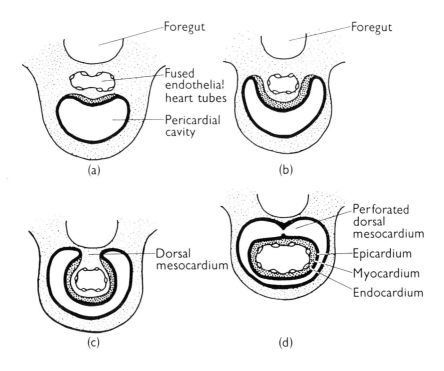

Fig. 12.1 The heart develops from a pair of endothelial tubes which fuse and invaginate the pericardial cavity. The dorsal mesocardium which is thus formed, becomes perforated so that the heart tube runs freely through the pericardial cavity.

The bulbus cordis leads into a short wide segment, the *truncus arteriosus*, the cranial end of which is dilated to form the *aortic sac* which gives rise to two vessels. These pass dorsally, on either side of the foregut, in the mesenchyme of the first branchial arch. These vessels are the *first aortic arches* and they join the corresponding dorsal aortae which lie in the roof of the pharynx. A cranial pro-longation of each dorsal aorta supplies the forebrain and will later form the internal carotid artery (Fig. 7.1). The paired dorsal aortae initially run the whole length of the embryo, but they soon fuse just caudal to the branchial region so that there is only a single midline vessel in the caudal part of the embryo.

The dorsal aorta distributes three main sets of branches (Figs. 7.1 and 12.3). From its dorsal aspect, a series of intersegmental arteries arise (p.197). Laterally, a number of branches supply certain structures derived from the intermediate cell mass (p.199) while, ventrally, a series of *vitelline arteries* (p.199) supply the yolk sac. The largest branches of the aorta are, however, the *umbilical arteries* which represent a pair of ventral branches to the allantois. These pass into the body stalk and enter the developing placenta (Fig. 7.1). They will later transfer their origins from the aorta to the developing internal iliac arteries.

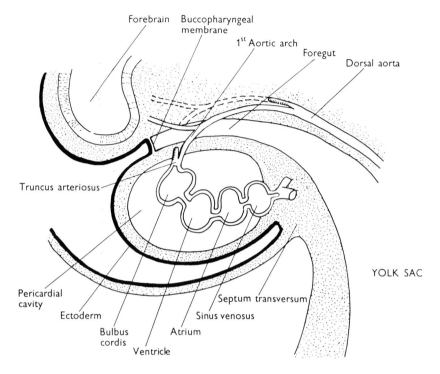

Fig. 12.2. The heart tube becomes subdivided into a number of chambers. From its cranial end a pair of aortic arches pass, one on either side of the foregut, to form the paired dorsal aortae. These fuse more caudally to form a single dorsal aorta.

The branches of the dorsal aorta(e)

This will be a convenient place to discuss further the branches of the dorsal aorta or aortae, above the level where the right and left aortae join.

The intersegmental arteries

As has been mentioned, these initially supply the neural tube, whose development precedes that of the muscles of the back or of the body wall. A little later, however, the intersegmental arteries give a branch that runs dorsally to the developing dorsal musculature (the *epimere*, p.127) and another that runs laterally to supply the body wall. These two branches become much larger than the neural tube branches so that the latter are, in adult terminology, known as the *spinal branches* of the intersegmental arteries (Fig. 12.4). In the thoracic and lumbar regions, the body wall branches become the posterior intercostal and the lumbar arteries, each of which has a posterior branch that supplies the extensor musculature, and a spinal branch that enters the vertebral canal. In both the embryo and the adult the spinal branch divides into ventral and dorsal branches (radicular arteries) that join the anterior and posterior spinal arteries respectively. In the

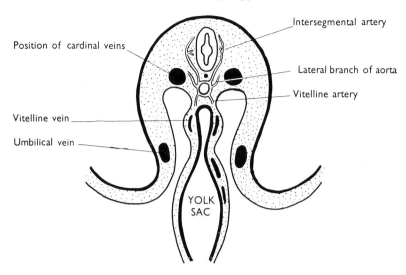

Fig. 12.3. A transverse section of the embryo to show the 3 sets of branches of the dorsal aorta and the 3 sets of veins.

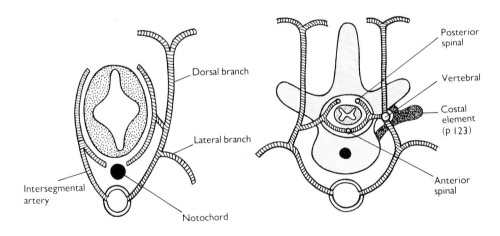

Fig. 12.4. The fate of the intersegmental vessels. On the left, the intersegmentals first supply the neural tube and then develop dorsal and lateral branches. The diagram on the right shows how the original intersegmental becomes the spinal branch. This diagram also shows the position of the longitudinal anastomosis that will form the vertebral artery.

cervical region, the first 7 intersegmental arteries are joined by a longitudinal anastomosis which forms the vertebral artery; the proximal segments of the first 6 disappear. The vertebral artery, therefore, comes to arise from the 7th inter-segmental artery which becomes the subclavian artery as described later. In the sacral region, the intersegmental arteries combine to form the later sacral arteries.

The lateral branches

These supply the nephrogenic ridge and its derivatives. At first there are a large number of such branches but eventually they are reduced to 4 in number — the phrenic, suprarenal, renal and gonadal arteries; with possibly some additional arteries to the kidney. Their further development will be described in Chapter 14.

The ventral branches

There are a number of ventral vitelline arteries that supply the yolk sac and then the gut but, again, these are reduced to three persisting arteries — the coeliac, superior mesenteric and inferior mesenteric arteries which supply respectively the fore-, mid- and hindgut. Their further development will be described in Chapter 16.

The venous system

The blood is drained back to the caudal 'venous' end of the heart by three sets of veins. The first of these comes from the placenta, which sends its oxygenated blood to the heart by means of paired *umbilical veins* running in the somatopleure (Fig. 12.3). The right vein is transient so that later in development only one vein, the left, is present although both umbilical arteries persist until term. Secondly, the vessels of the yolk sac drain into right and left *vitelline veins* which run in the splanchnopleure (Fig. 7.1). Finally, the tissues of the embryo itself drain into the *anterior* and *posterior cardinal veins* which are strategically placed as can be seen from Fig. 12.3. The anterior cardinal veins drain the cranial end of the embryo and the posterior cardinal veins the caudal end (Fig. 12.5a). They unite to form the *common cardinal vein* on each side (also known as the *duct of Cuvier*). The umbilical, vitelline and common cardinal veins all enter the septum transversum — this is possible because this is where the splanchnopleure and somatopleure meet (Fig. 6.14) and they finally drain into the sinus venosus on each side.

The superior vena cava

At this stage of development, the venous system of the embryo is bilaterally symmetrical but very soon the greater part of the venous drainage passes to the right side of the heart (Fig. 12.5b). This occurs as a result of the development of a new cross connection between the two anterior cardinal veins so that all the blood from the left side of the head and the left upper limb passes to the right anterior cardinal vein. Furthermore, as a result of changes in the umbilical and vitelline veins (p.285), the veins that drain the caudal part of the embryo become channelled to the right side, the posterior cardinal veins now becoming superseded so that only their terminal parts remain. The fate of the cardinal veins is shown

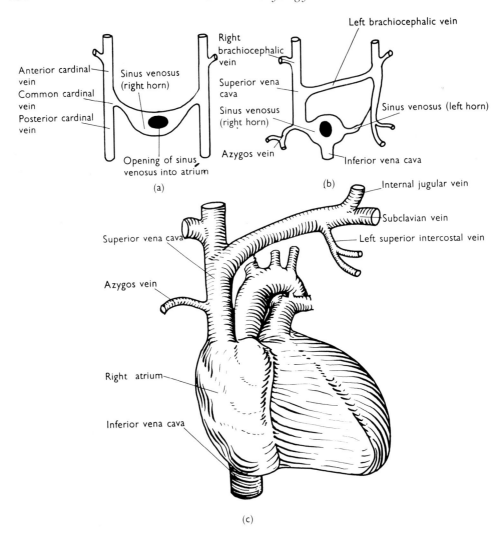

Fig. 12.5. (a) & (b) The development of the great veins. For explanation, see text. (c) The final arrangement of the great veins (branches of the arch of the aorta are not labelled).

clearly in Fig. 12.5. The new cross channel has become the left brachiocephalic vein, which joins the right brachiocephalic to form the superior vena cava. The terminal part of the right posterior cardinal becomes the terminal part of the azygos vein. As a result of these changes, the right horn of the sinus venosus becomes relatively large at the expense of the left horn, The latter, in fact, forms the coronary sinus of the adult while the cardinal veins system of the left side, caudal to the brachiocephalic vein atrophies in part, and also contributes to various small and unimportant veins. It can easily be understood that in rare cases in man (and normally in many animals such as the rat) there may be a left superior vena cava which ends in the coronary sinus.

The inferior vena cava

This vessel has a complex origin and only a simplified version of its development will be given here — in fact its development caudal to the origin of the renal veins is imperfectly understood. The initial venous drainage of the lower part of the body by the posterior cardinal veins has already been mentioned. Their role is taken over by a number of other longitudinally-running venous channels in the abdomen, of which only two will be mentioned here (Fig. 12.6). The bilateral veins of the *thoraco-lumbar line* (*supracardinal veins*) lie lateral and slightly dorsal to the aorta. Their largest tributaries are the common iliac veins and, as occurred in the formation of the superior vena cava, they soon become joined across the midline in the lower abdomen so that the left common iliac opens into the right thoraco-lumbar vein and the left thoraco-lumbar vein disappears. The other important longitudinal veins are the *subcardinals* which lie in the ventromedial part of the nephrogenic ridges and are therefore *ventral* to the plane of the aorta. The left and right subcardinals are connected across the midline by an *intersubcardinal anasto-*

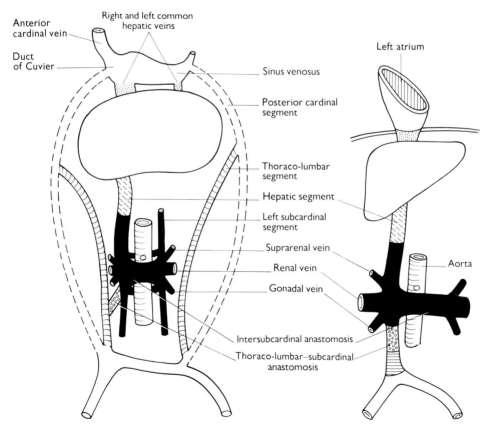

Fig. 12.6. Development of the inferior vena cava. The various segments that make up the adult vessel are shown on the smaller diagram. See text for description.

mosis just below the superior mesenteric artery and are also connected, slightly caudal to this, to the right thoraco-lumbar veins. The renal, suprarenal and gonadal veins drain into the subcardinal veins on each side at the level of the intersubcardinal anastomosis.

With the disappearance of the subcardinal and thoraco-lumbar veins on the left, the left renal, suprarenal and gonadal veins come to drain into the right subcardinal vein by means of the intersubcardinal anastomosis which thus represents that part of the left renal vein that crosses in front of the aorta. Cranially, the right subcardinal vein links up with the veins of the liver (see Chapter 16) and thus with the common hepatic vein. Caudally, it receives blood from the lower part of the right thoraco-lumbar vein by means of the anastomosis between them. The inferior vena cava is thus formed, from below upwards, by the right thoraco-lumbar vein (into which drain both common iliacs), the anastomotic channel between thoraco-lumbar and subcardinal veins, the right subcardinal vein (which receives the left renal vein via the intersubcardinal anastomosis), a venous channel that develops from a plexus joining the subcardinal vein to the common hepatic vein (*hepatic segment*) and finally the common hepatic vein itself (p.285) that opens into the right horn of the sinus venosus. The left common hepatic vein (a remnant of the terminal part of the left umbilical vein) disappears but its position is indicated in Fig. 16.9.

This complicated system of veins is not of purely academic interest. It explains the asymmetric drainage of the left and right gonadal and suprarenal veins, and the (rare) occurrence of a left inferior vena cava. Note that the post-renal segment of the inferior vena cava (i.e. that below the origin of the renal veins) develops from vessels that lie in a plane ventral to those giving rise to the pre-renal segment. Thus the right phrenic, suprarenal and renal arteries pass behind the inferior vena cava while the right gonadal and common iliac arteries pass in front of it. Finally, the various longitudinal veins are interconnected dorsal to the aorta as well as via the intersubcardinal anastomosis so as to form a complete venous ring — the *renal collar* — at the level of the renal veins. Thus the left renal vein may occasionally pass behind the aorta, or there may be a persistence of the complete renal collar.

The aortic arches

The first aortic arches develop very early and form an essential link in the primitive circulation. They are followed by second and third aortic arches which have a similar course but lie within the mesenchyme of the second and third branchial arches respectively. By the time the third aortic arch has formed fully, the first aortic arch has begun to break up and a short time later the fourth aortic arch develops and the second aortic arch disappears. Finally, the sixth aortic arch appears (it will be remembered that there is no fifth arch in the human embryo). As a result of this cranio-caudal gradient in development, the only aortic arches that contribute to the great vessels in the adult are the third, fourth and sixth. In fact, certain small vessels do develop from the first two arches, but they can be ignored.

To recapitulate, at this stage of development the aortic sac (p.196) which lies ventral to the pharynx is connected to the paired dorsal aortae by the third, fourth and sixth aortic arches. This may be seen in Figs. 12.7 and 12.8 which also show the cranial prolongation of the dorsal aortae towards the forebrain and a new vessel which grows cranially from the ventral end of the third arch on each side to form the external carotid artery. Another new vessel has also appeared on each side, running caudally from the sixth arch to supply the developing lungs (p.211). Before describing the subsequent fate of the aortic arches, it will now be necessary to discuss the concomitant development of the heart.

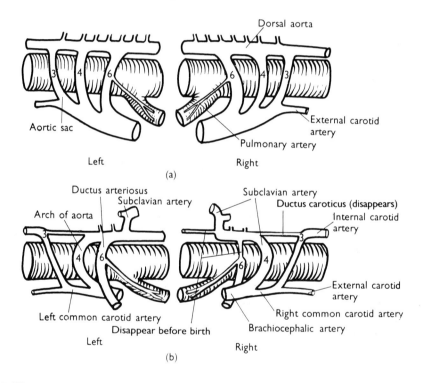

Fig. 12.7. The aortic arches. (a) The right and left 3rd, 4th and 6th aortic arches during the height of their development. (b) The subsequent fate of these arches.

The development of the heart

The heart tube, subdivided into its four chambers, grows much faster than the pericardium. Since it is fixed at its cranial and caudal ends, it must perforce become kinked and this occurs both in the anteroposterior and in the transverse planes. These acute bends of the tube are shown in Fig. 12.9. In the lateral view

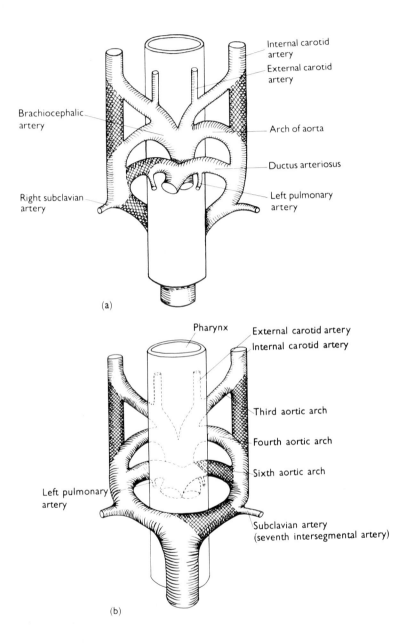

Fig. 12.8. The relation of the aortic arches to the pharynx, (a) viewed from in front and (b) viewed from behind. The cross-hatched vessels will later disappear. Diagram (b) will be found helpful in under-standing the congenital malformations that affect these vessels, particularly 'vascular rings'.

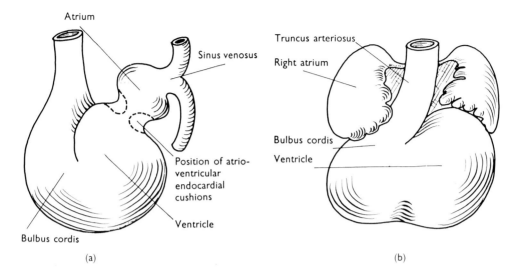

Atrium

Sinus venosus

Position of atrio-
ventricular
endocardial
cushions

Ventricle

Bulbus cordis

(a)

Truncus arteriosus

Right atrium

Bulbus cordis

Ventricle

(b)

Fig. 12.9. Lateral (a) and anterior (b) views of the developing heart after the formation of the acute bends in the heart tube. (a) is at a slightly earlier stage than (b).

(Fig. 12.9a) it will be seen that the bulbus cordis and the ventricle come to lie ventral to the atrium and the sinus venosus. The atrium leads into the ventricle through a narrow atrio-ventricular canal and in this, the endocardium proliferates to produce dorsal and ventral swellings, the *endocardial cushions*. Fig. 12.9b indicates how a further lateral twist of the tube brings the bulbus cordis to lie to the right of the ventricle so that the bulbus and ventricle soon form one common chamber in which a depression corresponding to the developing interventricular septum can already be seen. The thin-walled atrium, which is also showing signs externally of its subdivision into right and left atria, is growing rapidly so that it bulges forwards on either side of the truncus arteriosus (Fig. 12.9b). In order to follow the formation of the inter-atrial septum and the development of the individual atria it will be necessary also to study the further development of the sinus venosus.

The atria and the sinus venosus

As a result of the relative decrease in size of the left horn (*vide supra*) it is now the right horn of the sinus venosus that opens into the posterior wall of the atrium, rather towards the right side, by means of a slit-like opening which is guarded by a pair of *venous valves* (Fig. 12.10). These project like a pair of vertical lips into the atrium and, like lips, are fused with each other at either end. This may be seen diagrammatically in Fig. 12.11 which, together with Fig. 12.12, also shows how the dorsal and ventral endocardial cushions fuse with each other across the atrio-ventricular canal. This thus becomes divided into left and right canals. At about

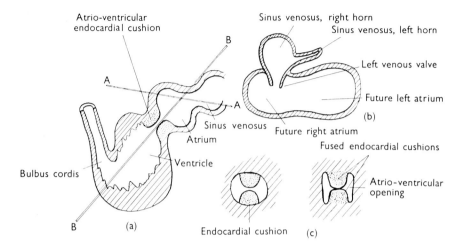

Fig. 12.10. (a) A longitudinal section through the developing heart. A section through A−A is shown at (b). The opening of the sinus venosus into the atrium is guarded by a pair of extremely thin venous valves. (c) The division of the atrio-ventricular canal into two, by means of the fusion of the atrio-ventricular cushions.

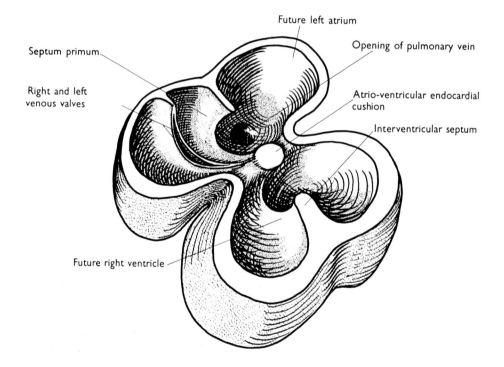

Fig. 12.11. The posterior part of a heart, opened along the line B−B in Fig. 12.10. The right and left sides of the heart are still in communication but the septum primum and interventricular septum are beginning to form.

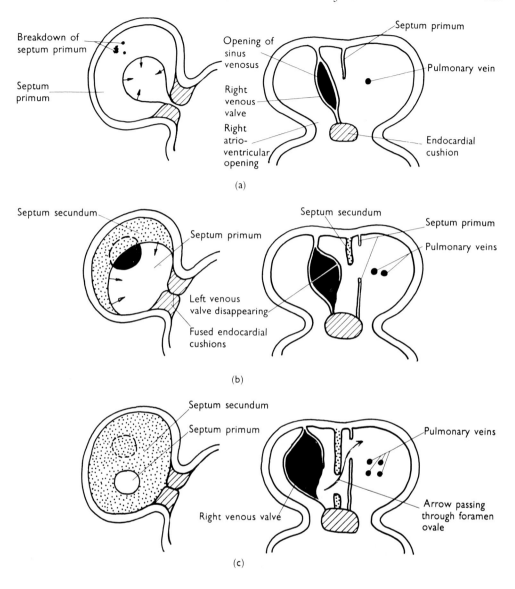

Fig. 12.12. Three stages in the development of the atrial septum. The left-hand diagrams show the right side of the developing septum and the right-hand diagrams show a section along the line B–B in Fig. 12.10. The septum secundum is dotted.

this time, too, a thin crescentic septum, the *septum primum*, begins to grow down into the atrium and thus initiates the division of the single chamber into right and left atria.

The subsequent development of the inter-atrial septum can be followed in Fig. 12.12. In the first pair of diagrams (Fig. 12.12a), the septum primum can be seen growing down towards the atrio-ventricular cushions. It must be remembered that oxygenated blood from the placenta (mixed with some venous blood, p.213) is being returned to the right atrium and it is essential that it should be possible for the majority of this blood to be passed through the inter-atrial septum to the left side of the heart as soon as possible so that it may pass from the left ventricle into the systemic circulation. At first, this takes place through the opening bounded by the down-growing crescentic edge of the septum primum — the *ostium primum*. Before the septum primum reaches the atrio-ventricular cushions, a new inter-atrial communication appears as a result of a perforation in the upper part of the septum — the *ostium secundum*. At the same time a new and thicker septum, the *septum secundum*, begins to grow down towards the atrio-ventricular cushions. This is also crescentic (Figs. 12.12 and 12.13) and it finally overlaps the opening in the septum primum (Fig. 12.12c). In this way, a flap-type valve is formed so that blood can pass freely from the right atrium to the left, but passage in the opposite direction is prevented by the apposition of the thin and mobile septum primum to the relatively rigid septum secundum.

Two other changes take place in the atria. In the left atrium, blood returning from both lungs enters through a single pulmonary vein. The walls of this vein become incorporated into the wall of the atrium, firstly as far as the bifurcation into left and right pulmonary veins, and finally as far as the next bifurcation, so that the originally single opening becomes two, and finally four, separate openings. On the right side, the sinus venosus becomes incorporated into the right atrium and the venous valves become relatively less prominent, the left valve usually disappearing completely (Fig. 12.12c). The adult right atrium is seen in Fig. 12.14. The sinus venosus (right horn) forms the smoother posterior portion of the atrium; into it opens the coronary sinus (originally the left horn of the sinus venosus, p.200), and the superior and inferior venae cavae. The part of the atrium derived from the embryonic atrium lies anterior to the crista terminalis from which the musculi pectinati pass forward. The septum secundum forms the thick *annulus ovalis* (*limbus fossa ovalis*) while the thin septum primum forms the floor of the fossa ovalis. The left venous valve disappears, but the right venous valve

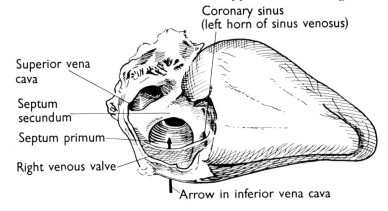

Fig. 12.13. A dissection of the right atrium in a fetus of about 5 months.

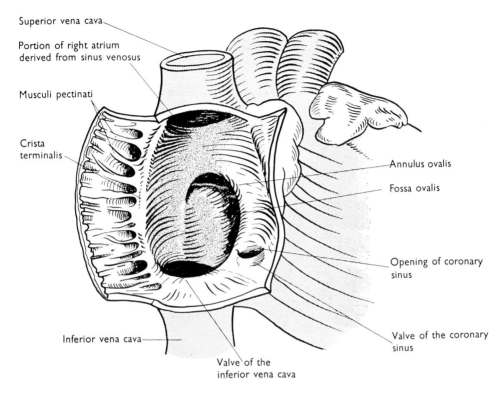

Superior vena cava

Portion of right atrium
derived from sinus venosus

Musculi pectinati

Crista
terminalis

Annulus ovalis

Fossa ovalis

Opening of coronary
sinus

Valve of the coronary
sinus

Inferior vena cava

Valve of the
inferior vena cava

Fig. 12.14. The interior of the adult right atrium, seen from in front.

forms the crista terminalis, the so-called valve of the inferior vena cava and the
valve of the coronary sinus.

The development of the ventricles and great arteries

Fig. 12.15 shows the early development of the interventricular septum which, at
this stage, is a crescentic structure with a large interventricular foramen above its
upper free border. Immediately cranial to the septum lies the bulbus cordis and
truncus arteriosus (p.196). The bulbus cordis in this region now becomes divided
into two canals by right and left *bulbar ridges*, which grow from each side and
ultimately fuse with each other to form a complete septum. This septum is prolonged distally into the truncus arteriosus, where it has a spiral form, so that the
two canals now spiral round each other (Figs. 12.15 and 12.16). Distally, one of
these canals becomes continuous with the sixth aortic arch (see p.211) while the
other joins the third and fourth arches. The former canal is destined to become the
pulmonary trunk and the latter the ascending aorta. The spiral form of the septum
explains why, in the adult, the pulmonary trunk is at first anterior to the aorta,
then on its left and finally behind it (compare Figs. 12.5 and 12.16). The tissue of
the bulbar ridges now grows down to close off the interventricular foramen,

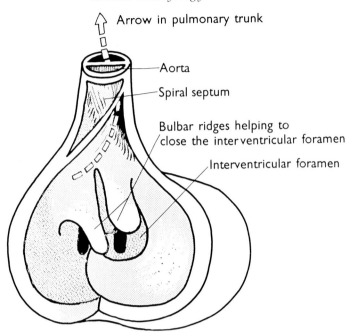

Fig. 12.15. The heart, opened from the front to show the spiral bulbar ridges.

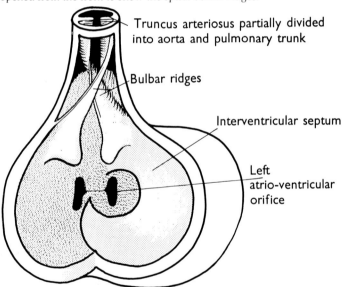

Fig. 12.16. A similar view to 12.15. Fusion of the right and left bulbar ridges has formed a separate aorta and pulmonary trunk. The interventricular foramen is partly closed and will later be closed completely by further development of the bulbar ridges and by proliferation of the tissue of the atrio-ventricular cushions. After closure of the interventricular foramen the right atrio-ventricular orifice will open exclusively into the right ventricle and the left orifice into the left ventricle.

together with a mass of tissue derived from the atrio-ventricular endocardial cushions (Fig. 12.16). This tissue forms the membranous part of the interventricular septum and growth takes place in such a way that the pulmonary trunk becomes continuous with the right ventricle and the aorta with the left. A part of

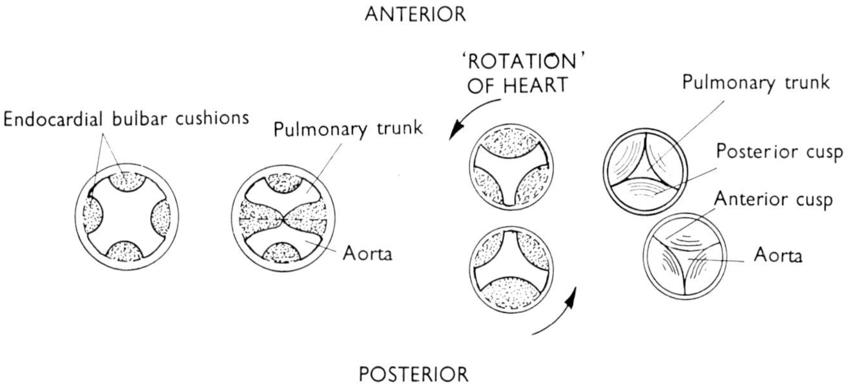

ANTERIOR

'ROTATION'
OF HEART

Fig. 12.17. The development of the aortic and pulmonary valves. The valves are depicted as being viewed from above.

each of the bulbar ridges, even before they meet across the lumen of the bulbus, becomes thickened to form the right and left *bulbar cushions,* and secondary anterior and posterior cushions also appear (Fig. 12.17). When the bulbus and truncus separate into aorta and pulmonary trunk, the right and left cushions also split so that each vessel contains three cushions, which become hollowed out to form three semi-lunar valves. A slight rotation of the heart occurs during development, so that the valves take up their adult positions.

It should be noted that it is not possible to determine the relative parts played by the bulbus cordis and the embryonic ventricle in the formation of the right and left ventricles of the adult.

Further development of the aortic arches

As has been mentioned, the only aortic arches that are of great importance are the third, fourth and sixth. These may be seen in Figs. 12.7 and 12.8. From the ventral end of the third arch the external carotid artery is growing forward into the region of the face while, from the middle of the sixth arch, another vessel is growing down to the developing lung. The dorsal aorta between the third and fourth arches (the *ductus caroticus*) becomes smaller and finally disappears (Fig. 12.7b). Blood passing into the third arch is, therefore, directed cranially towards the forebrain. The third arch, together with the cranial part of the dorsal aorta, thus forms the internal carotid artery while the common carotid is produced as a result of the elongation of the aortic sac just proximal to the junction of internal and external carotids.

On the left side, the fourth arch enlarges to form the arch of the aorta from which the left common carotid may now be said to arise. The sixth arch is also large; its proximal part, together with the vessel that passes down to the lung, forms the left pulmonary artery (it will be remembered that after the division of the truncus arteriosus by the spiral septum, the pulmonary trunk becomes continuous with the sixth arch). The distal part of the left sixth arch becomes the

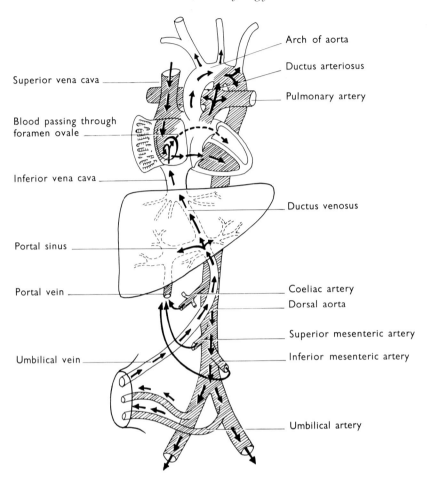

Arch of aorta

Ductus arteriosus

Pulmonary artery

Superior vena cava

Blood passing through
foramen ovale

Inferior vena cava

Ductus venosus

Portal sinus

Coeliac artery

Dorsal aorta

Portal vein

Superior mesenteric artery

Inferior mesenteric artery

Umbilical vein

Umbilical artery

Fig. 12.18. A diagram of the fetal circulation. The cross-hatching represents de-oxygenated or mixed blood but it is not possible, in a black and white diagram, to illustrate the precise degree of mixing. Further details are given in the text.

ductus arteriosus (p.214). The seventh intersegmental artery becomes greatly enlarged to form the subclavian artery and the subsequent 'descent' of the heart (p.176) causes it to undergo a relative ascent to its adult position.

On the right side the fourth arch persists and, together with a part of the right dorsal aorta and the seventh intersegmental artery, forms the right subclavian artery. The proximal part of the right sixth arch, together with the vessels which grew down from it to the lung, becomes the right pulmonary artery. The distal part of the sixth arch and the right dorsal area caudal to the seventh intersegmental aorta disappear completely.

The relation of the aortic arches, and their derivatives, to the pharynx are best understood from Fig. 12.8 which explains the semi-spiral course of the great vessels around the trachea and oesophagus in the adult. It will also be found useful in understanding some of the anomalies of development which will be described later.

The course in the adult of the nerves associated with the branchial arches can be appreciated when it is remembered that in each arch, except the sixth, the nerve lies cranial to the corresponding artery (p.174, Figs. 11.1 and 11.2). In the sixth arch, the nerve (recurrent laryngeal) lies caudal to the sixth aortic arch. During the 'descent' of the heart, this nerve becomes drawn caudally by the sixth arch so that in the adult the recurrent laryngeal nerve on the left side hooks under the ligamentum arteriosum. On the right side, however, where most of the sixth arch disappears, the nerve slips up to the fourth arch and therefore hooks under the subclavian artery.

The fetal circulation

The circulation in the fetus is so designed that oxygenated blood and nutrients can return to the heart from the placenta, the blood then being distributed throughout the body and returned in a de-oxygenated state to the placenta for re-oxygenation, elimination of carbon dioxide and other waste products of metabolism and further collection of nutrients. The lungs and the liver, in fetal life, are by-passed by three vascular short circuits or shunts — the *foramen ovale* in the inter-atrial septum, the *ductus arteriosus* between the left pulmonary artery and the aorta and the *ductus venosus* in the liver (Fig. 12.18).

Blood returning from the placenta through the umbilical vein has its haemo-globin about 80 per cent saturated by an oxygen tension (pO_2) of 30–40 mm Hg (such high saturation at a low pO_2 is made possible by fetal haemoglobin having a particularly high affinity for oxygen see p.105). When this blood reaches the liver, much of it passes through the hepatic sinusoids to the inferior vena cava. Between one third and two thirds of this blood, however, passes straight through the ductus venosus into the inferior vena cava, thus short-circuiting the liver. A sphincter mechanism in the ductus wall near the entrance of the umbilical vein serves to regulate this flow.

Upon entering the right atrium from the inferior vena cava, the stream of oxygenated blood meets the curved free border of the relatively rigid septum secundum which, like the bows of a ship, divides the stream into two parts and is, for this reason, often known as the *crista dividens*. About 60 per cent of this stream of blood is diverted by the crista dividens into the left atrium, from which it passes to the left ventricle for distribution via the aorta to the systemic circulation. The first branches of the aorta pass to the coronary circulation and then to the head and upper limbs. The privileged position in which the brain thus finds itself must undoubtedly contribute to the rapid early growth of this organ in comparison with the rest of the body.

The remaining 40 per cent of the inferior vena cava blood is deflected into the right atrium where it mingles with the venous blood returning from the heart and upper limbs via the superior vena cava. This blood, which has a much lower pO_2

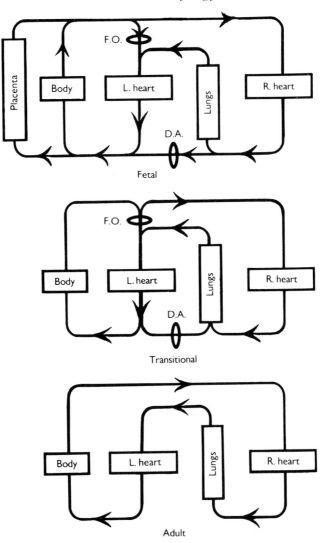

Fig. 12.19. A schematic representation of the changes which take place in the fetal circulation at birth. (After Barn, Davies, Mott & Widdecombe, 1954. From *Foetal and Neonatal Pathology* by Geoffrey S. Dawes, Copyright 1968. Year Book Medical Publishers, Inc. Used by permission.)

than that entering the left ventricle, passes into the right ventricle and pulmonary trunk. The muscular pulmonary arteries are in a constricted condition because of the low pO_2 of the blood within them and because the unexpanded nature of the lungs causes them to be tightly coiled. There is, therefore, a high resistance to perfusion of the pulmonary vascular tree and this coupled with the fact that vascular resistance in the placenta is low causes about 90 per cent of the pulmonary artery blood to pass through the ductus arteriosus into the descending aorta. The ductus itself is almost as large as the aorta, has a thick media of smooth muscle and in the later stages of development a number of muscular swellings or mounds beneath the intima. As might be expected from this vascular arrangement, the wall of the right ventricle is as thick as, or even thicker than, the wall of the left and it is only during the neonatal period that the left ventricle becomes by far the thicker of the two. The neonatal electrocardiogram clearly shows this right ventricular dominance.

Blood from the descending aorta passes to the gut (from which it is returned via the portal vein to the liver (p.285) and to the body wall and lower limbs (from which it is returned via the inferior vena cava). Most of the aortic blood, however, is conveyed to the placenta by the two umbilical arteries.

Changes in the fetal circulation at birth

These changes are shown diagrammatically in Fig. 12.19. When the baby is born, the thick muscular walls of the umbilical vessels contract as a result of thermal and mechanical stimuli (the umbilical vessels have no nerve supply in the cord) and pulsation in the umbilical arteries can no longer be felt. The falling pressure in the portal sinus (p.285) causes narrowing of the opening of the ductus venosus, aided by the contraction of the smooth muscle in its wall. There is some evidence, however, that closure of the ductus venosus begins even before birth. With the baby's first gasps, the lungs expand and improve the oxygenation of the blood. Under these influences, the tortuous pulmonary arterioles become uncoiled, allowing almost all the right ventricular outflow to enter the lungs. This progressive fall in pulmonary resistance continues for 3–4 weeks as a result of the dissolution of the thick muscular media, until it reaches about 20 per cent of the systemic resistance. The amount of blood returning to the left side of the heart is thus increased at the expense of that passing through the ductus arteriosus and the blood pressure in the left atrium rises above that in the right atrium. This causes the thin and flexible septum primum to be pressed against the more rigid septum secundum, thus closing the foramen ovale. These septa normally become adherent to form the fossa ovalis and its limbus.

With the establishment of regular respiration, the fluid in the lungs rapidly becomes resorbed and the pO_2 plateaus at a much higher level. This vital transition begins the closure of the ductus arteriosus. Initially, this is by contraction of the smooth muscle both of the media and of the subendothelial mounds. There is considerable evidence that prostaglandins of the E series are responsible for maintaining the patency of the ductus before birth and inhibitors of prostaglandin synthetase, such as indomethacin, may be used to effect its closure in cases where the normal closure has failed to take place (*vide infra*).

The closing down of the three vascular shunts in the embryo are rapid and, at first, 'physiological' rather than 'anatomical' closures. They depend on a number of factors, including the state of oxygenation of the fetus. Blood may still be shunted through the ductus venosus for hours or even days after birth and blood may also occasionally pass through the ductus arteriosus for up to 2 weeks after birth. Later, however, the 'short circuits' become permanently closed and their remnants, like those of the umbilical vessels, are represented only by fibrous tissue. The two umbilical arteries become the *medial umbilical ligaments* of the adult; the umbilical vein is represented by the *ligamentum teres* and the ductus venosus by the *ligamentum venosum*. The ductus arteriosus forms the *ligamentum arteriosum* round which, since it represents the sixth aortic arch, the left recurrent laryngeal nerve passes.

The lymphatic system

The lymphatic capillaries, like the blood capillaries, develop first as small spaces in the mesenchyme. These link up with each other to form a network of lymphatics and also link up with six *lymph sacs* situated in the lower part of the neck and in the abdomen in close relationship with, and (in the neck) opening into, the embryonic venous system. One of these sacs later forms the cisterna chyli, which gives origin to the thoracic duct. The development of the epithelial 'skeleton' of other parts of the lymphatic system are dealt with in other chapters (the tonsils and thymus in Chapter 11 and the spleen in Chapter 16) and it remains only to describe briefly the manner in which these structures, along with the lymph nodes, receive their population of lymphocytes.

   The primary origin of the lymphocytes is from primitive stem cells that are found in the yolk sac mesenchyme and later in the liver and spleen. These cells enter the bone marrow (the only source of stem cell proliferation after birth) and divide to form lymphoblasts and finally 'neutral' or 'uncommitted' lymphocytes. These pass into the blood stream and enter various organs where they undergo a process of maturation to form T- or B-lymphocytes. The T-lymphocytes mature in the thymus and the process of lymphopoiesis can be observed in the fetal thymus from a very early stage. A little later, lymphopoiesis is seen to be occurring in the lymph nodes and tonsils and later still in the spleen. The lymphocyte count in the blood is about $1000/mm^3$ at 3 months and $5000-10\,000$ at 6 months.

The immune system

Of the five classes of immunoglobulins that circulate in the maternal blood, only IgG is able to cross the placental barrier and at birth has the same level in both maternal and fetal blood. This is, therefore, able to provide a defence against infection during the first few weeks of post-natal life. The fetus' own immuno-globulins begin to appear in the blood at about 20 weeks when IgG and IgM can be found. The other immunoglobulins are only present at very low levels before birth. Some organisms, such as those of rubella (German measles) and syphilis, are able to cross the placenta and in such cases the fetus is able to respond by producing high levels of IgM and IgA in the serum.

After birth the levels of the immunoglobulins begin to rise, although at different rates. The rise in titre continues over a number of years — IgG, for example, does not reach the adult level until the age of seven. Nevertheless, even very young babies can respond to antigenic stimuli by the rapid production of antibodies so that immunization against certain organisms is feasible in the first few months.

As is mentioned in Chapter 16, it is doubtful whether the human infant can absorb immunoglobulins from colostrum as occurs in some other mammals, even though IgA is found at much higher levels in the colostrum than in the maternal serum. This IgA, however, is not digested and can thus act locally to prevent the multiplication of pathogenic organisms in the gut.

Developmental anomalies of the heart and great vessels

Structural abnormalities of the heart and great vessels are among the commonest of congenital defects and account for more deaths in infancy than all other congenital anomalies put together, with an incidence of approximately 8 per 1000 live born children. They occur either as isolated defects or in various combinations. Little is understood of the aetiology of these malformations. In most instances they are probably the consequence of an interaction between some undefined environmental agent(s) and hereditary factors. Genetic vulnerability is especially high for isolated atrial and ventricular septal defects. A minority of congenital heart defects are integral parts of well recognised syndromes, such as Down's (21 trisomy), Edward's (18 trisomy) and Turner's (XO), or those caused by specific external influences (for example, rubella or thalidomide). Of the individual cardiac anomalies, *ventricular septal defect* (VSD) is most frequent, occurring in about 30 per cent of infants with congenital heart disease; *patent ductus arteriosus* (PDA) is the next most common (15 per cent). The six other most often encountered defects are — *atrial septal defect* (ASD), *aortic stenosis, coarctation of the aorta, transposition, Fallot's tetralogy* and *pulmonary stenosis*. Bicuspid aortic valve (possibly asymptomatic) may also be very common.

The clinical features of congenital heart defects show great diversity. Babies may present within a few hours of birth with heart failure or cyanosis. Others may not declare these symptoms until a few weeks, or even months, after birth. Small defects may not be found until a routine medical examination, such as that which takes place at school entry. It is worthwhile noting that even the most severe of heart defects will, by themselves, rarely cause intra-uterine death (unlike many other congenital defects, such as neural tube abnormalities). This is because the primary function of the fetal heart is simply to drive blood round the body in order to distribute oxygen to, and remove waste products from, its organs and tissues. The lungs are not needed. It is only when the placenta is removed from the circulation at birth and respiration comes to depend upon an intact cardio-respiratory system that a structurally intact heart is required for continued survival.

Great advances have been made in the investigation and management of cardiac defects over the last 10–20 years. Defects which were previously incompatible with life (for example, transposition of the great vessels) are now amenable to surgical correction. An understanding of the embryology of congenital heart defects is essential for their functional consequences and principles of management to be understood. In this chapter only developmental anomalies which occur most often in clinical practice will be described and it should be remembered that they may appear in different combinations. The classification adopted here is clinical and is based on the age and the manner in which congenital heart defects present.

Anomalies of the changes at birth

In the first few days after birth, the closure of the foramen ovale is often reversible so that any rise in pressure in the right atrium will create a shunt of blood into the left atrium. This event underlines the benign cyanotic episodes which occasionally occur with crying (which causes an increase in pulmonary vascular resistance). Normally, the two components of the septum fuse completely in the first few years of life. Occasionally fusion does not occur so that a probe can be passed from the left atrium into the right (*probe patency*). As long as the septa overlap this condition will be symptomless, since the higher pressure on the left side of the septum will keep the septum primum pressed against the septum secundum. If, for any reason later in life, pressure should rise in the right atrium cyanosis may occur due to a right/left shunt through the patent opening.

Patent ductus arteriosus

Failure of the ductus arteriosus to close, or to remain closed, most commonly occurs in very small prematurely born babies with surfactant deficient respiratory difficulties (see *hyaline membrane disease* — Chapter 13). Hypoxia, together with other as yet ill-defined influences, causes prostaglandin E_1 to be produced locally and this keeps the ductus patent. Hypoxia also increases pulmonary vascular resistance and this leads to shunting of blood across the ductus in the first few days in the right to left direction (i.e. from the pulmonary artery to the aorta) and this lowers the oxygen supply to the tissues even further. As lung function gradually improves with treatment shunting becomes left to right in direction, the magnitude depending on the diameter and pressure gradient across the duct between the aorta and pulmonary artery. This, in turn, reflects differences in the vascular resistance of the two channels. An increased blood flow through the lungs decreases lung distensibility thereby increasing the work of the breathing and diminishing oxygenation even further. Unless the ductus can be closed the mortality is very high.

The principal clinical features of a patent ductus arteriosus include easily palpable collapsing pulses (due to a high pulse pressure), a loud systolic heart murmur often extending into the diastolic phase, and heart failure. Chest X-ray will show an engorged pulmonary vascular tree. Surgical ligation of the ductus can be undertaken but, in such tiny infants, it is a very hazardous procedure although, with improved surgical and anaesthetic methods, the surgical approach is now being more widely practised. 'Pharmacological' closure is currently preferred using the drug indomethacin to interfere with the synthesis of prostaglandins of the E series which are responsible for keeping the ductus open.

Congenital heart defects causing problems in the first few days after birth

Cyanosis as the principal symptom

Cyanosis refers to a dusky bluish appearance of the skin and mucus membranes. It is due to the presence of more than 5 g of reduced haemoglobin per 100 ml of blood and may be caused by insufficient oxygenation of the blood or to a right/left shunt, i.e. the shunting of venous blood into the arterial system. Its presence at, or soon after, birth is an ominous sign of a severe congenital heart defect.

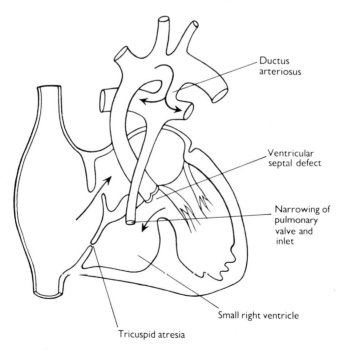

Fig. 12.20. Tricuspid atresia. Cyanosis is due to shunting de-oxygenated blood through the patent foramen ovale. The right ventricle is very small and pulmonary stenosis is often present. Blood reaches the lungs via a defect in the interventricular septum and a patent ductus arteriosus.

Atresia of the tricuspid and pulmonary valves (right heart hypoplasia)

Failure of either tricuspid or pulmonary valves and their corresponding orifices to develop normally (atresia) may be total or partial. Both cause different levels of obstruction to the flow of blood to the lungs. In tricuspid atresia (Fig. 12.20) there is obliteration of the right atrio-ventricular orifice and it is always associated with under-development of the right ventricle, patency of the foramen ovale and a small ventricular septal defect; narrowing of the pulmonary valve often exists. In pulmonary atresia (Fig. 12.21) the pulmonary artery and right ventricle are under-developed, the lungs receiving most of their blood through a patent ductus arteriosus.

The principal clinical feature associated with these defects is marked central cyanosis noted soon after birth. This is due to the desaturated blood that returns to the right atrium having to be shunted to the left side of the heart through an atrial septal defect. The left ventricle will, therefore, be ejecting a mixture of this desaturated blood and oxygenated blood returning from the lungs.

The prognosis for infants with tricuspid atresia and pulmonary atresia is poor. Immediate survival after birth for those with pulmonary atresia depends on the ductus arteriosus remaining open in order to allow blood to enter the lungs and, to this end, much interest is currently being shown in medical means for keeping the ductus patent by the administration of E type prostaglandins. These are potent relaxants of the ductus arteriosus, which maintains its patency until a palliative

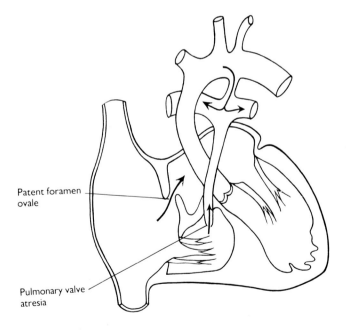

Patent foramen
ovale

Pulmonary valve
atresia

Fig. 12.21. Pulmonary valve atresia. Cyanosis is caused by the shunting of de-oxygenated blood through a patent foramen ovale. Blood can enter the lungs only through a patent ductus arteriosus.

surgical procedure can be undertaken to divert the systemic blood to the pulmonary circulation via a shunt usually created between the aorta and the right pulmonary artery. In tricuspid atresia immediate survival depends largely on the adequacy of the interatrial shunt which might require urgent enlarging by balloon septostomy (*vide infra*, transposition). If survival in infancy is achieved radical reconstructive surgery might later be undertaken to the right ventricle, pulmonary valve and pulmonary artery. Results of these procedures are, however, usually disappointing.

Transposition of the great arteries
(Fig. 12.22)

Transposition is the most common single cause of cyanotic heart disease in the newborn period. It is often associated with other cardiac anomalies. Its principal feature is that the aorta and pulmonary arteries arise on the wrong sides of the interventricular septum due to failure of the spiral septum to develop its normal configuration. The aorta, therefore, arises anteriorly from the morphological right ventricle and the pulmonary artery arises posteriorly from the morphological left ventricle. Because of the anatomical mis-matching, desaturated systemic venous blood returning to the right atrium passes into the right ventricle and thence to the body via the aorta: oxygenated pulmonary venous blood is routed via the left

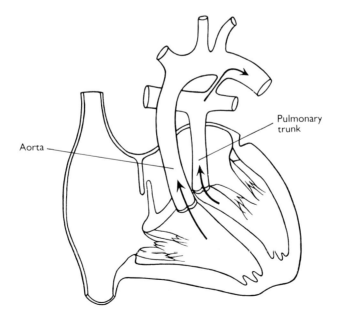

Fig. 12.22. Transposition of the great vessels. The aorta arises anteriorly from a morphological right ventricle, the pulmonary trunk from the left ventricle. A patent ductus arteriosus accompanies this anomaly and serves to increase the amount of oxygenated blood in the aorta.

ventricle back into the pulmonary circulation. Two parallel separate circulations therefore exist, an arrangement which is incompatible with life unless there is some mixing of blood. Initially this occurs through a stretched foramen ovale (*vide infra*). A patent ductus arteriosus will also invariably be present helping to increase systemic arterial pO$_2$. Without surgical treatment death will occur within a few months after birth.

Babies with transposition typically present with deep cyanosis immediately after birth. An early suspicion of the anomaly is essential in order that urgent cardiac catheterization can be undertaken to establish the diagnosis following which a palliative procedure can be undertaken to increase atrial mixing. This is the Rashkind manoeuvre of *balloon septostomy* in which a catheter with a balloon in its tip is passed via a peripheral vein into the right atrium and through the foramen ovale into the left atrium. The balloon is then inflated and pulled back sharply into the right atrium tearing a hole in the inter-atrial septum thereby improving mixing of circulations and increasing the available oxygen in aortic blood. If successful this procedure buys valuable time before definitive surgical correction is undertaken towards the end of the first year.

Heart failure as the principal symptom

Tachycardia (raised heart rate), tachypnoea (raised respiratory rate), an enlarged

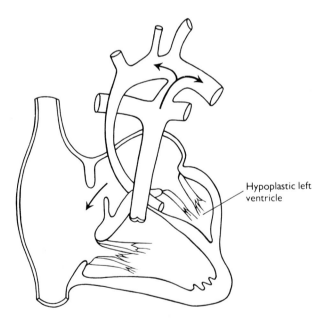

Hypoplastic left ventricle

Fig. 12.23. Hypoplastic left heart syndrome. Blood returning from the lungs can only reach the body by passing through a patent foramen ovale into the right atrium and thence via the right ventricle and a patent ductus arteriosus, into the aorta. Closure of the ductus will cause immediate death.

heart, hepatic enlargement and abnormal breath sounds (crepitations) are all symptoms of heart failure in infancy and, if they present within the early days after birth, are very ominous features.

Hypoplastic left heart syndrome

A wide spectrum of congenital cardiac anomalies cause heart failure. They include hypoplasia of the systemic outflow tract involving, in various degrees and combinations, the left ventricle, mitral valve, aortic valve and ascending aorta (Fig. 12.23).

Since there is an obstruction to the outflow of the left ventricle, oxygenated blood returning from the lungs can enter the systemic circulation only by passing through an atrial septal defect into the right side of the heart and then via a patent ductus arteriosus into the aorta. When the ductus closes after birth this outflow path is obstructed causing a fall in systemic output and pulmonary congestion. The baby soon dies in severe congestive cardiac failure. Babies with hypoplastic left heart syndrome are often normal for a few days after birth and even the peripheral pulses are normal due to the systemic circulation being fed by the ductus arteriosus. No re-constructive surgery is available.

Coarctation of the aorta

This is a narrowing of the lumen of the descending thoracic aorta at various sites below the origin of the left subclavian artery. It represents variations in the degree of maldevelopment of the fourth aortic arch. There are two principal types according to the site of the constriction in relation to the entrance of the ductus — pre-ductal and post-ductal. It is the pre-ductal (infantile) type which usually causes problems in the newborn period. (The post-ductal variety is described later on p.231).

Pre-ductal coarctation

In this variety the aortic narrowing is proximal to the site of the insertion of the ductus arteriosus and extends usually from the area of origin of the left subclavian artery (Fig 12.24). Sometimes it can extend backwards to the ascending aorta as part of the hypoplastic left heart syndrome (cf. above). A pre-ductal coarctation is usually a very severe type of malformation since, in about 40 per cent of cases, it is associated with other anomalies of the cardiovascular system, particularly patent ductus arteriosus and ventricular septal defect.

Pre-ductal coarctation usually presents in very early infancy. A soft systolic murmur might be the earliest sign detected at the routine examination of the newborn baby. Femoral pulses are usually normal since the patent ductus arteriosus allows blood to pass to the lower limbs. However, there will often be

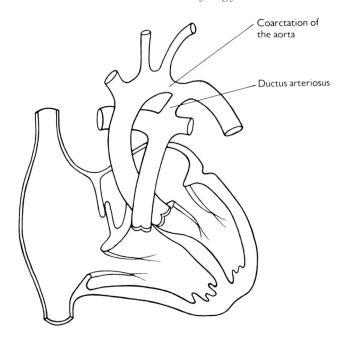

Fig. 12.24. Preductal coarctation of the aorta. The narrowed segment is immediately proximal to the ductus.

differential cyanosis with blueness in the lower part of the body (desaturated ductus blood) and pinkness in the upper part (supplied from the aortic arch). Sudden deterioration in the baby's condition will take place when the ductus closes causing an increase in pulmonary venous pressure and severe heart failure. A fall in systemic outflow leads to circulatory collapse and oliguria (inadequate production of urine). Urgent cardiac catheterization is indicated to confirm the diagnosis. Treatment requires the surgical resection of the coarctation with an end-to-end anastomosis or the use of part of the left subclavian artery to widen the circumference of the aorta (Hamilton flap).

Heart failure and cyanosis

Anomalous pulmonary venous drainage

These anomalies are due to failure of the common pulmonary vein and its immediate tributaries (usually two from each lung) to be absorbed normally into the left atrium. Drainage into some other part of the venous system has developed. Three patterns exist:
1 Supra-cardiac drainage via the innominate vein.
2 Cardiac drainage into the coronary sinus (incompatible with survival).
3 Infracardiac drainage into the portal vein and thence into the ductus venosus.

Whatever the type of the anomalous venous drainage, blood from the lung has to return via systemic veins into the right atrium. Initial survival depends, therefore, on the communication between atria (usually by an atrial septal defect of the ostium secundum or a stretched foramen ovale) to allow filling of the left side of the heart. With infracardiac venous drainage the return of blood from the lungs is often obstructed due to impedance to flow through the portal vein, Severe heart failure will usually present soon after birth and it is common for these babies to die early in the neonatal period. In supracardiac venous drainage, blood returns from the lungs in a common channel made up usually of a dilated left superior vena cava and left innominate vein. The typical clinical presentation is one of heart failure and cyanosis in the first few days after birth. The chest X-ray often shows a typical supracardiac shadow of the anomalous vein, the 'sugar loaf' appearance. Treatment is by surgical anastomosis of the left superior vena cava to the left atrium.

Miscellaneous presentations

As can be seen from Fig. 12.8, during normal development the pharynx (and, therefore, the oesophagus and trachea) are completely surrounded by the developing aortic arch system. Stridor (noisy breathing) from birth is an important symptom of a bilateral aortic arch caused by the persistence of a right aortic arch: the left and right arches together form a vascular ring around the oesophagus and trachea. Other anomalies emerging through maldevelopment of the aortic arch system are very rare. The diagnosis can be confused with the stridor due to a congenital soft larynx (p.241). Following confirmation by an aortogram, a bilateral aortic arch can be surgically corrected by dividing the narrower arch thereby releasing the pressure effects of the ring.

Abnormalities in heart position

Dextrocardia

If the heart is normal but all the thoracic viscera, including the heart, are reversed in position the complex anomaly is called *situs inversus*. This is not usually associated with significant heart defects and requires no further investigation.

Dextroversion

In this anomaly the heart is abnormally rotated — the other viscera are normal in position: this is nearly always associated with serious intracardiac congenital defects and is usually diagnosed as an incidental finding when investigating other major symptoms of suspected congenital heart defect.

Congenital heart defects presenting at 1−3 months

Heart failure as the principal symptom

Ventricular septal defect

This is the most common congenital heart anomaly. In 50 per cent of cases it occurs alone and in the remaining 50 per cent it is part of a more complex malformation. There are two types of abnormality:

1   a high defect in the membranous interventricular septum due to failure of the interventricular foramen to close beneath the aortic opening;

2   small defects, single or multiple, arising in the muscular septum itself.

There is a wide range of functional disturbance which depends mainly upon the size of the septal defect and the resulting left-to-right shunt (Fig. 12.25). Small defects allow some shunting of blood but are of little consequence. These might

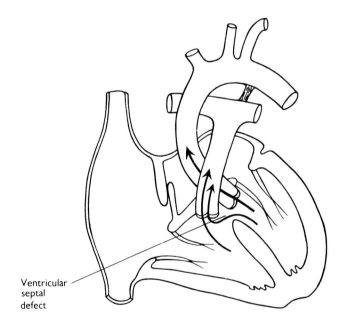

Fig. 12.25. Ventricular septal defect. This is due to failure of closure of the membranous part of the interventricular septum. Pulmonary blood flow is increased, the amount of increase depending upon the size of the shunt.

remain asymptomatic or be diagnosed as a soft heart murmur during routine examination — the 'innocent murmur'. Large defects allow large volumes of blood to shunt across the septum into the pulmonary vascular bed as the pulmonary vascular resistance falls below its high level at birth to reach 'adult' levels under normal circumstances by 2–3 weeks after birth. With large volumes of blood shunted into the pulmonary circulation lung compliance falls, the work of breathing increases, the left side of the heart becomes overloaded and heart failure results.

Symptoms of heart failure usually appear between 1 and 3 months. The infant will typically fail to thrive with tachypnoea (rapid breathing), increased respiratory muscle effort and feeding difficulty. Frequent chest infections might be a presenting symptom. The natural course of events for many ventricular septal defects is for spontaneous closure to take place during the first 6 years or so of life. This is especially the case with the single septal defect surrounded completely by muscle. The principal underlying management of the large defect is to control heart failure with drugs in anticipation of closure.

Irreversible pulmonary hypertension from a permanent elevation in vascular resistance can develop (though, fortunately, rarely) if the septal defect allows a large shunt which does not lessen over the first year. This can develop into a reversed shunt from right to left. Careful follow-up is needed for children with ventricular septal defects with regular clinical evaluation, chest X-ray and electrocardiography. If heart failure cannot be controlled, surgical closure of the defect usually with a pericardial patch will be indicated usually between the ages of 6 months and three years.

Small septal defects rarely cause functional changes. Often the accompanying murmurs are diagnosed, if not at birth then in early childhood during routine clinical examination. Such defects will usually undergo spontaneous closure. The only precaution required is to use antibiotic cover for dental extractions to prevent septic 'vegetations' (blood clots) forming on the endocardium — *subacute bacterial endocarditis*.

Ostium primum defect (Fig. 12.26)

The endocardial cushions of the atrio-ventricular canal contribute to the formation of the membranous part of the interventricular septum and the closure of the ostium primum (p.208) as well as to the atrio-ventricular valves themselves. If the endocardial cushions fail to develop normally, a complex lesion results — the *ostium primum defect (endocardial cushion defect; atrio-ventricular canal defect)*. It comprises defects of the atrial septum, ventricular septum, mitral valve and tricuspid valve. For unexplained reasons, about one third of all infants with ostium primum defect have Down's syndrome. The clinical features depend on the size of the cardiac defect, especially the extent of regurgitation through the cleft mitral

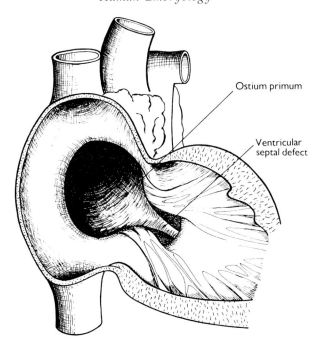

Fig. 12.26. Ostium primum defect. There is a combination of atrial and ventricular septal defects because of failure of normal development of the atrio-ventricular cushions.

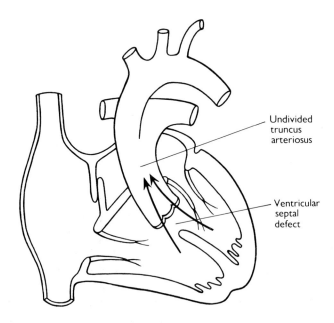

Fig. 12.27. Persistent truncus arteriosus. The trunk common to both aorta and pulmonary trunk overrides a ventricular septal defect. Pulmonary blood flow is increased.

valve. Typically a left-to-right shunt occurs at birth at both atrial and ventricular levels. Symptoms are usually similar to those of a ventricular septal defect with heart failure, failure to thrive and recurrent chest infections presenting usually in the first few months of life. It is a far more serious lesion than ventricular septal defect, however, since spontaneous closure is rare and definitive surgery technically more difficult. Pulmonary hypertension and vascular disease develop earlier than with an isolated ventricular septal defect. Surgical repair is technically very difficult with a high mortality.

Persistent truncus arteriosus

In this anomaly the ridges that form the spiral septum in the bulbus and truncus arteriosus fail in their fusion and growth to meet the interventricular septum. The pulmonary arteries will arise therefore from a large vessel common to the pulmonary and aortic trunks (Fig. 12.27). Severe heart failure develops early in the first few weeks after birth. The presentation is often similar to a severe type of ventricular septal defect. Banding of the pulmonary artery will be needed to protect the lungs against later irreversible vascular disease, allowing an attempt at total correction later in childhood. The long-term prognosis is very poor.

Cyanosis as the leading symptom

Fallot's tetralogy (Fig. 12.28)

In this anomaly a ventricular septal defect (membranous type) is associated with a narrow right ventricular outflow region (*pulmonary infundibular and valvular stenosis*), the aorta arises directly above the septal defect from both ventricular cavities (*over-riding aorta*) and there is right ventricular hypertrophy. It is primarily the result of anterior displacement of the spiral septum. Because of the right ventricular outflow obstruction, some of the blood expelled from the right ventricle flows through the septal defect into the aorta, resulting in varying degrees of cyanosis. The symptoms are, typically, shortness of breath on exercise and cyanotic episodes, later giving rise to extreme pallor. A major contributory factor to these attacks is spasm of the muscle of the infundibulum. The constant cyanosis leads to *polycythaemia* (an attempt on the part of the body to compensate by increasing the number of red blood cells) which, in turn, increases the viscosity of the blood and consequent risks of cerebral thrombosis. In young children squatting is a typical physical sign. This posture helps to reduce the right-to-left shunt.

Management is by surgery. Initially blood flow to the lungs has to be improved by a shunt — subclavian artery to pulmonary artery (*Taussig-Blalock shunt*) or ascending aorta to right pulmonary artery (*Waterston shunt*). These procedures are usually undertaken during the first year. After this age primary definitive correc-

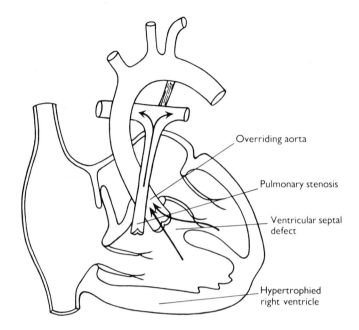

Fig. 12.28. Fallot's tetralogy. The four components are: pulmonary stenosis, overriding aorta, ventricular septal defect and hypertrophy of the right ventricle. The right-left shunt across the septal defect produces cyanosis.

tion is undertaken — resecting the infundibular stenosis, pulmonary valvotomy, closure of ventricular septal defect and removal of any shunt which has been undertaken. Prognosis is excellent.

Congenital heart defects presenting in later childhood

Patent ductus in older children

A patent ductus arteriosus can be diagnosed *de novo* in later childhood without there having been any neonatal illness. In babies this might present with failure to thrive and respiratory infections in the same manner as a ventricular septal defect. Diagnosis is confirmed by cardiac catheterization which will also exclude other anomalies. Surgical ligation is always indicated. It is interesting that the incidence of this later type of patent ductus increases with altitude due, it is believed, to lower oxygen tension in the blood relaxing the duct wall musculature.

Atrial septal defect (ostium secundum defect)

This results from the failure of the septum secundum to grow normally or to excessive resorption of the septum primum leading to a large communication between the left and right atria (Fig. 12.29). In contrast with the ostium primum defect, the secundum defect rarely presents problems in early childhood. It is usually diagnosed later in childhood, or early in adult life, during medical examination prompted by the hearing of a heart murmur which is due to increased flow through the pulmonary valve. Unlike a ventricular septal defect, pulmonary vascular resistance does not increase until early to middle adult life so that there is no real urgency to patch up the defect. If diagnosed in childhood the operation is optimally performed between six and ten years. Ostium secundum defect is sometimes accompanied by a partial anomalous pulmonary venous drainage usually affecting one or more veins from the right lung into the superior vena cava. Unlike total anomalous pulmonary venous drainage it is usually a chance finding and causes no symptoms on its own.

Aortic coarctation, post-ductal (adult) type

In this type of aortic coarctation the narrowing is at, or just distal to, the site of the insertion of the ductus arteriosus which is represented usually by a fibrous ligament (Fig. 12.30). In contrast with the pre-ductal variety it is less often associated with other congenital abnormalities. Sometimes post-ductal aortic coarctation is

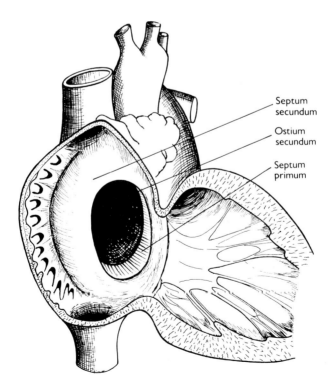

Septum
secundum

Ostium
secundum

Septum
primum

Fig. 12.29. Atrial septal defect of the ostium secundum type.

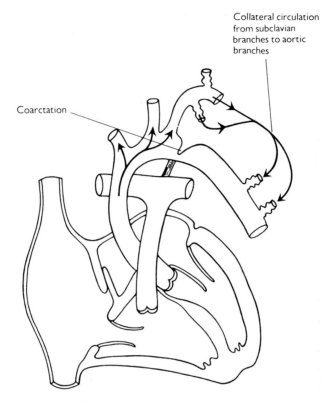

Fig. 12.30. Post-ductal coarctation of the aorta.

found with other defects, for example in Marfan's syndrome. It is commonly diagnosed during routine school medical examination when a systolic heart murmur, poor femoral pulses and hypertension in the arms are noted. X-ray of the rib cage will often show erosion of the lower borders of the ribs due to large collateral blood vessels which have been supplying the lower part of the body. These anastomoses are carrying blood from the subclavian artery to the aorta below the stenosis via the anastomosis around the scapula, the internal thoracic artery and the posterior intercostal arteries. Surgery is usually undertaken between the ages of five and ten years in order to avoid the complications of cerebral haemorrhage and dissecting aneurysm (a rupture of portions of the wall of the great vessels). The narrowed section is removed and end-to-end anastomosis performed. The outcome is excellent.

Pulmonary stenosis

Narrowing of the pulmonary valve as an isolated anomaly rarely presents a major problem in early childhood. It is usually discovered in the course of a medical examination when a heart murmur is heard in the pulmonary area. Following definitive investigation with cardiac catheterization surgery might, at some stage, be indicated. Very mild degrees of pulmonary stenosis are best left alone.

Aortic stenosis

This is a far more serious anomaly than pulmonary stenosis. It might be diagnosed on hearing a murmur during a routine examination. Another presentation in childhood is syncope (fainting) due to a transient interference with blood flow through the aortic valve. Following confirmation by cardiac catheterization, surgery will be needed involving valvotomy or even prosthetic valve replacement.

Development stages

21−22 days: First heart beats. Four primitive heart chambers (sinus venosus, atrium, ventricle, bulbus cordis).

25 days: Formation of bulbo-ventricular loop.

26 days: Aortic arches begin to develop sequentially.

32 days: Septum primum appears.

37 days: Common atrio-ventricular canal divided by fused atrio-ventricular cushions.

42 days: Aorta and pulmonary trunk separate.

46 days: Interventricular septum complete. Septum secundum develops.

Further reading

Congdon, E.D. (1922) Transformation of the aortic arch system during the development of the human embryo. *Contr. Embryol. Carnegie Inst.* **14**, 47.

Dawes, G.S. (1968) Changes in the circulation at birth. Chapter 13 in: *Foetal and Neonatal Physiology*, Year Book Medical Publishers Ltd, Chicago.

De Vries, P.A. & Saunders, J.B. de C.M. (1962) Development of the ventricles and the spiral outflow tract in the human heart. *Contr. Embryol. Carnegie Inst.* **37**, 87.

Fukuda, T. (1973) Fetal hemopoiesis. *Virchows Arch.B.,* **14**, 197.

Lie, T.A. (1968) *Congenital Anomalies of the Carotid Arteries.* Excerpta Medica Foundation, Williams & Wilkins, Baltimore.

Maron, B.J. (1974) The development of the semi-lunar valves in the human heart. *Am. J. Path.,* **74**, 331.

O'Rahilly, R. (1971) The timing and sequence of events in human cardiogenesis. *Acta Anat.* **79**, 70.

Padget, D.H. (1948) The development of the cranial arteries in the human embryo. *Contr. Embryol. Carnegie Inst.,* **36**, 205.

Rudolph, A.M. & Heymann, M.A. (1974) Fetal and neonatal circulation and respiration. *Ann. Rev. Physiol.,* **36**, 187.

Taussig, H.B. (1960) *Congenital Malformations of the Heart,* 2nd edn. Harvard University Press, Cambridge, USA

13
Coelom, Lungs, Diaphragm

At first, the intra-embryonic coelom is a continuous cavity that is destined to form, in the adult, the pericardial, pleural and peritoneal cavities. In the male, part of it also becomes separated off to form the tunica vaginalis of the testis (p.258). The general arrangement of the coelomic cavity, after the formation of the head fold, has been described in Chapter 6. To summarize, it consists firstly of an anterior transversely-orientated portion from which the pericardial cavity will develop. This lies ventral to the foregut and cranial to the septum transversum (Fig. 13.1). The caudal part of the heart tube is embedded in the septum trans-versum (p.195). On each side, the pericardial cavity is continuous with a pair of *coelomic ducts* (p.89) that pass caudally, lying on either side of the foregut and dorsal to the upper border of the septum transversum (Fig. 6.14). These open out into the future peritoneal cavity which surrounds part of the foregut, the whole of the midgut, including the dorsal part of the yolk sac, and much of the hindgut (p.277). Around the neck of the yolk sac the intra-embryonic coelom is continuous, still, with the extra-embryonic coelom (Figs. 6.10 and 6.13). This communication is important for, as will be described in Chapter 16, most of the midgut herniates out through this communication and undergoes a great deal of its development while lying right outside the embryo in the extra-embryonic coelom.

The relation of the coelomic ducts are difficult to visualize in three dimensions and are best understood by reference to the septum transversum.

The septum transversum

This is literally a transverse septum, composed of mesoderm, that forms the caudal limit of the pericardial cavity and separates it from the future peritoneal cavity. This may be seen in Figs. 13.1, 13.2, 13.3 and 13.4

In Fig. 13.2, which passes through the plane a—a in Fig. 13.1, the pericardial cavity can be seen to be forming the ventral aspect of the embryo in this region. It passes dorsally on each side to form the coelomic ducts which lie on either side of the foregut. The septum transversum forms the caudal wall of the pericardial cavity and the sinus venosus is partly embedded in it.

Fig. 13.3 is a section through the septum transversum itself (plane b—b in Fig. 13.1). The two coelomic ducts pass dorsal to the septum on either side of the foregut. From this it will be understood that, in the septum transversum, the

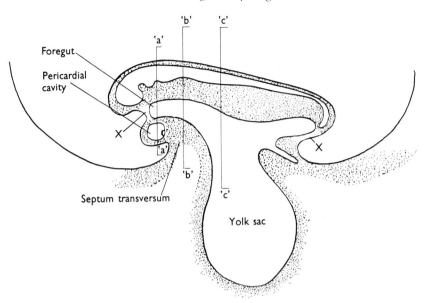

Fig. 13.1. A longitudinal section through an embryo to show the planes of section of Figs. 13.2, 13.3 and 13.4.

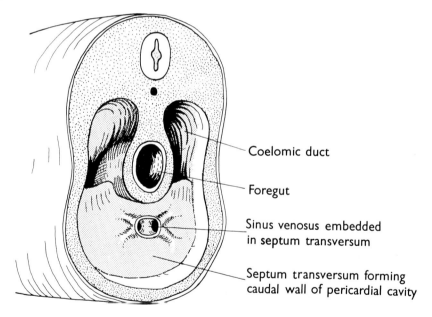

Coelomic duct

Foregut

Sinus venosus embedded in septum transversum

Septum transversum forming caudal wall of pericardial cavity

Fig. 13.2. A section through a−a in Fig. 13.1 seen from *in front*.

mesoderm of the somatopleure and of the splanchnopleure are transversely connected (Fig. 6.14). This is why it is possible for the umbilical veins (which lie in the somatopleure), the vitelline veins (which lie in the splanchnopleure) and the cardinal veins (which lie in the body wall dorsal to the coelomic cavity, see Fig. 12.3 for relative positions), all to converge and empty into the sinus venosus.

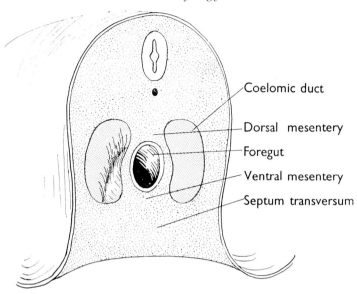

Fig. 13.3. A section through b–b in Fig. 13.1 seen from *in front*.

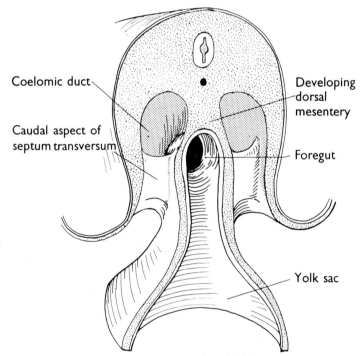

Fig. 13.4. A section through c–c in Fig. 13.1 seen from *behind*.

Finally, Fig. 13.4 (plane c–c in Fig. 13.1) shows how the coelomic ducts eventually open out around the neck of the yolk sac and communicate with the extra-embryonic coelom. (The section shown in this diagram is viewed from the caudal aspect.)

It will now be necessary to describe the way in which this continuous coelomic cavity becomes divided up to form the three serous cavities of the adult thorax and abdomen. This division is closely bound up with the early development of the lungs, which will be described next.

The development of the air passages and lungs

A linear groove first appears in the floor of the pharynx and future oesophagus (Fig. 11.2). This is known as the *laryngo-tracheal groove* and, as it deepens, the caudal end begins to separate off from the foregut and divides at its termination into right and left lung buds. This separation of the primitive pharynx into trachea and oesophagus gradually extends cranially until the only communication between the air passages and the pharynx is at the extreme upper end (Fig. 13.5)

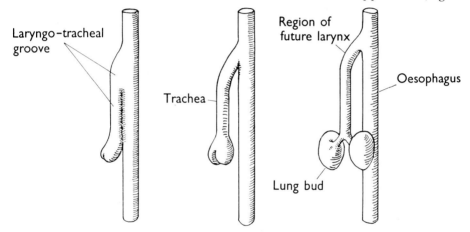

Fig. 13.5. Three stages in the development of the trachea.

around which the skeletal elements of the fourth and sixth branchial arches form the cartilages of the larynx. The hypobranchial eminence (p.173) becomes enlarged and frees itself from the surrounding tissue to form the epiglottis. The lung buds grow out into splanchnopleuric mesoderm which will form the connective tissue and blood vessels of the lung and the surface cells of the mesenchyme covering the lung buds form the visceral layer of the pleura. As the lung buds increase in size, they protrude into the coelomic ducts which become locally enlarged to accommodate them. In the account of the development of the lungs that follows later it should be borne in mind that, unlike the kidneys, liver, heart or other similar organs, the lung is totally functionless before birth so that the final stages in the 'embryology' of the lung are, in fact, post-natal.

The separation of the pleural cavities

As a result of the lateral growth of the lung buds and the consequent localized lateral bulging of the coelomic ducts, two transverse ridges are produced in the lateral wall of each duct — one cranial and the other caudal to the area of lung enlargement. Both ridges are continuous ventrally with the dorsal aspect of the septum transversum. The cranial ridge, the *pleuro-pericardial membrane*, contains the common cardinal vein, which is passing ventrally, lateral to the coelomic duct to reach the septum transversum and the sinus venosus (Fig 13.6). The phrenic nerve will also later pass through the mesoderm of this ridge (Fig. 13.7b) after the migration of the myotomes of the third, fourth and fifth cervical somites into the septum transversum region to form the musculature of the diaphragm (p.240).

As the heart undergoes its 'descent' (p.176), the common cardinal veins become increasingly vertical and the ridges to which they give rise correspondingly more and more prominent until they eventually fuse with the mesoderm covering the front of the oesphagus thus obliterating the canal in this region. The pericardial cavity is now cut off from the rest of the coelom (Fig. 13.7a and b).

The more caudal of the two ridges mentioned above (the *pleuro-peritoneal membrane*) becomes relatively more prominent as a result of the further growth of the lung above (Fig. 13.7c) and the liver (within the septum transversum) below. The communication between pleural and peritoneal cavities eventually becomes completely closed off by these mesenchymal ridges; this occurs first on the right side. Closure is assisted by the growth of myoblasts into the tissue (p.240).

The lungs

The lung becomes wedge shaped in transverse section and its thin anterior border begins to grow ventrally into the mesoderm of the body wall lateral to the pericardium (Fig. 13.7c). The mesoderm is thus split into an outer layer which forms the body wall and an inner layer which covers the pericardium. The latter will form the mediastinal pleura and the fibrous pericardium and contains the superior vena cava (the terminal part of the right common cardinal vein) and both phrenic nerves. These relations are shown in Fig. 13.7.

The lung buds are, at first, symmetrical endodermal outgrowths, each surrounded by a condensation of mesenchyme. At an early stage they become asymmetrical since the right bud divides into three and the left into two branches; these represent the lobar bronchi. Further subdivisions, both of the endodermal component and of the surrounding mesenchyme, give rise to the segmental bronchi; the segments are demarcated by faint grooves on the surface of the lung, although these soon disappear.

The subsequent development of the air passages may be divided into three stages. Firstly, the *glandular* stage when the segmental bronchi continue to divide until the smallest subdivisions represent the air passages down as far as the terminal bronchioles. The tubules end blindly and are lined by cuboidal epithelium so that a section of the lung at this stage (4 months) resembles a gland. After this the developing lung enters the second, or *canalicular*, stage when the smallest tubules become vascularised and the epithelium is thinned out; new peripheral

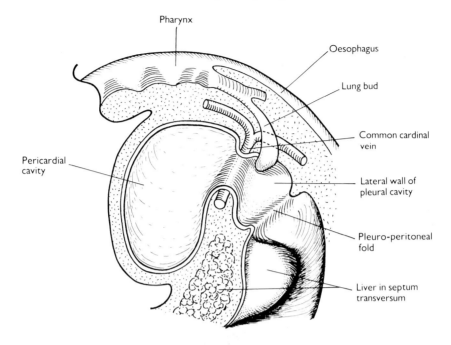

Fig. 13.6. A parasagittal section through the region of the septum transversum to show the lateral wall of the pericardial cavity and coelomic duct.

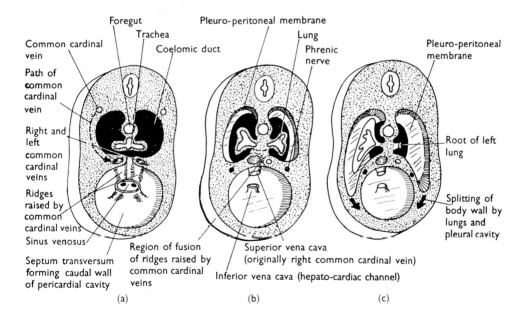

Fig. 13.7. Three sections showing the development of lungs and the pleuro-peritoneal membranes. The lungs grow ventrally in the direction of the arrows in (c).

tubules, also with a very thin epithelium, are added. At the end of this stage the lung can function. During the last three months of intra-uterine life the lung is said to be in the *alveolar* or *saccular* stage of development. The smallest bronchioles, now recognisable as respiratory bronchioles, end in saccules lined with thin respiratory epithelium and primitive alveoli can be recognised as shallow outgrowths; true alveoli, however, are not present before birth. In the last weeks before birth the respiratory passages become lined by a phospholipid material, known as *surfactant*, although it is at first present only in small amounts and does not reach its full development until just before birth. Its function is to reduce the surface tension of the fluid in the alveoli so that they do not collapse during expiration. The pressure required to inflate a cavity varies inversely with its radius so that the tiny developing alveoli have a tendency to collapse. The components of surfactant when isolated from the amniotic fluid following amniocentesis, are an important factor to be taken into account when deciding whether the baby is capable of an independent existence.

Breathing movements occur *in utero*, although these are not continuous. The air passages are filled with fluid and, because of the open ductus arteriosus, only a small proportion of the right ventricular output flows through the lung.

At birth, the pulmonary vascular bed opens up and the relatively thick arterial walls of the fetal pulmonary arteries begin to become thinner, a process that takes several months; the fluid in the respiratory passages is rapidly absorbed and, as a result of the presence of surfactant, they do not collapse but become air-filled. True alveoli develop — this is a gradual process and occupies several months. New alveoli are formed as the lungs grow and this continues up to the age of about 8 years, after which the alveoli grow in size but do not increase in number.

The development of the diaphragm

As will be described later (p.283), the septum transversum becomes extensively invaded by liver cells. Eventually only a very thin layer of it remains, separating the pericardial cavity from the liver, and this forms the central part of the diaphragm. When the lungs grow ventrally to split the body wall into two layers (p.239; Fig. 13.8a), they also grow caudally, again splitting the body wall into an outer layer — that will form part of the definitive body wall — and an inner layer that contributes to the periphery of the diaphragm (Fig. 13.8b). Dorsally the mesoderm, which forms a short mesentery for the caudal end of the oesophagus, also becomes incorporated into the diaphragm. These three main components form only the connective tissue framework of the diaphragm, including the central tendon. Primitive muscle fibres (myoblasts) grow into this tissue from the third, fourth and fifth cervical somites, bringing their nerve supply with them. The motor innervation of the diaphragm is, therefore, entirely by means of the phrenic nerve (C3, 4 and 5) which becomes elongated during the 'descent' of the septum transversum region. The phrenic nerve is also sensory to the central region of the diaphragm but the peripheral region, which is developed from the body wall

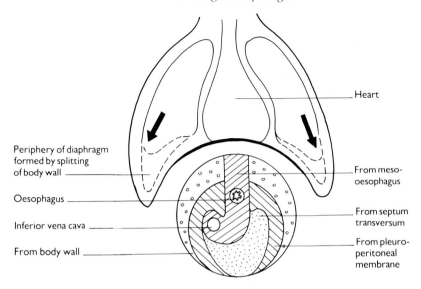

Fig. 13.8. Coronal section (a) shows how the lungs split the body to form the peripheral portion of the diaphragm. The arrows indicate the direction of lung growth in this plane. Inset, diagram (b) shows approximately the embryonic constituents of the adult diaphragm viewed from above.

(prior to its invasion by muscle), is innervated by the intercostal nerves as might be expected.

Developmental anomalies of the respiratory tract and diaphragm

Upper respiratory tract

Tracheo-oesophageal fistula

The most common developmental anomaly of the upper respiratory tract is a *tracheo-oesophageal fistula,* a complex abnormality which is due to the failure of the primitive trachea to separate completely from the oesophagus. As this anomaly is usually associated with oesophageal atresia, a foregut abnormality, it is considered elsewhere (Chapter 16). Other development anomalies of the upper respiratory passages are very rare; they include principally:

Choanal atresia

This is a narrowing of the posterior nares (often unilateral) which usually presents at birth with difficulty in breathing, variable cyanosis and feeding difficulties. Surgery is usually needed to restore patency to the narrowed respiratory passages.

Congenital laryngeal stridor

Several developmental anomalies can give rise to congenital laryngeal stridor, a

term given to the harsh sound produced usually during inspiration, often associated with breathing difficulties resulting from narrowing of the air passages
within the larynx. Several anomalies can cause the symptom — excessive laxity of
the small joints between the laryngeal cartilages (*laryngomalacia*) leading to a
tendency to collapse during inspiration; the presence of a web of tissue obstructing airflow (*incomplete atresia*) or the presence of cysts and *haemangiomata*
(vascular tumours). Surgery is usually needed for webs, cysts and haemangiomata.
Most cases of laryngomalacia present little difficulty in management, tending to
recover spontaneously within the first two years of life.

Lungs

Primary developmental anomalies of the lungs are so rare as to require only brief
mention. They include *lung cysts* (fluid or air-filled) and *lobar emphysema* (over-
inflation of a lung lobe due to deficiency of bronchial cartilage) usually of the right
middle lobe or left upper lobe. These anomalies will usually be diagnosed in the
investigation of respiratory symptoms, most commonly in the older child and
most will require surgical removal.

Secondary interference with lung growth, causing *lung hypoplasia*, is more
common. This can result from:

1 Abdominal viscera herniating into the pleural cavity, as occurs in congenital
diaphragmatic hernia (*vide infra*);

2 Restricted growth of the thoracic cage, due to:

   (a) diminished volume of amniotic fluid as, for example, occurs with renal
   agenesis (Potter's syndrome, see p.317), or chronic leakage of amniotic fluid;

   (b) rare skeletal dysplasias (e.g. asphyxiating thoracic dystrophy), which lead
   to a very small deformed rib cage.

Whatever the cause, lung hypoplasia is characterised by a markedly reduced
lung weight (individual lungs can weigh as little as 5 g, compared with 30 g in the
normal lung) due to a major reduction in the number of bronchial divisions and a
poorly developed pulmonary vascular tree. Other than in late onset diaphragmatic
hernia (see below) the prognosis of babies with lung hypoplasia is very poor, as
the lungs are unable to sustain adequate ventilation.

Diaphragm

Congenital diaphragmatic hernia

This abnormality is an important (albeit rare) cause of life-threatening breathing
difficulties immediately after birth. Abdominal viscera, small intestine, colon,
stomach, spleen and liver in various combinations prolapse into the pleural cavity
through an opening in the postero-lateral opening of the diaphragm (Fig. 13.9).
As a result the heart is pushed towards the opposite side. The left side

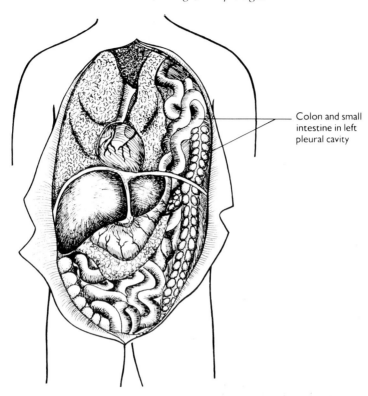

Colon and small
intestine in left
pleural cavity

Fig. 13.9. A case of diaphragmatic hernia.

is involved in 80 per cent of cases. The defect in the diaphragm is due to failure of the pleuro-peritoneal canal to close early in embryonic development, usually between the second and third months of intra-uterine life. This failure might be an isolated primary defect or secondary to a premature return of the physiological midgut hernia, the latter association accounting for the frequent association of congenital diaphragmatic hernia with malrotation of the intestines. An important consequence of the prolapse of viscera into the thorax is lung hypoplasia. Both lungs are affected, the one ipsilateral to the hernia especially so. The growth of the contralateral lung is affected by the heart and mediastinum which are pushed over by the hernia.

Most babies with a diaphragmatic hernia present as an acute emergency soon after birth, with difficulty in establishing ventilation due to failure of the lungs to expand. The abdomen appears flat and empty, bowel sounds may be heard in the thorax on auscultation and the heart apex is displaced. Confirmation of the diagnosis is by X-ray which shows gas-filled loops in the thoracic cavity and, in the case of a left-sided hernia, a heart shadow displaced to the right. Less frequently the diagnosis is made towards the end of the first week in the process of investigating cyanosis and dyspnoea. Even more rarely might it be diagnosed later in childhood in the course of a routine X-ray examination of the chest.

Treatment is by laparotomy, the intestines and other viscera being gently pulled out of the chest and returned into the abdominal cavity. The defect in the diaphragm is then repaired.

The earlier a diaphragmatic hernia presents, the worse is the prognosis. In babies who present in the first hours' after birth, the mean survival rate is less than 20 per cent; presentation after 24 hours of age is associated with a much improved survival rate (about 90 per cent). The reason for the poor prognosis of the baby who shows symptoms soon after birth is that early presentation indicates severe lung hypoplasia which fails to allow the lungs to function adequately. Even if the lungs are able to expand there is often such marked unevenness of this expansion that alveoli rupture at the lung surface, causing air to escape into the pleural cavity (*pneumothorax*), adding a further complication to operative management. Failure of the pulmonary vascular tree to develop together with the lung hypoplasia adds to the disordered cardio-respiratory function. For babies who survive early surgery the long-term outcome in regard to lung function is excellent. Some residual defects in ventilatory function can be discovered on detailed investigation with functional exchange volume and vital capacity being below normal. This lung dysfunction does not, however, interfere with the child's development or physical activities.

Eventration of the diaphragm

This rare anomaly can sometimes be mistaken for a congenital diaphragmatic hernia. In this condition one of the leaves of the diaphragm is weakened by a diminution in the amount of muscle, which is replaced by fibrous tissue. The whole hemi-diaphragm can be involved or only a small part of it. In contrast with a diaphragmatic hernia, the herniated abdominal viscera will be contained in a thin-walled fibrous sac.

Clinical presentation can be similar to that of diaphragmatic hernia but usually it is diagnosed much later in childhood, diagnosis usually being prompted by radiological investigation for recurrent chest infection. An elevated leaf of the diaphragm is easily observed. Treatment is by plicating the diaphragm. A muscular flap (usually from the latissimus dorsi) is sometimes used to reinforce the thin diaphragm. Long-term outcome is excellent with little, or no, residual defect in ventilatory function.

Development stages

22 days: Laryngo-tracheal groove appears, followed by lung buds
24–26 days: Head and tail folds complete. Coelomic duct fully developed
4–5 weeks: Trachea separates from oesophagus. Lobar bronchi recognisable
5 weeks: Pericardium closed off (right side first)
6 weeks: Segmental bronchi forming in lung

7 weeks: Pleuro-peritoneal openings closed (right side first)
4 months: Glandular stage of lung development
4–6 months: Canalicular stage of lung development
6–9 months: Alveolar stage of lung development, continuing after birth.

Further reading

Boyden E.A. (1971) Human growth and development, *Am J. Anat.* **132**, I.

Nelson N.M. (1970) On the etiology of hyaline membrane disease. *Pediatric clinics of North America* Vol. 17, No. 4, 943

O'Rahilly, R. & Boyden, E.A. (1973) The timing and sequence of events in the development of the human respiration system during the embryonic period proper. *Z. Anat. Entw.-Gesch.,* **141**, 273.

Reid L. (1967) The embryology of the lung. In: *Ciba Foundation Symposium, 'Development of the Lung'* A.V.S.Reuck & R.Porter (Eds). J. & A. Churchill Ltd., London.

Wells L.J. (1954) Development of the human diaphragm and pleural sacs. *Contr. Embryol. Carnegie Inst.* **35**, 107.

14
Urogenital System:1
Mesonephros, Cloaca, Suprarenal
Gland, Kidney

It will be recalled (Chapter 6) that prior to the formation of head and tail folds, when the embryo consists of a flat tri-laminar disc, the chorda mesoderm lies everywhere between the ectoderm and endoderm except in two regions, one cranial to the notochord and the other caudal to the primitive streak (Figs. 6.7 and 6.11). At the cranial end, the membrane formed by the close apposition of endoderm and ectoderm is known as the *buccopharyngeal membrane* (p.81) while that formed caudally and lying behind the remnants of the primitive streak is the *cloacal membrane*. As a result of the formation of the lateral folds and the tail fold, the hindgut is formed and the cloacal membrane now lies on the ventral aspect of the embryo (Figs. 6.12, 6.14 and 13.1) separating the hindgut from the amniotic cavity. The proximal end of the allantois will now open into the cloaca just anterior to the cloacal membrane (Fig. 14.1b). The allantois is relatively small in the human embryo and it does not extend far into the extra-embryonic tissues, as occurs in many of the lower animals in which the allantois acts as a functional bladder. The proximal end of the human allantois, however, takes part in the formation of the adult bladder and during an early stage of development, after the formation of the tail fold, it becomes taken into the embryo so that the cloacal membrane may now be said to form a closing membrane for a chamber, the *cloaca* (p.250) which is thus common to both the hindgut and a portion of the allantois (Fig. 14.1). Later in development the urinary system will also open into the aptly named cloaca (Latin: a sewer) so that this region of the human embryo resembles conditions seen in the adult state in many lower orders such as reptiles. In the human embryo, however, the cloaca will later become divided into two parts by a urorectal septum (p.250).

The nephrogenic ridge

In the dorsal body wall, the mesoderm of the intermediate cell mass of each side (Fig. 6.13) proliferates and forms two long ridges lying one on either side of the midline. Each ridge extends from the region of the cervical somites right down to the caudal end of the embryonic coelomic cavity. It is known as the *nephrogenic ridge* and, from it, will develop not only parts of the urinary system but also the stroma of the gonads and some of their associated ducts. On the lateral and ventral aspects of the ridge a longitudinal duct develops. This is the *mesonephric* or *Wolffian duct* (Fig. 14.2) which extends downwards along almost the whole length

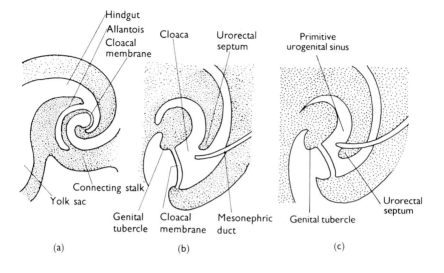

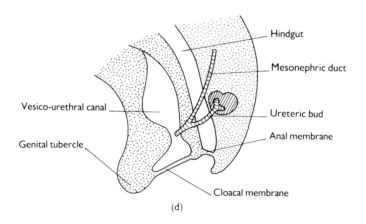

Fig. 14.1. The splitting of the cloaca by the urorectal septum to form the primitive urogenital sinus; also shown is the ureteric bud.

of the nephrogenic ridge and then passes medially to open into the ventral part of the cloaca on each side (Figs. 14.1 and 14.2). In the male, it plays an important part in the development of the genital system and in both sexes its lower end will form part of the bladder.

The cranial end of the nephrogenic ridge is displaced laterally because of the suprarenal gland which develops between the ridge and the root of the gut mesentery. This gland is not part of the urogenital system but, owing to its geographical location, a description of its development may conveniently be given at this point.

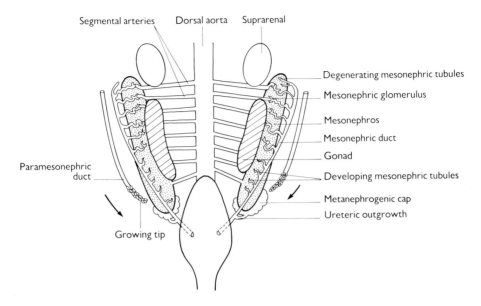

Fig. 14.2. The mesonephros and its relations. The glomeruli are functional at this stage but will disappear later.

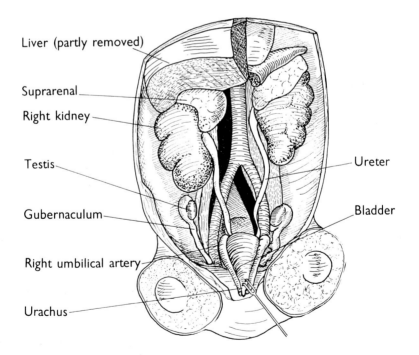

Fig. 14.3. A dissected fetus to show the urogenital system. Note the relatively large suprarenals, the lobulated kidneys and the testes which are still fairly high in the abdomen. The vas deferens (mesonephric duct) is not shown.

The suprarenal gland

In many animals this gland is multiple and, in man, it consists of a cortex and medulla which have quite different functions. The gland develops from two different sources. The medulla is derived from cells of the neural crest (p.143) which migrate ventrally to take up their position on either side of the root of the midline mesentery of the gut (p.277) near the cranial end of the nephrogenic ridge. The clump of neural crest cells becomes surrounded by layers of cells which are derived from the mesodermal epithelium (mesothelium) lining the coelomic cavity. The latter group of cells are destined to form the suprarenal cortex which, at first, consists of two distinct layers. Immediately in contact with the medulla is a very thick layer of eosinophilic cells which is known as the *fetal cortex* while, outside this, is a thinner rind of cells which will form the permanent cortex. The fetal cortex is largely responsible for the relatively huge size of the fetal suprarenal (Fig. 14.3) Its function is not yet known but it seems to be under fetal pituitary control. After birth the fetal cortex regresses and the suprarenal actually shrinks in size, at three months weighing only one half of its birth weight. When the fetal cortex has finally disappeared the adult cortex lies immediately in contact with the medulla.

The mesonephros

The nephrogenic ridge undergoes a number of changes which result in the formation of the *mesonephros*. This is an embryonic excretory organ which functions until it is replaced by the permanent kidney or *metanephros*.

As was mentioned previously, the development of the suprarenal gland causes the nephrogenic ridge (and, therefore, the mesonephros) to assume an oblique position. This is shown in Fig. 14.2 in which the position of the mesonephric duct can be seen. This diagram also indicates that the mesonephros consists of a series of glomeruli and tubules which are similar to, but less complicated than, those of the adult kidney. The glomeruli are relatively large; they lie medially in the mesonephros and they are supplied with blood by a series of lateral branches of the dorsal aorta. The tubules are tortuous but lack anything resembling a loop of Henle; they open laterally into the mesonephric duct. The development of these tubules follows a cranio-caudal gradient so that the mature tubules at the cranial end of the mesonephros are beginning to degenerate while, at the same time, new tubules are being added to the caudal end. In the very early stages of development of the nephrogenic ridge a few rudimentary tubules at the cranial end represent the *pronephros*, a primitive form of kidney found in certain simple vertebrates. In the human embryo, however, this form of excretory apparatus can be disregarded except that it acts as an organizer for the mesonephric duct.

A second longitudinal duct (Figs. 14.2 and 15.1) soon develops immediately lateral to the mesonephric duct. This is the *paramesonephric* or *Müllerian duct* which is particularly important in the female. The fate of this duct will be described in Chapter 15. The whole complex of mesonephros and the two ducts separates itself to some extent from the dorsal body wall so that it is suspended from the latter by a mesentery, the *urogenital mesentery* (Fig. 15.1).

The urogenital sinus

Meanwhile, various changes have been taking place in the cloaca. The mesodermal tissue which separates the allantois from the hindgut extends caudally to form a *urorectal septum* so that a gradual separation of the urogenital system from the alimentary canal occurs (Fig. 14.1). The urorectal septum grows downwards and finally reaches the cloacal membrane; the original cloaca is now divided into a dorsal region which forms part of the hindgut and a ventral *primitive urogenital sinus* (Fig. 14.1d). Similarly, the cloacal membrane becomes subdivided into an anterior *urogenital membrane* and a posterior *anal membrane*. The primitive urogenital sinus is further subdivided, for descriptive purposes, by the entrance of the mesonephric ducts. Above this level the allantois and the upper part of the primitive urogenital sinus together make up the *vesico-urethral canal* from which will develop the bladder and part of the prostatic urethra (probably the whole urethra in the female). Below this level lies the *definitive urogenital sinus* in which a short, narrow cylindrical portion, the *pelvic portion*, lies above a laterally compressed and elongated *phallic portion* (Fig. 15.4). As can be seen from Figs. 14.4 and 15.4 the phallic portion of the urogenital sinus extends forwards onto the ventral surface of a mesodermal swelling (covered by ectoderm) which lies in the midline. This is the *genital tubercle* and is, at this stage, similar in both male and female. Fig. 14.4 shows that the genital tubercle is interposed between the urogenital membrane, which is soon to break down, and the attachment of the umbilical cord which is relatively enormous at this stage. The genital tubercle begins as an ingrowth of mesoderm between the endoderm and ectoderm of the urogenital membrane immediately caudal to the umbilical region. This forms a pair of

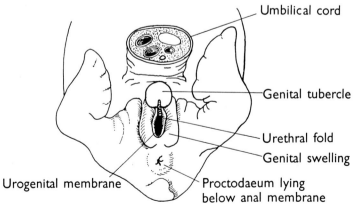

Umbilical cord

Genital tubercle

Urethral fold

Genital swelling

Urogenital membrane

Proctodaeum lying below anal membrane

Fig. 14.4. The external genitalia. There is little development of the infra-umbilical abdominal wall at this stage, the genital tubercle reaching as far up as the umbilical cord.

swellings on either side of the midline which rapidly fuse to produce the tubercle. As a result of the ingrowth of mesoderm and the development of the genital tubercle, the plane of the urogenital and anal membranes becomes rotated and, instead of facing ventrally, they come to face downwards between the legs so that their plane corresponds to that of the adult perineum (Fig. 14.1). On either side of the urogenital membrane lies a ridge of ectoderm-covered mesenchyme known as the *urethral fold*. Outside this lies a less well defined elevation which is the *genital swelling*. Anteriorly is the genital tubercle.

Further growth in the region between the genital tubercle and the umbilicus leads to the development of the infra-umbilical abdominal wall, the mesoderm of which will be invaded by dermato-myotomes from the somites so that the musculature of the abdominal wall will finally develop.

The metanephros

The lower end of the mesonephric duct develops a distinct angulation as it bends forwards and medially to enter the urogenital sinus. From this point a small outgrowth grows dorsally and cranially towards the lower end of the nephrogenic ridge. This is known as the *ureteric bud* and the slightly dilated *ampulla* at its upper end becomes surrounded by a mass of cells from the ridge. These cells will later form the greater part of the permanent kidney (the *metanephros*) and the cluster of cells is, therefore, known as the *metanephrogenic cap* (Fig. 15.4). The presence of a ureteric bud is necessary for the induction of the metanephrogenic cap so that, in cases of congenital absence of a ureter, the kidney will also be missing.

As the tip of the ureteric bud ascends it begins to divide dichotomously, each subdivision terminating in an *ampulla*. The whole metanephrogenic cap also partially divides so that each ampulla is capped by a mass of cells. The proliferation of the branches of the ureteric bud proceeds rapidly at the periphery but the first 3−5 generations will later dilate and coalesce as the metanephros begins to secrete urine and these form the pelvis of the kidney and the major calices. The next few generations form the minor calices and the main collecting ducts. The remaining subdivisions will become the smaller collecting ducts. Their associated clumps of metanephrogenic cap cells will form the *nephrons*. Each ampulla induces the formation of a hollow nephrogenic vesicle, to which it is closely adherent. A cleft develops in the vesicle, into which mesenchymal cells penetrate, so that the whole resembles the letter 'S' (Fig. 14.5). This *S-shaped body* will form the parietal and visceral layers of Bowman's capsule and the whole tubular system of the nephron. The mesenchymal cells in the cleft proliferate and form the capillary tuft of the glomerulus, while the two layers of cells adjacent to this form the visceral and parietal layers respectively. The other limb of the S elongates to form the proximal and distal tubules while the part of the tubule that intervenes between these will push its way down into the medulla to form a loop of Henle (arrowed in Fig. 14.5).

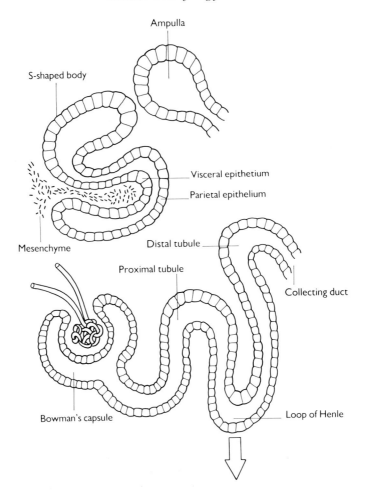

Fig. 14.5. The upper figure shows an S-shaped body in close proximity to an ampulla. The lower figure illustrates the fusion of the two and the differentiation of the S-shaped body into the various parts of the nephron.

Thus the distal tubule develops immediately adjacent to the glomerulus and remains so placed while the loop itself grows down. Therefore, in the adult kidney, each ascending limb of Henle's loop continues into a distal tubule, whose macula densa is in contact with its own glomerulus. This feature is important from the point of view of the physiology of the nephron.

In the early stages of branching of the ampullae, each ampulla divides into two. Of the two divisions, one induces the formation of a nephrogenic vesicle while the other divides again. One of the latter branches induces another nephron, while the other divides into two. This process repeats itself and continues peripherally until a large number of nephrons have been formed (Fig. 14.6). Thus, at a stage

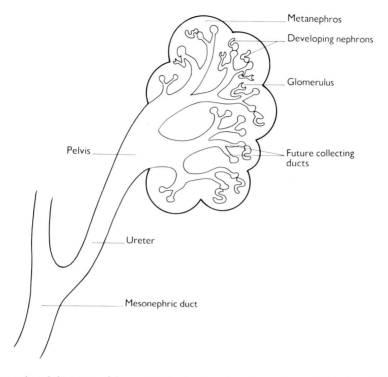

Fig. 14.6. The early subdivisions of the ureteric bud and metanephrogenic cap. Note that the first glomeruli to develop are those of the future juxtamedullary region.

when the first formed glomeruli are well advanced, the more peripheral are in the early stages of development so that the outermost layer of the cortex contains only rudimentary nephrons and is known, therefore, as the *nephrogenic zone*. The later stages of ampullary branching develop in a slightly different way, but a detailed account need not be given here. Full histological maturation of all the nephrons is not complete until a long time after birth and the neonatal kidney is functionally, as well as structurally, immature. It cannot produce very concentrated urine nor can it excrete excessive amounts of fluid and this is of great importance in the care of premature infants.

As a result of the coalescence of a number of early divisions of the ureteric bud to form major and minor calices and of growth changes in the calix itself a number of collecting ducts, each draining a much larger number of nephrons, comes to open into each minor calix at the summit of a papilla. The kidney is thus subdivided into lobes and, in the fetal kidney, these are visible on the surface as broad elevations separated by grooves (Fig. 14.3). In the human kidney this *fetal lobulation* of the surface of the kidney becomes lost so that the surface is smooth, although occasionally in the human kidney and always in certain animal kidneys, it may persist into adult life. It is of no pathological significance.

In the early stages of their development the two developing kidneys are very close to each other and not far away from the urogenital sinus. (Do not forget that diagrams, like Fig. 14.2, depict very small fetuses only about 10 mm long altogether). As the abdomen grows, the kidneys undergo a relative ascent and become further apart as they ascend. They also rotate so that the hilum faces medially instead of forwards. During its ascent, the kidney receives its blood supply from the lateral mesonephric branches of the aorta (p.199), picking up ever higher branches and relinquishing the lower ones. It finally reaches the suprarenal gland where the ascent stops and the kidney retains its highest aortic branch which becomes the permanent renal artery. Frequently, however, more than one artery persists, so that one or more aberrant renal arteries may be present. These enter the cortex directly rather than through the hilum and it is important to remember that they are end arteries so that, if they are damaged, the portion of kidney that they supply will become ischaemic.

Since the ureteric bud is responsible for inducing the development of the permanent kidney, developmental anomalies of the latter are closely related to anomalies of the ureteric bud itself. Consideration of these will be deferred to the next chapter.

The bladder and urethra

The development of the kidney represents one of the few exceptions to the general embryological rule that a gland that is connected to a hollow viscus by a duct, develops as an outgrowth from that viscus (e.g. liver, pancreas, prostate). The ureter, as has been seen, first starts as an outgrowth from the mesonephric duct but this relationship soon changes. The lower ends of the mesonephric ducts up to, and beyond, the ureteric buds become taken into the endodermal vesico-urethral canal so that part of the wall of the canal becomes mesodermal. At the same time, complicated growth changes occur so that the ureters come to open into the definitive bladder while the mesonephric ducts open lower down into the pelvic part of the definitive urogenital sinus (Fig. 15.4). Thus the whole trigone of the bladder and the posterior wall of the urethra, down as far as the openings of the mesonephric ducts, are mesodermal in origin. As will be seen in Chapter 15, this portion of the urethra corresponds to the upper half of the prostatic urethra in the male and probably the whole urethra in the female; the openings of the mesonephric ducts in the male will become the openings into the prostatic urethra of the ejaculatory ducts (p.260).

The bladder is thus derived mainly from the endodermal vesico-urethral canal and from the lower end of the mesodermal mesonephric duct. The allantois may make a contribution to the apex but the major part of the allantois regresses and becomes converted into a fibrous cord, the *urachus*, which passes from the apex of the bladder to the umbilicus.

In the infant the bladder is an abdominal rather than a pelvic organ. At birth, the bladder neck is at the level of the upper border of the pelvis and it does not reach its adult position until puberty.

Further reading

The list at the end of Chapter 15 relates also to this chapter.

15

Urogenital system:2
Gonads, Internal and
External Genitalia

The gonads

The gonads which, at first, have a similar appearance in both sexes, are first seen as thickenings of the coelomic epithelium along the medial aspects of part of the nephrogenic ridge (later, essentially, the mesonephros—p.249). At this stage, the thickenings extend along about the middle two quarters of the nephrogenic ridge (Fig. 14.2) and are known as *genital ridges*. Each genital ridge increases in size to become an elongated swelling which is covered by coelomic epithelium. It gradually frees itself from the mesonephros by developing a mesentery of its own (Fig. 15.1) which will later be called the *mesorchium* in the male and the *mesovarium* in the female. At the same time, some workers maintain that cells of the coelomic epithelium which cover the genital ridges (the *germinal epithelium*) proliferate to form solid cords of cells which grow into the substance of the developing gonads. Included in these cellular cords are a number of special cells which are destined eventually to give rise to the ova or spermatozoa. They are known as *primordial germ cells*. Animal experiments and special staining techniques show that in both sexes they originate in the yolk sac wall, having been segregated there at an early stage of development. They then migrate via the innermost layers of the dorsal body wall and thence into the developing genital ridge.

Up to this stage, the development of the male and female genitalia has been similar and the sex of the embryo cannot be differentiated except by karyotyping or by the presence or absence of Barr bodies in the cell nuclei. It will now, however, be necessary to deal separately with the two sexes.

Development in the male

The development of the testis

The cords of cells supposedly derived from the germinal epithelium, which include the primordial germ cells, become cut off from the surface by the development of a dense layer of connective tissue which forms the *tunica albuginea*. Septa grow in from the tunica to divide the testis into compartments and the cellular cords within them become canalized to form seminiferous tubules. Inside the tubules the primordial germ cells differentiate into the precursors of the sperma-

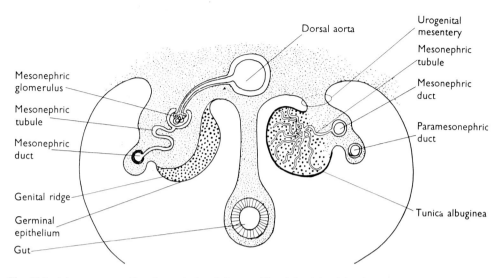

Fig. 15.1. A transverse section through the abdomen. The right side of the diagram shows a more advanced stage of development than the left.

tozoa (p.34) and the remaining cells form Sertoli cells. Masses of interstitial cells form between the tubules; they are functional in the fetus (p.39) as well as in the adult and the Sertoli cells, too, secrete a hormone (p.39). Near the future posterior border of the testis the canalized cell columns anastomose to form a network of tubules, the *rete testis*.

The mesonephric duct in the male

The male mesonephric duct, after the mesonephros has ceased to function, becomes taken over by the genital system under the influence of androgens secreted by the fetal testis (see Chapter 3). The majority of the mesonephric tubules disappear but those in the region of the testis link up with the rete testis and so form a series of communications between this and the mesonephric duct. They thus become the efferent ductules which constitute much of the caput epididymis and are continued into that part of the mesonephric duct which becomes tightly coiled to form the body and tail of the epididymis and the ductus deferens (Figs. 15.1 and 15.2). A few remaining mesonephric tubules form various remnants around the testis and epididymis and these can sometimes give rise to cysts in later life.

When the lower end of the mesonephric duct becomes taken into the bladder to form its trigone (p.254), the ureter and the mesonephric duct will open separately. By complex growth changes in the wall of the developing bladder the ductus deferens, which develops from the mesonephric duct (*vide supra*), comes to open into the middle of the pelvic portion of the definitive urogenital sinus (Fig. 15.4).

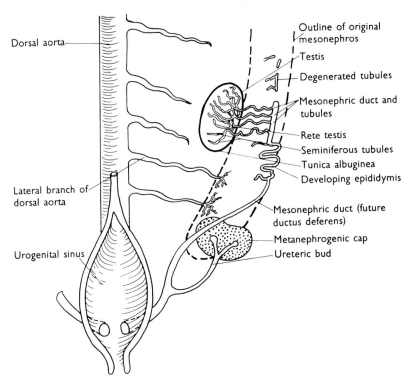

Dorsal aorta

Lateral branch of
dorsal aorta

Urogenital sinus

Outline of original
mesonephros
Testis
Degenerated tubules
Mesonephric duct and
tubules
Rete testis
Seminiferous tubules
Tunica albuginea
Developing epididymis
Mesonephric duct (future
ductus deferens)
Metanephrogenic cap
Ureteric bud

Fig. 15.2. A diagram to shown the take-over of the mesonephric duct by the testis, and the development of the metanephros.

The descent of the testis

By the time the testis and epididymis have become recognisable, a thick column of mesodermal tissue has partly separated itself from the dorsal body wall to form the *gubernaculum*. When fully differentiated this consists of a cylinder of loose tissue with much interstitial ground substance, bearing considerable resemblance to Wharton's jelly in the umbilical cord. The lower pole of the testis and the tail of the epididymis are embedded in its upper end in a manner which has been compared to an acorn in its cup. The lower part of the gubernaculum extends through the inguinal canal, around which the abdominal muscles are differentiating, and down to the genital swelling (p.251) which will later form the scrotum. The 'descent' of the testis within the abdomen is largely a relative movement and is due to the growth of the upper part of the abdomen away from the future pelvic region, leaving the testis behind. True descent occurs only from the region of the internal ring down into the scrotum. This usually takes place during the seventh or eighth month of intra-uterine life and is preceded by marked swelling of the gubernaculum which has the effect of dilating both the inguinal canal and the scrotum. The gubernaculum then seems to shorten and, accompanied anteriorly by an outpouching of peritoneum known as the *processus*

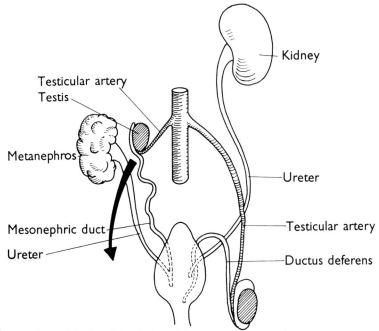

Fig. 15.3. A diagram to explain the adult relation of the testicular artery and ductus deferens to the ureter. The arrow shows the path of testicular descent.

vaginalis which grows into the substance of the gubernaculum, it retracts into the scrotum. The testis and epididymis retain their relationship to the upper end of the gubernaculum and follow it down. The coverings of the cord, including the cremaster muscle, differentiate around the gubernaculum. It must be said, however, that all the forces responsible for testicular descent are not yet fully understood. After full descent has occurred the processus vaginalis becomes sealed off from the general peritoneal cavity, this process usually being completed at or shortly after birth. It now forms the *tunica vaginalis* of the testis. The process of testicular descent is under androgenic control, the production of androgens being stimulated by maternal or chorionic gonadotrophins.

The testicular artery is a lateral branch of the aorta which enters the testis before descent has commenced. After descent has occurred, the testis still retains its original blood supply together with its venous and lymphatic drainage. The testicular vessels in the adult, therefore, have a long course on the posterior abdominal wall and the lymphatic drainage of the testis is to the lateral aortic glands. The relationships of the vessels and of the vas to the ureter can readily be explained on an embryological basis (Fig. 15.3).

The internal genitalia in the male

From the lower end of the ductus deferens a diverticulum grows out into the surrounding mesoderm to form the seminal vesicle (Fig. 15.4). A number of outgrowths from the pelvic portion of the definitive urogenital sinus, both above and below the opening of the ductus, form the prostate gland; the endodermal

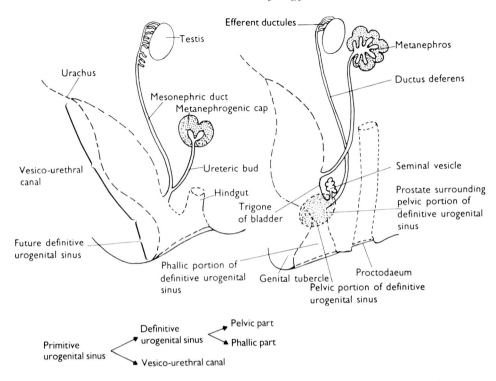

Fig. 15.4. A diagram to show the development of the male bladder and internal genitalia. The endodermal derivatives are dotted. The lower end of the mesonephric duct forms the trigone of the bladder and the upper half of the posterior wall of the prostatic urethra. The ureter and mesonephric duct (ductus deferens) now open separately. The 'flow chart' below shows how the primitive urogenital sinus becomes divided.

lining forms the walls of the alveoli and the surrounding mesoderm develops into the fibro-muscular stroma of the gland. In adult terminology, the duct of the seminal vesicle is said to join the ductus deferens to form the ejaculatory duct which then opens into the prostatic urethra on the urethral crest. The paramesonephric ducts disappear almost completely in the male although some remnants remain in the form of the *appendix testis* which is occasionally subject to painful torsion. Regression is induced by the presence of an anti-Müllerian hormone, secreted by the Sertoli cells of the fetal testis, to which the ducts are sensitive for a short time. The upper end of the ducts persists as the appendix of the testis while the fused lower ends (*vide infra*) contribute to the prostatic utricle.

Development in the female

The development of the ovary

The ovary, at first, cannot be distinguished from the testis until the latter develops a thick tunica albuginea; indeed, it remains histologically in an indifferent state of

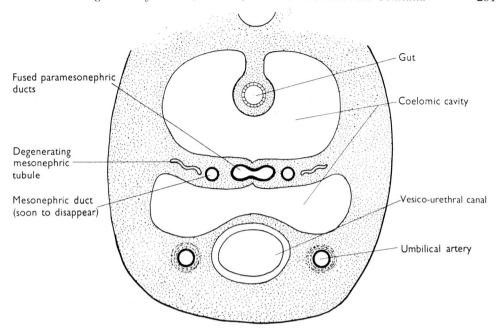

Fused paramesonephric ducts

Degenerating mesonephric tubule

Mesonephric duct (soon to disappear)

Gut

Coelomic cavity

Vesico-urethral canal

Umbilical artery

Fig. 15.5. A transverse septum is formed in the lower abdomen as a result of the swinging across toward the midline of the paramesonephric ducts and their mesenteries. They fuse to form the utero-vaginal canal.

development until the fourth month of pregnancy. In the ovary, the cords of cells which are thought to grow into the interior of the gonad from the germinal epithelium break up into clusters in which the primordial germ cells form the primitive ova or *oogonia*. The oogonia are surrounded by other cells of germinal epithelium origin and also by cells arising from the ovarian stroma. The whole complex eventually gives rise to the Graafian follicle (p.42). The ovary, like the testis, develops its own mesentery, the mesovarium, which connects it to the mesonephros.

The mesonephric and paramesonephric ducts in the female

Lateral to the ovary lie the mesonephric tubules and the mesonephric and para-mesonephric ducts. The latter are, at first, the most lateral structures in the nephrogenic ridge (Fig. 15.1) but towards the caudal end of the ridge the two paramesonephric ducts pass medially, ventral to the other structures in the ridge, and meet each other in the midline (Figs. 15.5 and 15.6). They then run down together and end up in close relation to the dorsal wall of the urogenital sinus. Unlike the mesonephric ducts they do not open into the sinus but they produce an elevation, the *Müllerian tubule*, on the dorsal wall, halfway down the pelvic part of the sinus (Fig. 15.8a). As a result of the paramesonephric ducts meeting in the midline, their mesenteries also swing across and produce a transverse septum

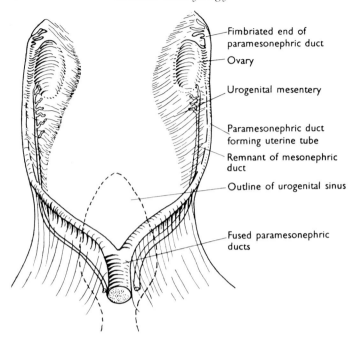

Fimbriated end of
paramesonephric duct

Ovary

Urogenital mesentery

Paramesonephric duct
forming uterine tube

Remnant of mesonephric
duct

Outline of urogenital sinus

Fused paramesonephric
ducts

Fig. 15.6. The mesonephros together with its ducts and its tubules have almost disappeared.
The urogenital mesentery now contains principally the ovary, the paramesonephric duct and the
gubernaculum (not shown).

between the hindgut and the vesico-urethral canal (Fig. 15.5).

The paramesonephric duct originally began as an ingrowth from the surface
epithelium near the upper end of the mesonephros. The duct so formed then grew
caudally. The original opening is retained permanently so that, even after the
complete development of the ducts, their upper ends communicate with the
coelomic cavity. The opening of the duct lies in close relation to the ovary on each
side and, after the development of fimbria, it can be recognised as the ostium of
the uterine tube. The lower portions of the ducts, where they lie alongside one
another, soon fuse to produce a single midline structure known as the *utero-
vaginal canal* which forms the uterus although it does not give rise to the whole
vagina (Fig. 15.8).

The broad ligament of the uterus

The ovary, like the testis, is embedded in the upper end of a gubernaculum which
lies in a similar position to that of the male and ends in the genital swelling. Like
the testis, too, the ovary undergoes a relative descent but it only reaches the
pelvic region and never (or, at least, very rarely) passes through the inguinal canal
to reach the exterior. The mesonephros, meanwhile, undergoes degeneration just
as it does in the male and normally it disappears almost completely except for a

few tubules and a small part of the mesonephric duct. These form inconspicuous remnants found within the broad ligament and are of interest only because they may form cysts in later life. Occasionally almost the whole of the mesonephric duct persists and it is then known as *Gärtner's duct,* which runs alongside the uterus and vagina, and may also produce cysts in later life.

After the disappearance of the mesonephros the urogenital mesentery, which originally suspended all the derivatives of the nephrogenic ridge from the dorsal body wall, now supports only the paramesonephric duct in its free border and the ovary, which is attached to it by the mesovarium (Fig. 15.6). After the 'descent' of the ovary, this mesentery becomes orientated transversely and forms the double peritoneal fold which is known as the broad ligament of the uterus (Figs. 15.7 and 15.8). The gubernaculum gains a secondary attachment to the side of the uterus and then becomes converted into a fibrous cord. It thus becomes two ligaments, one passing from the lower pole of the ovary to the uterus and the other from the uterus to the genital swelling (p.251). The latter will later become the labium majus. These ligaments are, respectively, the *ligament of the ovary* and the *round ligament of the uterus* (Fig. 15.7).

The uterus and vagina

The utero-vaginal canal (formed from the fused paramesonephric ducts) at first comes into contact with the dorsal wall of the urogenital sinus and its lower end

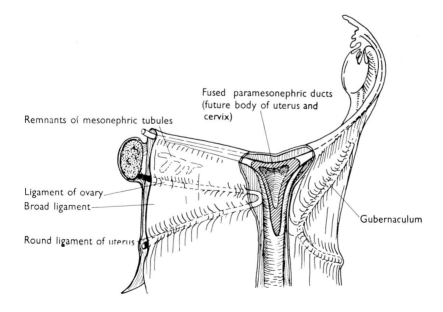

Fused paramesonephric ducts
(future body of uterus and
cervix)

Remnants of mesonephric tubules

Ligament of ovary
Broad ligament

Round ligament of uterus

Gubernaculum

Fig. 15.7. A diagram to show how the gubernaculum becomes the round ligament and the ligament of the ovary.

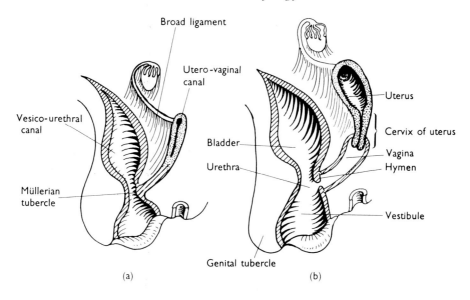

Fig. 15.8. The development of the female internal genitalia.

which is not fully canalized at this stage, produces therein the *Müllerian tubercle* (p.261). Soon, however, the solid end of the canal becomes pushed away from the urogenital sinus by a proliferation of cells which appear to be derived from the endoderm of the sinus (Fig. 15.8). This solid mass of cells, the *sinus upgrowth*, together with the utero-vaginal canal, will between them form the vagina, the cervix and the body of the uterus. Opinions differ as to the relative importance of the endodermal and mesodermal components of these structures and only a simplified version need be given here. It seems probable that the lining of the whole vagina is derived from the sinus upgrowth which soon becomes canalized. The surrounding mesoderm forms the connective tissue and muscle which are found in the wall of the vagina. At the upper end of the vagina, slight dilations occur which push up around the developing cervix of the uterus and form the vaginal fornices. At the lower end, the area of contact between vagina and urogenital sinus increases and becomes more extensive than the opening of the vagina into the sinus. The opening is the hymeneal orifice and the annular shelf which surrounds it becomes the hymen. As can be seen from Fig. 15.8 most of the definitive urogenital sinus will later form the vestibule, from which small diverticula are given off to form the greater vestibular (Bartholin's) glands.

Like the bladder, the uterus in the child is an abdominal rather than a pelvic organ and the cervix is approximately the same length as the body of the uterus. It is only at puberty that the adult position and proportions are attained.

The external genitalia

Female external genitalia

Up to the seventh week of development the appearance of the external genitalia is similar in both sexes (Fig. 14.4). The female genitalia undergo some changes similar to those in the male (*vide infra*) but these are not very marked and can be disregarded. Both urethra and vagina open into the common vestibule which is widely open to the exterior after the disappearance of the urogenital membrane. The opening is flanked by the urethral folds and the genital swellings which become, respectively, the minor and major labia. The genital tubercle enlarges to form a *phallus* and this, in the female, becomes bent back on itself to develop into the clitoris.

Male external genitalia

The phallus, developed from the genital tubercle, becomes much larger in the male, a process controlled by the secretion of androgens from the fetal testis. A proliferation of endodermal cells from the anterior extremity of the phallic part of the urogenital sinus, extends forwards into the phallus as a sagittally placed *urethral plate*. This was originally in contact ventrally with the ectoderm of the urogenital membrane and, as might be expected, it is also in contact with the ectoderm of the ventral surface of the phallus (Fig. 15.9), even after the urogenital membrane has disappeared. The urethral plate lies above a *urethral groove* on the under surface of the phallus; the groove is continuous posteriorly with the region lying between the urethral folds (Fig. 15.10).

After the disappearance of the urogenital membrane the urethra is widely open in the perineum but the urethral folds soon begin to fuse with each other to close off the opening and form a floor to the posterior part of the urethra. This fusion takes place from behind forwards (Fig. 15.10). When the process reaches the phallus the urethral plate splits ventrally and forms an endodermal lining to the deeper part of the urethral groove. The ectoderm then fuses across the midline

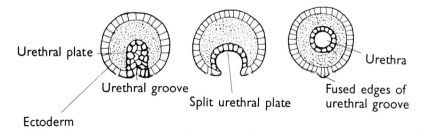

Fig. 15.9. Transverse sections through the phallus of a male embryo to show the development of the urethra from the urethral plate.

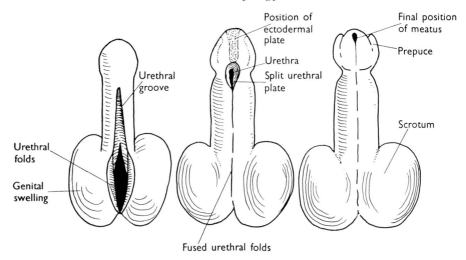

Fig. 15.10. Development of the male external genitalia.

leaving the endoderm-lined urethra within the phallus, in a manner reminiscent of the closure of the neural tube (Figs. 15.9 and 15.10). As a result of these changes the external urethral opening is carried forward towards the tip of the phallus although it still opens on the under surface. A plate of ectoderm then grows backwards from the tip to meet the urethra. This becomes canalized and, with the closure of the previous opening, forms the terminal part of the urethra. A circumferential invagination of ectoderm invades the phallus for a short distance from its tip and when this breaks down it separates the prepuce from the glans penis. Finally the descent of the testis into the genital swellings, which thus form the scrotum, completes the development of the external genitalia. The line of fusion of the urethral folds is clearly seen as a midline raphe on the scrotum (Fig. 15.10).

The determination of sex

In the first instance, the *chromosomal sex* of the embryo is determined at fertilization, when the normal zygote will contain either two X chromosomes or an X and a Y (p.8). The main factor concerned with producing 'maleness' is the presence of a Y chromosome (rather than the absence of a second X chromosome), since individuals with chromosomal abnormalities (such as Klinefelter's Syndrome (47XXY)) show male characteristics in spite of the presence of two X chromosomes. In recent years it has been shown that the masculinizing effect of the Y chromosome is probably due to a Y-linked antigen known as the *H-Y antigen* (since it is the same antigen that causes the histo-incompatibility of skin grafts from male to female in certain strains of mice). The presence of the H-Y antigen apparently leads to the transformation of the neutral gonad into a testis, thus establishing the *gonadal sex* of the fetus. At about the eighth week, the fetal testis begins to secrete testosterone and Müllerian-inhibiting hormone from the inter-stitial and Sertoli cells respectively and these, in turn, cause the development of the male genitalia and the establishment of *somatic sex*. The full development of male genitalia is also dependent upon the presence of a steroid *5-reductase* that converts some of the testosterone to dihydrotestosterone as well as upon the presence of receptor sites for this hormone in the genital primordia.

Anomalies in any of these stages in sexual development, as well as abnormal development of other endocrine glands such as the suprarenal, can cause various types of 'ambiguous sex' in the fetus and careful diagnosis at birth is essential in these conditions in order to determine the true sex.

Developmental anomalies of the urogenital system

As has been seen, the development of the urogenital system is complex and many of the processes concerned depend upon the proper completion of previous stages so that abnormalities of one viscus are very liable to be associated with those of another. In consequence, developmental abnormalities are extremely common and it has been estimated that about 10 per cent of the population are affected if minor and usually unnoticed degrees of anomaly are taken into account; however, the number of anomalies requiring treatment is very much smaller than this.

Certain associated abnormalities that may be found in the neonate may sug-gest the presence of maldevelopment of the urinary tract. A good example is a peculiar facial appearance — *Potter's facies* — in which the eyes are widely separated, the nose curved strongly and the ears low-set.

Abnormal development of the kidney

Abnormalities of structure

One or both kidneys may be absent (*agenesis*) and this is usually associated with absence of the ureter and of all, or part, of the trigone. If both kidneys are absent, there will also be a diminution in the amount of amniotic fluid (*oligohydroamnios*) (p.316) which gives rise to associated defects, such as pressure deformities of the lower limbs and Potter's facies (*vide supra*, and Chapter 17). Clearly, bilateral agenesis is incompatible with life.

If the ureteric bud develops but fails to induce the proper differentiation of the metanephrogenic cap, the kidney may be small and poorly developed (*hypoplasia*), or it may develop abnormally (*dysplasia*) showing bizarre histological appearances.

There are a number of different forms of *cystic disease of the kidney* and the commonest, *adult polycystic disease*, affects about 1 in 1000 individuals and is inherited as an autosomal dominant. Typically, both kidneys are enormously enlarged because of the presence of a large number of fluid-filled cysts which may replace most of the kidney tissue (Fig. 15.11). The cysts are formed as a result of dilatation of various portions of the nephron, particularly of the loops of Henle.

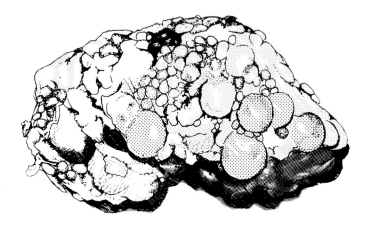

Fig. 15.11. A specimen of polycystic kidney. Very little functioning kidney substance remains.

The cause of the condition is uncertain. At one time it was thought that it was due to failure of the ureteric bud derivatives to link up with the tubules derived from the metanephrogenic cap but, since the cysts are continuous with other parts of the same nephron and since the condition is also frequently associated with a cystic condition of the liver, this seems unlikely. It may be that the distensibility of a part of the nephron is abnormally increased for some reason and there may be some element of partial obstruction of the affected nephrons.

Clinically, the condition may remain 'silent' for many years until some complication — such as hypertension or cerebral aneurysm (a localised dilatation of one or more intracranial arteries) — draws attention to the renal condition. The average age of death is 50 years.

The infantile variety of *cystic disease* is quite a different condition, being inherited as a recessive trait and usually causing death in childhood, although an increasing number of these children are now surviving as a result of haemo-dialysis and transplants. The cysts are derived from collecting ducts and are small and fusiform, the kidney retaining its normal shape.

Abnormalities in the early stages of development of the ureteric bud may cause faulty development of the caliceal system. If one of the divisions, for example, fails to induce the development of the corresponding portion of the metanephrogenic cap the result will be a *caliceal cyst* or *pyelo-caliceal diverticulum. Congenital hydronephrosis* is not uncommon. This is a dilatation of the pelvis and calices which may be enormous and is often associated with other developmental anomalies. The cause is obscure but it may be due to abnormal folds or constrictions of the ureter, or to muscular inco-ordination at the pelvi-ureteric junction, thus stressing the importance of peristalsis in the ureter, possibly arising from a 'pacemaker'.

Abnormalities of position

The 'ascent' of the kidney that occurs during development has already been mentioned, although it is not such a spectacular event as a consideration of adult anatomy would suggest, being largely due to differential growth of neighbouring structures. However, abnormalities of the process of ascent are common and are often associated with fusion of the two kidneys at an early stage of their development (Fig. 15.12).

Simple ectopia of the kidney is a condition in which the normal ascent has not occurred so that the ureter is short and the kidney is found low down in the abdomen or even in the pelvis. It usually retains its fetal lobulation and does not rotate normally, so that the hilum faces forwards (*malrotation*). The kidney retains its embryonic blood supply so that the renal artery arises from the lower part of the aorta or from the common iliac vessels.

In *crossed ectopia* one kidney (usually the left) crosses the midline during its ascent and comes to lie near the opposite kidney, although the ureteric orifice in the bladder is in its normal position. The two kidneys usually fuse and the ectopic kidney (and sometimes the contra-lateral kidney) is usually malrotated so that its hilum does not face medially. The commonest form of ectopic kidney is that in which the left kidney has crossed the midline and has fused with the lower pole of the right, both hila facing forwards. Sometimes the two hila face in opposite directions — the so-called *S-shaped* or *sigmoid kidney*.

Malrotation can also occur in kidneys which are in the normal position.

A particular form of fusion and malrotation of the kidney is that in which the two kidneys have fused at their lower poles across the midline, the hila facing

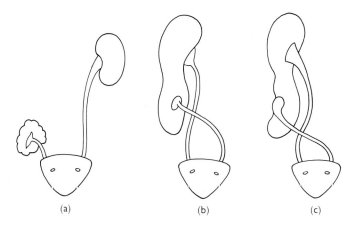

(a)   (b)   (c)

Fig. 15.12. Ectopia of kidney. (a) Failure of ascent. The kidney lies in the iliac region and is distorted with the hilum facing forwards (non-rotation). (b) Crossed ectopia. The ectopic kidney has crossed the midline and fused with the normal kidney. In this illustration one hilum faces medially and the other faces forwards. Often both face forwards. (c) S-shaped or sigmoid kidney.

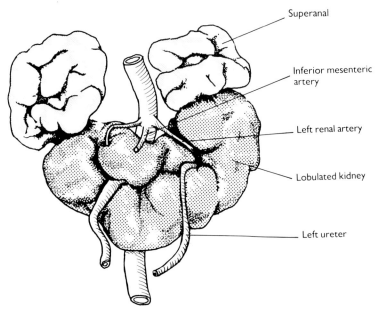

Superanal

Inferior mesenteric
artery

Left renal artery

Lobulated kidney

Left ureter

Fig. 15.13. Horseshoe kidney. This specimen was from a full term fetus so the suprarenals are large.
Note the relation of the isthmus to the inferior mesenteric artery.

more or less forwards. This condition is known as a *horseshoe kidney* (Fig. 15.13)
and the deformity presumably occurs at a very early stage in ascent when the two
kidneys are close together. During the ascent, the isthmus usually rises to the level
of the inferior mesenteric artery, which prevents further ascent. The ureters cross
in front of the isthmus and may be obstructed in this region. The condition is
fairly common (1 in 400 postmortems) and may remain unsuspected throughout
life.

Anomalies of the ureter

Agenesis (failure of development) of the ureter must necessarily be associated
with agenesis of the kidney since, in the absence of a ureteric bud, the metanephrogenic cap cannot form. Congenital narrowing of the ureter may occur,
usually at the pelvi-ureteric junction or at the lower end near the bladder.

More commonly, the ureter is duplicated and this anomaly takes various forms.
The most common variety is that in which the kidney has two pelves and ureters
and the ureters unite to form a Y-junction so that there is only one ureteric orifice
in the bladder on that side. It seems probable that this anomaly is due to an early
bifurcation of the ureteric bud so that the two divisions of the ureter pick up a
common metanephrogenic cap. The ureter may also be completely duplicated so
that there are two ureteric orifices, one in more or less the normal position in the
bladder while the other, the 'ectopic ureter', opens either into the bladder, the
urethra, the vagina or even the ductus deferens. In the male, the ectopic opening

is above the sphincter urethrae but, in the female, it may be below the sphincter so that incontinence may be a distressing feature.

The anatomical features of duplicated ureters may be understood by considering the normal development, even though the mechanism of absorption of the lower end of the mesonephric duct into the urogenital sinus is not properly understood (p.254). Duplication of the ureter is due to the development of more than one ureteric bud, the two buds picking up a common cap of metanephrogenic tissue (Fig. 15.14). When the lower end of the mesonephric duct is taken into the primitive urogenital sinus to form the trigone, the lower of the two buds (which drains the lower part of the metanephros) is 'fed into' the developing bladder first and migrates upwards towards the normal position of the ureteric orifice. The upper bud (which drains the upper part of the metanephros) follows later and so opens lower down in the bladder or, in the case of a very high ureteric bud, may not reach the bladder at all but may open into the definitive urogenital sinus below the vesico-urethral canal and so, in the fully developed fetus, will open into one of the extra-vesical situations mentioned above. Thus, when two ureters are present, the upper part of the kidney drains via the lower of the two ureteric orifices (the *Weigert–Mayer law*).

Sometimes, although only one ureteric bud is present, it arises from the mesonephric duct in an abnormal situation so that it may open into the bladder or lower urinary tract in an abnormal situation. Such *ectopic ureters* (or the ectopic member of duplicated ureters) are often associated with a poorly developed or dysplastic kidney and it has been suggested that this is due to its having picked up a metanephrogenic cap from the wrong portion of the nephrogenic ridge on

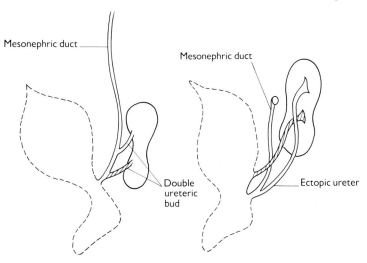

Fig. 15.14. Duplication of the ureter. (a) This condition is caused by duplication of the ureteric bud. The lower bud is shaded. (b) When the lower end of the mesonephric duct is taken into the urogenital sinus, the shaded ureter comes to occupy the normal position, while the upper (ectopic) ureter opens lower down, in this case into the mesonephric duct (later the ductus deferens).

account of its abnormal position. It may be, however, that the renal abnormality is due to *vesico-ureteric reflux*, a condition in which the normal valvular mechanism at the opening of the ureter into the bladder is not properly developed so that, when the detrusor muscle of the bladder contracts, urine is forced back up the ureter to the kidney as well as down the urethra. After birth this can give rise to recurrent urinary tract infection and, with severe reflux, to kidney damage.

Anomalies of the bladder

The urachus

In the embryo the vesico-urethral canal extends up to the umbilicus but, as the bladder forms, the lumen of the upper part of the canal becomes obliterated to form the urachus. A localised part of the urachus may retain its lumen and form a *urachal cyst*, or the lumen may persist at either end to form a *urachal sinus* or a *bladder diverticulum*. Rarely, the whole length of the urachus may posses a lumen so that urine may be discharged from the umbilicus. Any of these conditions is likely to be complicated by infection.

Exstrophy

An early and important step in the development of the infra-umbilical part of the abdominal wall is the ingrowth of mesoderm of somite origin between the umbilicus and the cloacal membrane (p.250). If this fails to occur, the cloacal membrane will remain adjacent to the umbilical region and, when it ruptures, the inside of the urogenital sinus will be exposed. Furthermore, the muscle sheets derived from the myotomes will not reach the midline. This developmental failure results in the condition of *exstrophy* (ectopia vesicae) in which the lining of the bladder is exposed below the umbilicus with the two ureteric orifices discharging urine onto its surface (Fig. 9.8). Below this, in the male, there is a small penis which has a deep groove in the midline on its upper surface (*epispadias*). This is the result of the original two halves of the genital tubercle being unable to fuse. The recti are widely separated and X-ray shows a wide gap between the pubic bones. Treatment of this condition is difficult.

Anomalies of the urethra

Epispadias

Epispadias can occur without exstrophy, so that the groove on the upper surface of the penis leads into a dorsal cleft in the upper urethra and, thence, through a small defect in the abdominal wall into the bladder. Its cause is not known for certain but it is probably due to failure of the two precursors of the genital tubercle (p.250) to fuse in the midline, leaving a small area of original cloacal membrane between them. The condition is, therefore, closely allied to that of exstrophy.

Hypospadias

While epispadias is uncommon, *hypospadias* occurs relatively frequently. This is a condition in the male in which the ventral part of the urethra is imperfectly developed. It is due to a fault in the fusion of the urethral folds to form the penile urethra or to a failure of canalization of the ectodermal ingrowth at the tip of the penis (refer to Fig. 15.10). The condition may be due to a lack of secretion of testosterone from the fetal testis or to inadequate receptor sites on the urethral folds. It may be present in various degrees of severity.

In the simplest type, the urethral folds fuse but the distal part of the urethra fails to develop so that the urethra opens on the under surface of the glans (*glandular hypospadias*), often by a very small opening. In *penile hypospadias* there may be one or more openings on the under surface of the shaft of the penis; a groove may lead forward from the abnormal opening to the glans. The glans itself is flattened and spread out and the prepuce is hooded. The shaft of the penis is often bowed with a ventral concavity (*chordee*).

In the more severe degrees of this deformity, the opening of the urethra is still further back and failure of the urethral folds to fuse leads to the scrotum being cleft in the midline and, since the penis is small and strongly curved ventrally and the testes often undescended, it may be difficult to determine the somatic sex at birth. Occasionally the resemblance to a female somatotype may be increased by persistence of the lower end of the fused Müllerian ducts so that the prostatic utricle is replaced by a small uterus. The various conditions of severe hypospadias, in which the somatic sex is ambiguous, are sometimes referred to as *pseudohermaphroditism*. The chromosomal and gonadal sex is, however, obvious, unlike the very rare conditions of *true hermaphroditism* in which there may be a testis on one side and an ovary on the other or, occasionally, both gonads may be mixed in type — *ovotestes*.

Cryptorchidism

Failure of descent of the testis and *maldescent*, in which the testis may descend to an abnormal position, are the most common anomalies of the male genital system. In failure of the process of descent (*cryptorchidism*) the testis may remain at any position between the scrotum and the pelvis. The final stages of normal descent may sometimes take place after birth so that it is necessary to wait for 3–4 months before finally making a diagnosis. A powerful cremasteric reflex may also simulate the condition by dragging the testis upwards when stimulated during examination or by external factors (e.g. a low temperature). If the testis remains in the abdomen near the deep ring it is impalpable but it may be palpated if it is

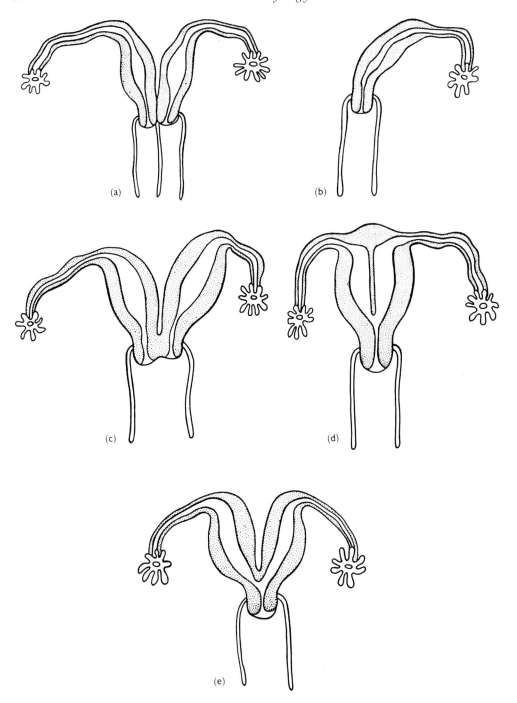

Fig. 15.15. Various forms of duplication of the uterus. (a) Vagina duplex and corpus and cervix duplex (b) Uterus unicornis (c) Uterus duplex (d) Uterus subseptus (e) Uterus bicornis.

retained within the canal or in the inguinal region. It often feels softer than a normal testis. The maldescended (ectopic) testis may lie in the perineum, over the pubis, in the thigh or in other even more unlikely positions.

Cryptorchidism is often associated with abnormalities of the epididymis since the gubernaculum is attached to both testis and epididymis.

The undescended testis shows histological and histochemical abnormalities and normal spermatogenesis is not possible. It is also more liable to trauma, and to torsion (a condition in which the testis and epididymis rotate so that twisting of the spermatic cord may lead to obstruction of the vessels) and is more likely to develop malignant tumours than the normal testis. Treatment is, therefore, necessary in infancy. Descent may be achieved by treatment with gonadotrophins but surgical intervention may sometimes be necessary.

Anomalies of the uterus and vagina

Since development of the single, midline uterus and vagina depends upon the fusion of the two paramesonephric (Müllerian) ducts, it is not surprising that various forms of duplication may occur (Fig. 15.15). Thus, complete failure of fusion of the ducts will give rise to a duplication of the whole genital tract in which the vagina is in two halves separated by a septum with a separate cervix and with a unilateral uterine body associated with each half (*vagina duplex* and *corpus* and *cervix duplex*). Rarely, one of the Müllerian ducts may not appear at all, giving rise to a *uterus unicornis*. Less severe grades of failure of fusion of the ducts may give rise to a single vagina into which lead two cervices, each associated with one horn of a uterus (*uterus duplex*). A single vagina and cervix may be associated with a uterus subdivided into separate halves (*uterus bicornis*) or a single uterine body may be partly subdivided by a septum (*uterus subseptus*). All these conditions usually lead to sterility.

A failure of canalization at the lower end of the developing vagina may produce an *imperforate hymen*, a condition which may be symptomless until the menarche when the vagina and uterus will become distended with the retained products of menstruation.

Finally, remnants of the mesonephric ducts and tubules (epoöphoron paroöphoron and Gärtner's duct) may give rise to various forms of cysts in the broad ligament which may become infected or rupture giving acute abdominal symptoms.

Developmental stages
(Chapters 14 and 15)

23–24 days: Nephrogenic ridge formed
   Pro/mesonephric duct appears
24–26 days: Mesonephric tubules appear

28 days: Primitive germ cells demonstrable

Mesonephric ducts join cloaca

5 weeks: Ureteric bud and metanephrogenic cap present

Gonads present

Genital tubercle apparent

5—6 weeks: Paramesonephric duct develops

7—8 weeks: Sex of gonad apparent

Cloacal membrane perforates

3—4 months: External genitalia recognisable as male or female

Prostate develops

Male urethra complete

Müllerian tubercle apparent

7—9 months: Process of descent of testis.

Further reading (Chapters 14 and 15)

Forsberg, J-G. (1973) Cervico-vaginal epithelium: its origin and development *Am. J. Obs. Gynae.* **115**, 1025.

Guraya, S.S. (1980) Recent progress in the morphology, histochemistry, biochemistry and physiology of developing and maturing human testis. *Int. Rev. Cytol.* **62**, 187—309.

Jones, H.W. & Scott, W.W. (1971) *Hermaphroditism, Genital Anomalies and Related Endocrine Disorders.* Williams & Wilkins, Baltimore.

Kissane, J.M. (1974) Congenital malformations in: *Pathology of the Kidney*, (ed.) Heptinstall, R.H. Little, Brown & Co., Boston. 51—119.

Moffat, D.B. (1982) 'Development of the urogenital system in the male' and 'Developmental abnormalities of the urogenital system'. Chapters 44 and 45 in: *Scientific Foundation of Urology* (eds.) Chisholm, G.D. & Innes Williams, D. Heinemann, London.

O'Rahilly, R. & Muecke, E.C. (1972) The timing and sequence of events in the development of the human urinary system during the embryonic period proper. *Z. Anat. Entw.-Gesch.*, **138**, 99—109.

Potter E. (1972) *The Normal and Abnormal Development of the Kidney.* Year Book Medical Publishers, Chicago.

Short, R.V. (1979) Sex determination and differentiation. *Brit. Med. Bull.* **35**: 121—127.

16
Digestive System

As a result of the formation of the head, tail and lateral folds (Chapter 6), the embryo develops a recognisable alimentary system. The *foregut* extends from the buccopharyngeal membrane back to the plane of the anterior wall of the yolk sac (Fig. 6.12); it passes dorsal to the free border of the septum transversum and between the coelomic ducts (Figs. 6.14, 13.3 and 13.4). Caudally, the *hindgut* extends from the plane of the caudal wall of the yolk sac to the cloacal membrane and near its termination it will later join with the allantois to form the *cloaca*. The midgut is not well defined since at the stage shown in Figs. 6.12 and 6.14 it is represented mainly by the roof and part of the lateral wall of the yolk sac. Soon, however, the yolk sac becomes very much smaller and its neck becomes con-stricted to form the vitello-intestinal duct (p.286) so that the *midgut* becomes recognisable (Fig. 6.13). At the same time the midgut pulls away from the dorsal body wall, to form a mesodermal dorsal mesentery. Eventually this part of the gut becomes a well marked loop (Fig. 16.1) with the remains of the yolk sac attached to its most ventral point. Figs. 16.1, 16.2 and 16.3 show that the foregut is attached by a mesentery to the septum transversum. This is the *ventral mesentery* and it has a caudal free border since it is only found in the region of the foregut. It must be mentioned here that embryonic mesenteries bear no resemblance to the thin, double layers of peritoneum that are found in the adult. Instead they are very thick slabs of mesoderm, the surface cells of which form the future peritoneum. The foregut, then, has both dorsal and ventral mesenteries while the midgut and hindgut have only a dorsal mesentery.

In the midline of the dorsal body wall, and therefore at the root of the dorsal mesentery, is the dorsal aorta. In the early stages of development this has a number of ventral branches which are known as *vitelline arteries* (p.199) since they supply the yolk sac. These arteries soon become reduced to three main vessels in the future abdominal region. They are the *coeliac artery*, which supplies most of the foregut, the *superior mesenteric artery*, which supplies the midgut, and the *inferior mesenteric artery* which supplies the hindgut. It will be seen later that the junction between fore- and midgut in terms of adult anatomy lies near the middle of the second part of the duodenum and, as might be expected, there is here in the adult an anastomosis between a branch of the coeliac artery (the superior pancreatico-duodenal) and a branch of the superior mesenteric artery (the inferior pancreatico-duodenal). Similarly, towards the left side of the transverse colon, the

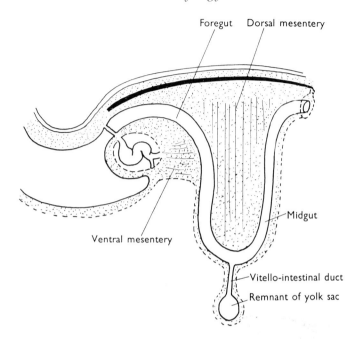

Fig. 16.1. The gut pulls away from the dorsal body wall mesoderm to form a dorsal mesentery and away from the septum transversum to form the ventral mesentery.

middle colic artery (from the superior mesenteric artery) anastomoses with the superior left colic artery (from the inferior mesenteric artery).

Histogenesis of the gut

The endodermal cells of the fore-, mid-, and hindgut give rise to the epithelial lining (stratified squamous in the oesophagus, columnar elsewhere). A condensation of mesenchyme around the epithelium will later differentiate into the connective tissue, muscle and blood vessels of the gut wall while the outermost layer of mesenchyme forms the visceral layer of peritoneum. During development, the lining epithelium undergoes proliferation so that the lumen becomes partly, or wholly, occluded for a time — the lumen, anyway, is very small relative to the thickness of the gut wall. It is only at a much later stage of development that the lumen becomes fully established. Failure to do so results in *atresia* — a localised constriction or complete occlusion which will be discussed later.

Some activity goes on in the alimentary canal before birth. Amniotic fluid is swallowed and some secretion occurs from various glands, including the liver. Peristalsis probably begins just after the 10th week of intra-uterine life.

At full term the ileum and the large intestine contain dark green *meconium*, which consists of swallowed amniotic fluid, glandular secretions and bile. During a part of intra-uterine life, the epithelium of the fetal small intestine shows

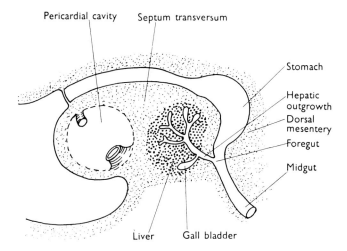

Fig. 16.2. The hepatic outgrowth grows into the ventral mesentery from the end of the foregut. The columns of liver cells invade and replace the cells of the septum transversum.

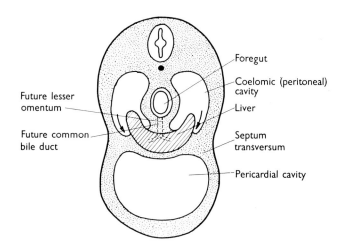

Fig. 16.3. A transverse section through the peritoneal and pericardial cavities to show the position of the liver within the septum transversum. To a large extent the liver becomes separated from the diaphragm except for the region lying between the arrows (the bare area).

marked pinocytotic activity. In this way meconium is taken into the cells to form *meconium corpuscles.* In many species of mammals immunoglobulin molecules from the milk enter the cells in this way after birth. The animals concerned (e.g. the rat) receive some of their passive neonatal immunity in this way but, in the human fetus, passive immunity is mainly the result of the passage of immunoglobulins across the chorio-allantoic placenta (see Chapter 8).

The foregut

The foregut is, at first, a simple tubular structure but a dilatation soon marks the site of the future stomach which is initially orientated in the sagittal plane. Between the caudal end of the pharynx and the proximal end of the stomach the foregut forms the oesophagus; as already mentioned, the endoderm becomes the lining epithelium and the surrounding mesoderm condenses to form the muscle and connective tissue of the oesophageal wall. The mesentery of the oesophagus remains very short and eventually disappears, except at its caudal end where it makes a small contribution to the diaphragm (see Chapter 13).

The distal end of the foregut is marked by the *hepatic outgrowth*. This is an endodermal diverticulum which grows out from the gut into the ventral mesentery very close to its free border (Fig. 16.2). The diverticulum divides into two, one division becoming the cystic duct and gall bladder and the other dividing again and again to form the biliary ducts and hepatic cells of the liver. The columns of liver cells thus produced invade the septum transversum until the greater part of the septum has been replaced by liver tissue and only a thin layer, separating the liver from the pericardial cavity, remains (Fig. 16.3). Further details of the development of the biliary system will be given later (p.283).

The dorsal mesentery in the region of the stomach (often known as the *dorsal mesogastrium*) becomes hollowed out from its right side by an ingrowth from the coelomic cavity known as the *bursa omentalis* (Fig. 16.4). The bursa omentalis increases in size and extends caudally, dorsal to the stomach, and cranially along the right border of the oesophagus and behind the liver. The latter extension is known as the *pneumato-enteric recess* and will form the upper recess of the lesser sac, the bursa omentalis itself forming the main part. As a result of the formation of the bursa omentalis and of different rates of growth in different parts of the stomach wall, the stomach comes to lie transversely and it now has anterior and posterior walls instead of left and right. Hence in the adult, the left vagus is

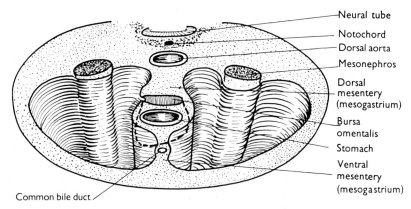

Common bile duct

Neural tube
Notochord
Dorsal aorta
Mesonephros
Dorsal mesentery (mesogastrium)
Bursa omentalis
Stomach
Ventral mesentery (mesogastrium)

Fig. 16.4. The bursa omentalis grows into the dorsal mesentery from the (embryo's) right. Its lower part is indicated by the dotted line.

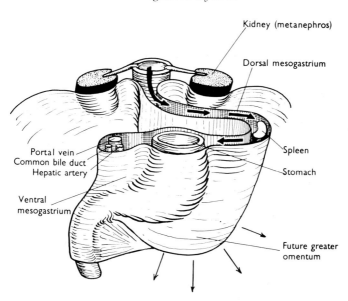

Fig. 16.5. As a result of the ingrowth of the bursa omentalis and of the rotation of the stomach, the dorsal mesentery is thrown over to the left. It also grows in the direction of the small arrows. The larger arrows show the course of arteries which pass to the spleen and stomach.

concerned mostly with supplying the front of the stomach and the right with the back (Fig. 16.5). Owing to the resulting change in disposition of the dorsal and ventral mesenteries, it can now be seen that the dorsal mesentery is attached to the greater curvature of the stomach and the ventral mesentery to the lesser. The free edge of the latter has now become more or less vertical. Fig. 16.5 also shows how the spleen develops, as a mesodermal condensation of the mesenchyme together with a contribution from the coelomic epithelium, in the dorsal mesentery. This becomes invaded by lymphocytes (see Chapter 12). The splenic artery, coming from the coeliac artery, must necessarily traverse the dorsal mesentery to reach the spleen, while branches from the splenic artery to the stomach will have to continue along the dorsal mesentery between spleen and stomach. The part of the dorsal mesentery that is attached to the greater curvature of the stomach hangs down as a pouch-like structure which can be seen in Fig. 16.6. The two double layers of peritoneum which form its anterior and posterior walls become the four layers of the *greater omentum*. Like the kidney, the spleen is lobulated in the fetus and the notches which are found on its anterior border in the adult are vestiges of the grooves which separated the lobules in the fetus.

Extensive fusion occurs between the dorsal mesentery and the posterior abdominal wall and this has the effect of carrying the attachment of the mesentery from the midline to the anterior surface of the left kidney (Fig. 16.7). The portion of the dorsal mesentery between the kidney and the spleen thus becomes the *lieno-renal ligament* and that between the spleen and the stomach, the *gastro-splenic ligament*. It can thus be seen that the lieno-renal ligament, the gastro-splenic

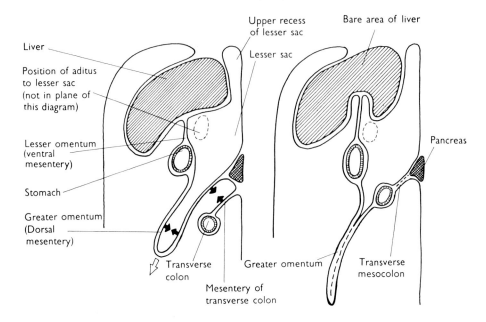

Fig. 16.6. Midline sagittal sections to show the formation of the lesser sac.

ligament and the greater omentum are really all parts of the same structure, namely the dorsal mesentery; the three parts of this become recognisable as soon as the spleen develops. As will be seen later, the transverse colon with its own mesentery later comes to lie just below the stomach (Fig. 16.6). Fusion occurs between the posterior leaves of the greater omentum and the transverse colon and its mesentery and, to a variable degree, between the layers of the omentum itself. The adult transverse colon thus appears to be embedded in the posterior surface of the greater omentum.

The ventral mesentery, which originally connected the lesser curvature to the septum transversum, becomes so altered by the large size of the liver that it now appears to join the lesser curvature to the liver (Fig. 16.6) and can be recognised as the lesser omentum. The coelomic cavity burrows around the convex surface of the liver (arrows in Fig. 16.3) but, centrally, the liver remains in contact with a part of the septum transversum which will form the central part of the diaphragm (p.240). This part of the liver is destined to become the bare area while remnants of the original ventral mesentery around this area form the falciform, right and left triangular and coronary ligaments.

The pneumato-enteric recess forms the upper recess of the lesser sac and is related anteriorly to the liver. The original site where the bursa omentalis invaded the dorsal mesentery remains small and becomes the *aditus to the lesser sac*. As will be understood by reference to Figs. 16.5 and 16.7, it is bounded anteriorly by the right free edge of the lesser omentum in which lies the common bile duct (*vide infra*). The hepatic artery and portal vein also lie in the free border of the lesser omentum.

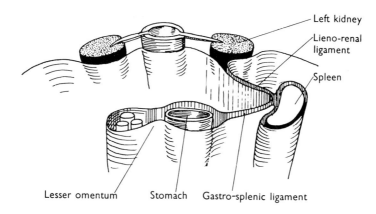

Fig. 16.7. A similar view to Fig. 16.5, after fusion of the dorsal mesentery with the dorsal body wall.

Liver, biliary apparatus and pancreas

As has been mentioned, the columns of liver cells derived from the endodermal foregut diverticulum invade the mesoderm of the septum transversum so that the latter is no longer recognisable as a thick mass of mesoderm but is reduced to a thin layer which forms the caudal wall of the pericardial cavity. Remnants of the mesoderm of the septum transversum also form the connective tissue components of the liver. Running into the septum transversum and thence into the sinus venosus (p.199) are five (originally six) major veins, but only three of these approach it from the abdominal aspect. These are the right and left vitelline veins, which drain the yolk sac and lie in the splanchnopleure, and the left umbilical vein which returns blood to the embryo from the placenta and lies in the somato-pleure. The right umbilical vein disappears early in embryonic life. In the septum transversum these three veins lose their identities as the liver increases in size and comes to resemble a vascular spongework since there are large vascular spaces between the columns of liver cells. The whole liver, therefore, has a very red and vascular appearance and it is, in fact, an important site of haematopoietic (blood forming) activity during fetal life. The further development of the vascular system in the vicinity will be described later (p.284).

The pancreas

The pancreas develops from two endodermal outgrowths from the foregut. The *ventral pancreatic outgrowth* appears in the caudal angle between the hepatic diverticulum and the foregut. The *dorsal pancreatic outgrowth* appears a little cranial to the ventral outgrowth. It is found on the dorsal aspect of the foregut and therefore grows into the substance of the dorsal mesentery (Fig. 16.8a). Growth follows the usual embryological pattern of glands, the original endodermal outgrowth giving rise to numerous subdivisions which form the duct system and

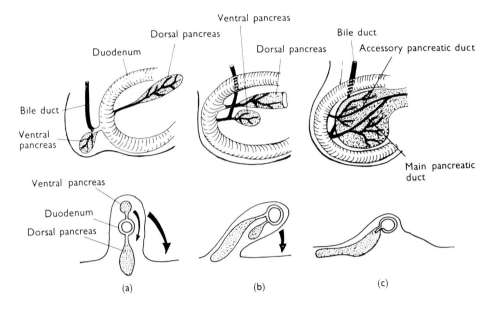

Fig. 16.8. The development of the pancreas. The upper diagram shows the pancreas and bile duct seen from in front; the lower row represents a series of cross sections viewed from above.

glandular alveoli; while the surrounding mesoderm forms the connective tissue and blood vessels.

The stem of the hepatic diverticulum is now recognisable as the common bile duct and this, and the duct of the ventral pancreas, have a common opening into the duodenum on its ventral aspect. Owing to differential growth in the gut wall the whole complex of ventral pancreas and common bile duct appears to migrate dorsally around the duodenum until it meets the dorsal pancreas (Fig. 16.8b). The ducts of the two pancreatic outgrowths now come into communication in such a way that most of the dorsal pancreas drains via the duct of the ventral pancreas into the duodenum (Fig. 16.8c). This composite duct becomes the main pancreatic duct, opening in common with the common bile duct. Before opening into the duodenum the ducts dilate to form an hepato-pancreatic ampulla (*ampulla of Vater*). The opening of the dorsal pancreas may persist to become the *accessory pancreatic duct* which therefore opens cranial to the normal duct. The greater part of the dorsal mesentery of the foregut eventually fuses with the posterior abdominal wall and the pancreas becomes a retroperitoneal structure, as does the C-shaped curve of the duodenum (Fig. 16.8c).

Portal vein

Of four veins which originally entered the septum transversum from the abdominal region (Figs. 12.3 and 16.9) only three persist in the late embryo and only two into post-natal life. The right umbilical vein disappears completely at a

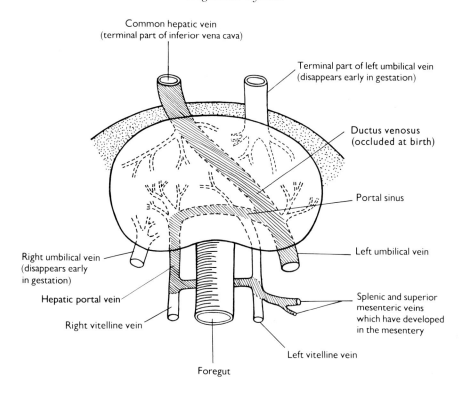

Common hepatic vein
(terminal part of inferior vena cava)

Terminal part of left umbilical vein
(disappears early in gestation)

Ductus venosus
(occluded at birth)

Portal sinus

Left umbilical vein

Right umbilical vein
(disappears early
in gestation)

Hepatic portal vein

Right vitelline vein

Splenic and superior
mesenteric veins
which have developed
in the mesentery

Left vitelline vein

Foregut

Fig. 16.9. The vessels in the region of the liver. The cross-hatched vessels persist, at least until birth, while the others disappear.

very early stage (p.199), leaving only a single vein to return blood from the placenta. The two vitelline veins are joined together by a cross connection which passes dorsal to the gut (Fig. 16.9). Blood drains into the left vitelline vein from a new vessel (the superior mesenteric vein) which appears in the mesentery and then passes via the dorsal connection into the right vitelline vein. These vessels become straightened out to form the *hepatic portal vein* which thus enters the liver towards its right side, having passed dorsal to the duodenum. This explains why the adult portal vein passes behind the first part of the duodenum. The veins which originally entered the sinus venosus from the septum transversum become reduced to one which is now a short wide vessel leading from the liver to the right side of the sinus venosus. This vessel is known as the *common hepatic vein (hepato-cardiac channel)*; it forms the terminal part of the inferior vena cava; the part of the sinus venosus into which it opens will become the posterior part of the right atrium (p.208). In early development a left hepato-cardiac channel, matching that on the right, was present but this disappears when the inferior vena cava becomes delineated (p.201). Within the liver, some of the vascular spaces become particularly large in the regions where the blood flow is brisk and these form the main venous channels within the liver. The hepatic portal vein and the (left) umbilical vein open into a large space known as the *portal sinus*, and they also

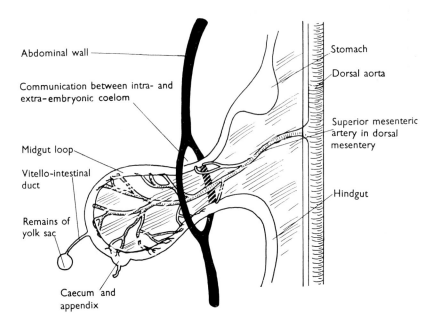

Abdominal wall

Communication between intra- and
extra-embryonic coelom

Midgut loop

Vitello-intestinal
duct

Remains of
yolk sac

Caecum and
appendix

Stomach

Dorsal aorta

Superior mesenteric
artery in dorsal
mesentery

Hindgut

Fig. 16.10. A diagrammatic side view of the midgut loop herniated out into the extra-embryonic coelom.

supply large branches to the liver substance. Blood is collected from the vascular spaces of the liver into a number of large veins (later to become the hepatic veins) which enter the common hepatic vein, but a good deal of the umbilical vein blood (⅓ to ⅔ of the total volume) passes straight through a wide oblique channel, known as the *ductus venosus*, which runs from the left side of the portal sinus to the common hepatic vein, thus short-circuiting the hepatic sinusoids. The ductus venosus is thin-walled and only has small amounts of smooth muscle in its wall. The changes which occur in the ductus venosus at birth are described on p.215.

The small intestine and colon

The most noticeable feature of the midgut is that it develops a large ventrally directed loop. This is so long that the midgut actually passes outside the embryo into the extra-embryonic coelom. (It will be remembered (p.89) that the intra- and extra-embryonic parts of the coelom communicate around the neck of the yolk sac (Fig. 6.13).) The dorsal mesentery in this region thus becomes very extensive and contains, within its substance, the superior mesenteric artery (the midgut artery) and vein. At the apex of the midgut loop, the original communication between the yolk sac and the midgut becomes reduced to form the long narrow *vitello-intestinal duct*, at the distal end of which the shrivelled remains of the yolk sac can still be recognised (Fig. 16.10). Just distal to the vitello-intestinal duct the midgut shows a slight dilatation which is the future caecum.

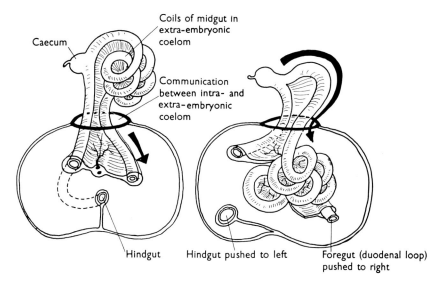

Fig. 16.11. The return of the midgut loop into the abdomen seen from above. The right (proximal) limb returns first; the caecum is the last to return and comes to lie high in the abdomen on the right side.

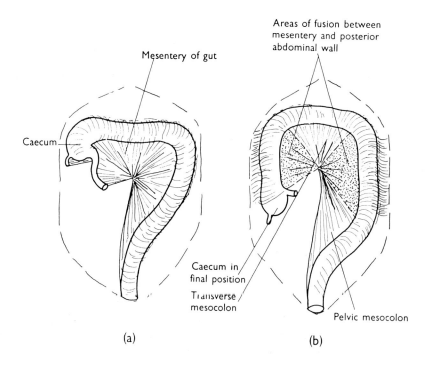

Fig. 16.12. (a) The colon and its mesentery immediately after the return of the midgut loop to the abdomen. (b) The final stage of rotation of the gut, the caecum has attained its final position and the ascending and descending colon have become retroperitoneal.

The whole loop of the gut now undergoes a series of changes in position during the course of which the herniation of the gut into the extra-embryonic coelom is reduced so that the gut is returned into the abdomen, space being provided for this by a relative diminution in the size of the liver. The first stage of this rotation of the gut occurs when the midgut loop turns anti-clockwise through 90° about the axis of the superior mesenteric artery (Fig. 16.11) so that the proximal limb of the loop comes to lie to the right and the distal limb to the left. The proximal limb now increases greatly in length to form most of the jejunum and ileum. When the midgut loop is returned to the abdomen, the proximal (right) limb returns first, possibly because the caecum impedes the return of the distal limb. As a result of the feeding back into the abdomen of the long and bulky small intestine, the C-shaped duodenal loop is pushed to the right and flattened up against the dorsal body wall to which its mesentery fuses (Fig. 16.8). Similarly, the greater part of the hindgut, together with its mesentery, is pushed to the left (Fig. 16.12). Finally, the caecum returns to the abdomen and comes to lie on the right side of the embryo below the liver, now much reduced in size (Fig. 16.12a). In the final stage of rotation of the gut, the caecum appears to descend to the right iliac region and thereby brings into being the ascending colon. It is possible, however, that this 'descent' of the caecum is purely relative to the abdominal parietes since immediately after the return of the midgut to the abdomen the caecum lies near the supracristal plane so that the ascending colon apparently comes into being as a result of the general growth of the abdomen.

The mesentery of the jejunum and ileum remains more or less unchanged but, in the region of the colon, portions of the mesentery fuse with the posterior abdominal wall (Fig. 16.12b) so that, as can be seen in this diagram, the ascending and descending parts of the colon become retroperitoneal structures while the transverse and pelvic parts retain a mesentery — the transverse and pelvic meso-colons respectively. The transverse mesocolon undergoes fusion with the dorsal mesogastrium to form the posterior wall of the lower part of the lesser sac (Fig. 16.6, p.281).

The appendix is, at first, developed at the apex of the caecum which is conical in shape. One side of the caecum grows faster than the other so that the attachment of the appendix moves over to one side.

The colon and the anal canal

The hindgut extends from about two thirds of the way along the transverse colon down to the site of the original cloacal membrane, i.e. down as far as the junction between endoderm and ectoderm. On the ectodermal side, the cloacal membrane lies at the bottom of a small depression known as the *proctodaeum* (Fig. 14.4). The hindgut forms part of the transverse colon, the whole of the descending and pelvic colon, the rectum and the upper part of the anal canal. The lower part of the anal canal is ectodermal in origin. The extent of the hindgut in adult terms will be appreciated when it is remembered that the hindgut artery is the inferior mesenteric. This therefore supplies a large part of the colon and, as the superior rectal artery, the whole rectum and the upper part of the anal canal. The lower part of the anal canal is supplied by the inferior rectal artery. The dual origin of the anal canal is also reflected in its venous drainage (upper part to the portal system; lower part to the systemic system), its lymphatic drainage (upper part to intra-abdominal nodes; lower part to inguinal nodes), its nerve supply (upper part, autonomic; lower part, sacral plexus) and its lining epithelium (upper part, columnar; lower part, stratified squamous). The anal canal is one of the important sites of portal-systemic anastomoses.

Developmental anomalies of the digestive system

Atresia

As was mentioned earlier, during development the lumen of the gut becomes partly or wholly occluded by a proliferation of the lining epithelial cells. Atresia of the bowel is often the result of a failure of vacuolisation of this epithelium at about 8 weeks. The resulting obstruction will be partial or complete. The aetiology is unknown, although interference with the blood supply to segments of the

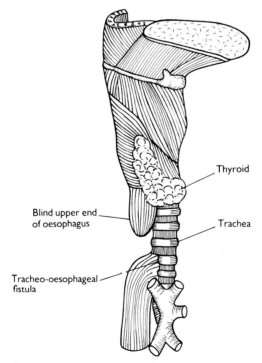

Fig. 16.13. The commonest form of tracheo-oesophageal fistula in which the upper segment of the oesophagus ends blindly while the lower segment has a fistulous communication with the trachea.

bowel is a widely quoted hypothesis. Those parts of the bowel most commonly affected are, in order of frequency: the oesophagus, duodenum, ileum, jejunum and rectum.

Oesophageal atresia

This condition is usually associated with a *fistula* (an abnormal communication between two epithelial surfaces) between the oesophagus and trachea, the whole complex malformation being due to an incomplete separation of the early laryngo-tracheal groove from the foregut early in embryonic development (p.237). There are several varieties of the oesophageal atresia/tracheo-oesophageal fistula malformation, the commonest being that in which the upper part of the oesophagus terminates as a blind pouch at the level of the thoracic inlet with the lower part communicating with the trachea via a fistula, usually 0.5−1 cm above the carina (Fig. 16.13). Oesophageal atresia is often associated with other congenital abnormalities, the most important being atresia of the lower bowel (especially ano-rectal), congenital heart defects and abnormalities of the genito-urinary tract. From the point of view of treatment, the most important feature is the distance separating the two segments of the oesophagus — this is, on average, about 1 cm with a maximum of 5 cm.

Clinically, oesophageal atresia is sometimes suspected before birth because the fetus is unable to swallow amniotic fluid. Since this is an important link in the circulation of amniotic fluid, there is an excessive amount of fluid in the amniotic cavity (*hydramnios*).

After birth the baby often produces an abundance of frothy saliva which may cause choking and cyanotic episodes. If fed before a diagnosis is made, the baby will cough and become cyanosed because of aspiration of milk into the lungs from the distended blind-ended upper pouch. Lung problems can be further compounded by aspiration of gastric juice from the associated tracheo-oesophageal fistula.

The diagnosis is confirmed by passing a fine radio-opaque catheter through the nose into the oesophagus. If an obstruction is met at about 10 cm, oesophageal atresia is almost certainly present. An X-ray of the chest and abdomen will confirm the diagnosis and further define the type of malformation according to whether or not there is air in the stomach — the presence of air is proof of a fistula between the trachea and distal segment of the oesophagus. Treatment is by surgery, ligating the fistula and establishing continuity (*anastomosis*) between upper and lower segments of the oesophagus. A segment of colon may be transplanted later in the first year to bridge a large gap. The long-term outlook is usually excellent unless a colon transplant has been used, when it is less favourable.

Duodenal atresia

The second part of the duodenum is most frequently involved in this anomaly, usually below the hepato-pancreatic ampulla (*ampulla of Vater*). The obstruction may be complete, a thin diaphragm with a hole in the centre or a segment of narrowing (*stenosis*) (Fig. 16.14). For ill-understood reasons, about 30 per cent of all cases occur in association with Down's syndrome. There is no similar association with atresia of other parts of the gut but there is a very high (about 50 per cent) incidence of other abnormalities of heart, urinary tract and bowel — an important feature whenever outcome of management is being considered. About 50 per cent of all babies with duodenal atresia weigh less than 2.5 kg at birth.

Whatever the nature of the obstruction, the clinical features are similar. Presentation is in the first few days after birth and, as with oesophageal atresia, prenatal diagnosis is sometimes suggested by hydramnios. Vomiting, usually of fluid containing bile (unless the obstruction is proximal to the ampulla) is associated with a characteristic X-ray appearance (the *double bubble sign*). This is caused by the presence of both fluid and gas in the stomach and in the duodenum, forming fluid levels. Sometimes the stomach is distended and peristalsis may be visible on inspection of the upper abdomen.

Treatment is by removing the obstruction and anastomosing the distended proximal duodenum to normal bowel distal to the obstruction. Prognosis is excellent if there are no associated abnormalities.

Atresia of the jejunum and ileum

These are less commonly associated with other anomalies and there is no associa-

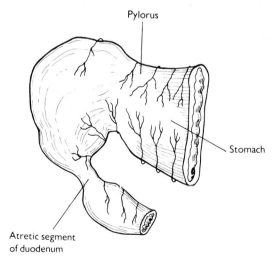

Fig. 16.14. Atresia of the second part of the duodenum. The duodenum is dilated above the constriction and poorly developed distal to it.

tion with Down's syndrome. The symptoms are those of intestinal obstruction. Bile-stained vomiting and abdominal distension are the cardinal features which usually occur later than those of duodenal atresia — on the second or third day after birth. Sometimes no meconium is passed. Diagnosis is confirmed by X-ray of the abdomen, which shows dilated segments of small intestine with multiple fluid levels. Distension of the proximal part of the gut may interfere with the blood supply, so early diagnosis and treatment are imperative. Treatment, as with duodenal atresia, is by laparotomy (opening the abdomen) to identify the site of the obstruction, to excise the dilated segment of bowel and to anastomose the two portions, proximal and distal, of healthy bowel.

Meckel's diverticulum

This malformation results from failure of a part of the communicating channel between the yolk sac and the midgut (vitello-intestinal duct) to disappear. It is usually in the form of a finger-like blind sac projecting from the anti-mesenteric border of the ileum and, in adults, is approximately 2 feet (60 cm) from the ileo-caecal junction. It is about 2 inches (5 cm) long and present in about 2 per cent of individuals. Its wall is similar in structure to the wall of the intestine but, in about 20 per cent of cases, the mucosa contains heterotopic epithelium, most commonly gastric in type. Meckel's diverticulum often remains entirely symptomless throughout life but, when symptoms are present, they are usually attributable to haemorrhage, with or without abdominal pain, due to the corrosive effects on the mucosa of the acid produced by the gastric mucosa lining the diverticulum. Treatment is by surgical removal of the diverticulum.

Other less common forms of persistence of the vitello-intestinal duct take the form of a fibrous band connecting a Meckel's diverticulum to the umbilicus, a small area of exposed mucosa at the umbilicus and (very rarely) a complete fistula between the ileum and the surface, so that intestinal contents may be discharged at the umbilicus. A fibrous band may cause intestinal obstruction as a result of kinking of a loop of small intestine over the band.

Abdominal wall

Exomphalos

This is a condition in which the midgut fails to return to the abdominal cavity from the extra-embryonic coelom at the 8th–10th week of gestation. Coils of intestine protrude from the umbilicus, covered only by a thin transparent layer of amnion (Fig. 16.15). The neck of the protrusion may be quite narrow in which case the 'hernia' may be pushed back into the abdomen and kept there by means of strapping on the abdominal wall. In other cases the protrusion is hemispherical,

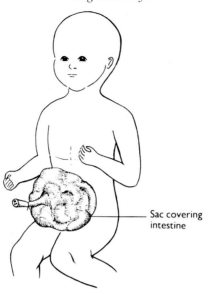

Sac covering
intestine

Fig. 16.15. Exomphalos. The umbilical cord is attached to the apex of the thin-walled sac. Compare with Fig. 9.9.

with a large defect in the abdominal wall due to failure of dermatome and myotome migration (p.127). Such cases must be treated surgically.

Gastroschisis

Although similar in appearance to an exomphalos at first sight, gastroschisis (Fig. 9.9) is anatomically distinct and has a different aetiology. The abdominal contents herniate through a defect in the abdominal wall musculature usually to the right of a normally inserted umbilical cord. In contrast with exomphalos, organs other than stomach and small intestine rarely herniate and there is no covering sac. The prolapse is thought to occur in the last trimester of pregnancy. The aetiology is unknown; one hypothesis is that the abdominal wall defect is vascular in origin. Because of the interaction of amniotic fluid and serosal secretions loops of the prolapsed gut, often much shorter than normal, are often matted together. Management is by surgical reduction and patching up the defect in the abdominal wall. Unlike exomphalos, associated malformations are much less common and mainly involve the intestines, malrotation being especially common.

Malrotation (arrested rotation)

This congenital malformation results when the midgut loop does return to the abdominal cavity at 8–10 weeks but does so in an abnormal fashion. The condition may take various forms but the commonest is that in which the caecum is found in the left hypochondrium and a peritoneal band runs from the caecum to the right side of the abdomen across the second part of the duodenum (*Ladd's transduodenal band*). This arrested rotation also predisposes to a *volvulus* (twisting) of the midgut around a very short mesentery, a condition with interferes with the blood supply of the affected loop.

Malrotation usually presents with the features of intestinal obstruction in the early weeks after birth. This is usually due to Ladd's band or, less commonly, to a volvulus. Diagnosis is made at laparotomy, when tight fibrous bands must be severed and the caecum placed in its normal position.

Other clinically 'silent' anomalies occurring during the return of the midgut to the abdomen are a high sub-hepatic caecum and the presence of a mesentery on parts of the gut which are usually retroperitoneal such as the duodenum and the ascending or descending colon. This is due to failure of the original dorsal mesentery to fuse with the parietal peritoneum.

Meconium ileus

Although not a true congenital abnormality of the intestine, meconium ileus is an early mechanical presentation of *cystic fibrosis* (p.344). It is worthy of consideration in this chapter as cystic fibrosis is the most common of all autosomal recessive disorders (1:1,600 live births). About 80 per cent of babies with cystic fibrosis have pancreatic insufficiency which can exert an effect in prenatal life. Viscid meconium, the result of lack of trypsin activity, passes sluggishly through the bowel causing obstruction at the level of the ileum.

The clinical features are similar to those of ileal atresia — abdominal distension, vomiting which becomes bile stained and failure to pass meconium. Sometimes perforation of the gut has taken place before birth causing meconium peritonitis. Diagnosis is usually made on X-ray of the abdomen, which shows the features of intestinal obstruction. However, because of the viscid meconium, there are fewer fluid levels; instead, the combination of gas and meconium gives a 'snowstorm' appearance. The large bowel is often smaller than normal due to its lack of functional activity in fetal life.

Management is by laparotomy in which the grossly dilated segment of ileum is resected and an end-to-side anastomosis performed, together with an ileostomy (creating an opening from the ileum to the outside) to decompress the bowel; 80 per cent of patients survive the neonatal period. The ultimate outcome depends on the severity of the underlying disease and the incidence of associated respiratory and alimentary problems.

This very rare malformation results from the ventral pancreatic outgrowth failing to migrate dorsally around the duodenum to meet the dorsal pancreas. It becomes adherent to the adjacent gut to form a sleeve of pancreatic tissue around the second part of the duodenum. Usually symptomless, it can occasionally cause duodenal obstruction.

The biliary system

Just as an abnormal form of division of the ureteric bud may give rise to various forms of duplication of the ureter (see Chapter 15) so variations in branching of the hepatic outgrowth may give rise to various patterns of the extra-hepatic biliary system. In fact, fewer than 50 per cent of individuals show the pattern of bile ducts that is described as 'normal' in anatomy textbooks. Although these variations are symptomless, they are of importance to surgeons. Commonly, the cystic duct descends side by side with the common hepatic duct and may join the latter behind, or even below, the first part of the duodenum. The two ducts are bound together by fibrous tissue, giving the appearance of a single common bile duct. An accessory right hepatic duct is commonly present. Partial or complete atresia of the bile ducts may occur although it is not altogether certain that the cause is similar to that of atresia of the intestine. Complete atresia of the biliary duct cannot be corrected and is incompatible with survival.

Ano-rectal anomalies

These constitute the largest group of congenital anomalies of the gastro-intestinal tract (Fig. 16.16). They result from deviant development of the mesenchymal uro-rectal septum (p.250) that normally grows down to divide the cloaca into primitive urogenital sinus and rectum or from failure of the endodermal hindgut to become continuous with the ectodermal proctodaeum. There are several classifications of ano-rectal anomalies. The simplest, and most satisfactory from a clinical point of view, is into two principal categories — high and low — depending on whether the bowel terminates above or below the puborectalis sling.

High malformations (Fig. 16.16(c),(d))

These anomalies account for approximately two-thirds of ano-rectal anomalies. The rectum ends as a blind pouch above the sling of the levator ani muscle of the pelvic floor. High malformations are commonly associated with fistulae which might be viewed as remnants of the original cloaca (or defects in the uro-rectal septum). In the male these connect anteriorly with the bladder (*recto-vesical*) or membranous part of the prostatic urethra (*recto-urethral*). In girls the fistulae are into the vagina (*recto-vaginal*) or the vestibule (*recto-vestibular*).

Inspection of the perineum is part of the routine examination of the newborn baby so that recto-anal malformations will be discovered soon after birth when the absence of an anal canal is observed. The external sphincter is incompletely

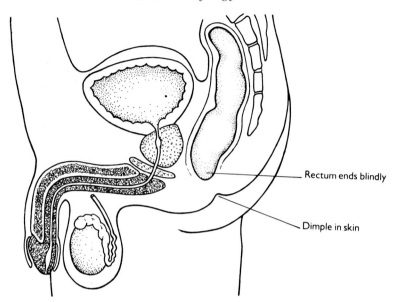

Rectum ends blindly

Dimple in skin

(a)

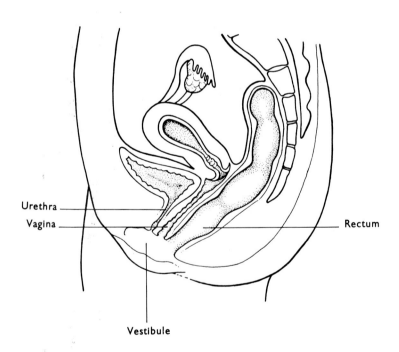

Urethra

Vagina

Rectum

Vestibule

(b)

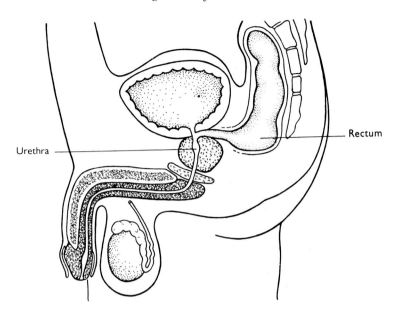

(c)

Urethra

Rectum

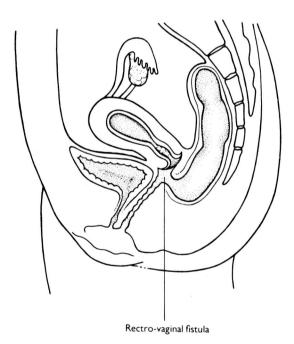

(d)

Rectro-vaginal fistula

Fig. 16.16. Ano-rectal anomalies.
(1) *Low anomalies* (a) Imperforate anus (b) 'Ectopic anus' with a superficial fistual in the vestibule.
(2) *High anomalies* (c) The rectum ends above the level of levator ani and there is a recto-urethral fistula. (d) The rectum ends above levator ani and there is a recto-vaginal fistula.

formed. Sometimes meconium will be noted in the urine (in boys) or in the vaginal introitus in girls, if a fistula is present. In the unusual event of the diagnosis being missed, the presenting symptoms will be those of intestinal obstruction with vomiting and failure to pass meconium in the latter part of the first week. In girls with a large recto-vaginal fistula meconium will, however, be passed. Babies who also have associated malformations (*vide infra*) have an increased likelihood of premature birth and low birth weight.

Treatment is by surgery in two stages. Intestinal obstruction must first be relieved by a colostomy (the creation of an artificial opening of the colon on the anterior abdominal wall) usually in the right half of the transverse colon. Towards the end of the first year (6−9 months) definitive surgery is undertaken. Any fistulae are divided and the rectum mobilised and pulled through the muscle sling of the pelvic floor into the anal sphincter. When bowel continuity has been established in this way the colostomy is closed. The long-term prognosis is excellent. However an important, though fortunately infrequent, residual problem is later soiling due to abnormal or absent sphincters.

Low malformations — imperforate anus

In these abnormalities the muscles of the pelvic floor and the internal sphincter are normal and the uro-rectal septum has developed normally. The aetiology of imperforate anus is probably a failure of the proctodaeum to become continuous with the endodermal hindgut. The anal canal is usually separated from the outside by a thin covering of skin (Fig. 16.16a). As with the high rectal anomalies, fistulous communications are usually present. These are often present as a superficial tract in the midline raphe of the perineum passing forward into the urethra or vulva. These fistulae may be considered as an 'ectopic anus' although this is not strictly correct since the anal canal is usually normally situated.

The clinical features that alert suspicion of imperforate anus are varied and include anal dimple, perineal fistula and anteriorly displaced anus. Treatment is by surgical excision of the membrane with suture of the rectal mucosa to the perianal skin at the site of the external sphincter. The long term outcome is, on the whole, better than with high ano-rectal anomalies. Continence is usually satisfactory since the internal sphincter is normal and rectal sensation intact.

Other malformations associated with ano-rectal anomalies

In babies with ano-rectal anomalies there is a high incidence of associated congenital malformations which may have a greater effect on the final outcome than the primary anomaly. They occur particularly in association with the high type of anomaly. Genito-urinary malformations are the commonest, including especially renal hypoplasia, cysts, congenital hydronephrosis (dilatation of the renal pelvis and ureter associated with destruction of renal tissue) and hypospadias (p.273).

Vertebral body anomalies are also common — hemivertebrae, absence of vertebrae and even extra vertebrae occurring in any segment of the spine. When these anomalies affect the sacrum (*sacral agenesis*), faecal and urinary incontinence are likely consequences. Other anomalies to occur with great frequency include those of the cardio-vascular system and of other parts of the alimentary system. There is a particularly interesting combination of anomalies mnemonically called the *VATER* syndrome — Vertebral defects, Anal atresia, Tracheo-esophageal (American spelling) fistula, Renal and Radial dysplasias. Another non-random combination of anomalies has been called the *VACTER* syndrome to draw attention to the association of cardiac and other anomalies — Vertebral, Anal, Cardiac, Tracheal, Esophageal and Renal anomalies. When the limbs are also involved some authors speak of the *VACTERL* syndrome. The extensive nature of these associated defects is not surprising when it is borne in mind that the process of cloacal division occupies a considerable span of time in the embryonic period so that a teratogen (p.313) acting over this period could affect a number of maturing systems.

Hirschsprung's disease

In this condition the primary congenital defect is an absence of ganglion cells of both Auerbach's and Meissner's plexuses in a segment of the gut. The cause of the condition is not known; the most acceptable hypothesis is that there is a failure of migration of neuroblasts which normally enter the cranial part of the alimentary canal during the 5th−7th weeks and migrate caudally within the muscle layers. The affected segment extends cranially from the most distal part of the rectum at the level of the internal sphincter for a variable distance. In about 25 per cent of cases the rectum alone is involved, in 50 per cent the sigmoid colon is also affected and in the remaining 25 per cent the aganglionic zone extends even further proximally. Associated anomalies are much less common than with abnormalities of the rectum and anal canal mentioned above.

There is a considerable spectrum of clinical presentation. Symptoms of intestinal obstruction in the newborn period (bile-stained vomiting, abdominal distention) can occur due to the failure of peristalsis to pass meconium beyond the aganglionic segment. However, since the obstruction is 'functional' and often incomplete, symptoms may not be present until early childhood, when constipation and soiling may occur.

Diagnosis is usually made by barium enema which clearly defines the aganglionic segment, often with proximal bowel dilatation. Further confirmation of the diagnosis comes from biopsy of the wall of the rectum which shows the typical absence of ganglion cells. In some centres ano-rectal manometric studies are used — in Hirschsprung's disease the internal spincter fails to relax in response to rectal distension.

Management of the condition is in two stages. The obstruction is initially relieved by a colostomy in the ganglionic segment of the bowel proximal to the narrowing. At a later stage, usually 6−9 months later, the aganglionic segment of the bowel has to be excised and normally innervated bowel anastomosed to the rectal stump which is distal to the aganglionic segment.

Developmental stages

21−22 days: Head and tail folds developing.
    Foregut and midgut forming.
24−26 days: Liver and pancreatic buds present.
    Buccopharyngeal membrane ruptured
5 weeks: Midgut recognisable as neck of yolk sac becomes constricted.
    Later, midgut herniates into extra-embryonic coelom.
6 weeks: Liver large enough to produce external bulge, above large midgut hernia.
    Spleen develops
7−8 weeks: Cloacal membrane disappears
8−9 weeks: Midgut hernia reduced into abdomen
10th week: Peristalsis begins.

Further reading

Fitzgerald, M.J.T. Nolan, J.P. & O'Neill, M.N. (1971) The position of the human caecum in fetal life. *J. Anat. (Lond.)* **109**, 71.

Grand, R.J., Watkins, J.B. & Torti, F.M. (1976) Progress in Gastroenterology. Development of the human gastrointestinal tract. A review. *Gastroenterology*, **70**, 790.

Kanagasuntheram, R. (1957) Development of the human lesser sac. *J. Anat. (Lond.)*, **92**, 188.

McLean, J.M. (1979) Embryology of the Pancreas. In: *The Exocrine Pancreas*, eds. Howat, H.T. & Sarles, H. W.B. Saunders.

Meyer, W.W. & Lind, J. (1966) The ductus venosus and the mechanism of its closure. *Arch. Dis. Childh.* **41**, 597.

Severn, C.B. (1971) A morphological study of the development of the human liver. 1. Development of the hepatic diverticulum. *Am. J. Anat.* **133**, 85.

Stephens, F.D. (1963) *Congenital Malformations of Rectum, Anus and Genito-urinary Tract.* Livingstone, Edinburgh.

Tench, E.M. (1936) Development of the anus in the human embryo. *Am. J. Anat,* **59**, 333.

Trier, J.S. & Moxey, P.C. (1979) Morphogenesis of the small intestine during fetal development. *Ciba Found. Symp.* **70**, 3.

Wilkinson, A.W. (1972) Congenital anomalies of the anus and rectum. *Arch. Dis. Childh.,* **47**, 960.

17
Growth and Development from Conception to Adolescence

The principal purpose behind the growth (increase in size) and development (maturation of physiological processes) of any organism is to allow it to achieve sexual maturity thereby ensuring continued survival of the species. The human is no exception to this broad biological principle. Birth — the end of the intra-uterine phase of existence — is obviously a most important event, especially in regard to changes which have to take place in cardio-respiratory and gastro-intestinal function but the growth programme itself is little affected by it. Growth and development is a continuum from prenatal through to postnatal life and the stage in development at which birth occurs varies widely between species. For example, if the period of rapid brain growth (the brain growth spurt) is taken as one marker of development remarkable variations are found. The guinea pig can be considered very mature at birth, the brain having completely undergone its growth spurt in prenatal life. The rat, in contrast, is very immature at birth — the brain growth spurt not yet having started. The human occupies an intermediate position with the brain undergoing its growth spurt in the period covering the last trimester (three months) of pregnancy and the first few years of postnatal life.

Normal growth and development

Human growth and development can conveniently be considered to take place in six periods, each with its own distinctive characteristics:

Embryonic: Conception—8 weeks
   (Mainly concerned with differentiation of systems and organs)
Early fetal: 12—28 weeks
Late fetal: 28 weeks—birth
   (these two mainly concerned with growth)
Infancy and early childhood: Birth—2 years
Childhood proper: 2 years—onset of puberty
Puberty (adolescence)

This chapter describes the principal features of growth and development of the human in each of these periods. It is first necessary, however, to give a general description of the nature of growth and its control.

301

Measurement of growth

It is necessary to realise that various ways of measuring growth exist. The simplest is, of course, one in which the relevant parameter, such as weight or height, is plotted directly against time. Such simple curves of growth usually have the form shown in Fig. 17.1a. Fig. 17.1b is a measure of the growth rate, i.e. the rate of change (dW/dt) with time. It shows clearly that a maximum growth rate is characteristic of most biological systems. If we consider a culture dish of bacteria (and the same applies to a clone of growing embryonic cells) we can understand the curve of specific growth show in Fig. 17.1c. The first cell in such a culture gives rise to two daughter cells each of which will divide giving rise successively to 4, 8, 16, 32, 64 etc. cells. This constitutes a logarithmic progression with the rate of cell division, and therefore the increase in weight, gradually slowing down when the food reserves in the bacterial culture dish begin to run low or the optimal size of a particular organ is approached. This aspect of growth may be appreciated by measuring the logarithm (log W) of the dimension being studied against time. Finally, Fig. 17.1d converts the curve of specific growth into a curve of the specific growth rate by again measuring the rate of change (d log W/dt) of specific growth. This demonstrates that the greatest rate of specific growth occurs early in biological systems such as those presented by the developing organism.

We often wish to compare the growth of one part of the body with that of another. For this we use the allometric equation $y = bx^k$. This may be plotted graphically in a linear form as:

$$\log y = \log b + k \log x$$

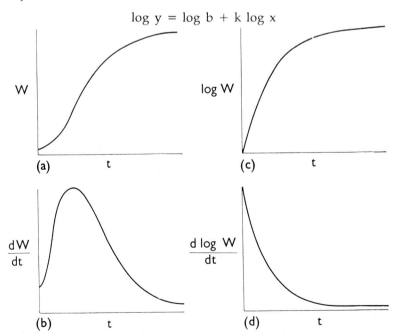

Fig. 17.1. Some methods of measuring weight changes. W = body weight, t = time. (a) Simple growth curve. (b) Curve of growth rate (c) Curve of specific growth (d) Curve of specific growth rate. For explanation see text. (From *Essays on Growth and Form*, edited by W.E.Le Gros Clark and P.B. Medawar, Clarendon Press, Oxford, 1945).

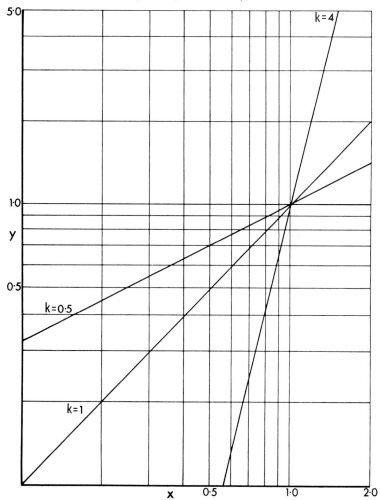

Fig. 17.2. The allometric equation ($y = bx^k$) plotted as log y against log x. Three examples are given; in one k = 1.0 and in the others k = 0.5 and 4.0. For further explanation see text. (From *Dynamics of Growth Processes* edited by E.J. Boell, Princetown University Press, Copyright 1954).

where y is the dimension of the part under study, x is a general dimension measured in the same terms (for example the length of the femur compared to the whole body length) and k is the ratio of:

$$\frac{\text{specific growth rate of x}}{\text{specific growth rate of y}}$$

Since K is a constant the allometric equation assumes that the two parts being compared bear a constant relationship to each other as growth occurs, i.e. one part constantly grows at (say) twice the rate of the other, b is the value of y when x = 1, it is not a biologically significant parameter. Examples of allometric relationships are given in Fig. 17.2.

It is occasionally useful to express a number of simultaneously changing values such as the relative lengths of various parts of the body during postnatal deve-

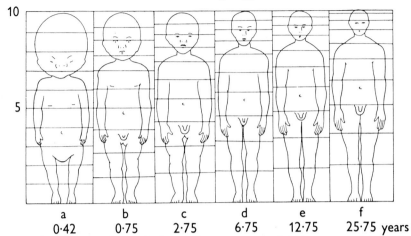

a   b   c   d   e   f
0·42   0·75   2·75   6·75   12·75   25·75 years

Fig. 17.3. Method of depicting changes in the relative proportions of different parts of the body by alteration of the form of a superimposed co-ordinate grid related to fixed points on the body surface. (From *Essays on Growth and Form* edited by W.E. Le Gros Clark and P.B. Medawar, Clarendon Press, Oxford 1945).

lopment. One method is to make an outline drawing of the organism or structure under study superimposed upon a co-ordinate grid. The co-ordinates can then be distorted in such a way that the object of study adopts another form. Complex algebraic functions can describe the distortion but these are beyond the scope of this book. For example, changes in human form can be illustrated with reference to certain fixed midline points (Fig. 17.3).

Mammalian growth

Two important principles are integral to mammalian, and especially human, growth. The first is that the brain undergoes its growth spurt before the rest of the body: the second is that for the body to grow to its maximum potential the brain has to undergo normal growth. The brain, therefore, plays a key role, though so far ill-understood, in the control of growth and development. Some knowledge of how the brain grows is, therefore, important. There are three principal phases. In the first, complete by about 16 weeks in the human fetus, the neuronal cell complement is almost totally acquired. The second phase is termed the principal brain growth spurt, beginning at about 20 weeks of gestation, reaching a maximum at 40 weeks and being complete by about the 5th year after conception. This spurt involves initially rapid multiplication of glial cells (principally oligodendroglia) which later take on the role of laying down myelin sheaths around the axons of neurones. These cells also serve as vital links in the chain by which neurones receive their nutrition. The final phase of brain growth, which occupies the remainder of childhood and extends into adulthood, involves the elaboration of the incredibly intricate system of inter-neural connections which probably lay the foundations for high intellectual function. This pattern of brain growth results in the brain at birth being already 25 per cent of its adult weight and, by the age of four, about 75 per cent of its adult weight. The importance of understanding these broad principles of brain growth is that vulnerability of the brain to insults from under-nutrition is greatest when its growth is proceeding most rapidly. The human infant is, therefore, vulnerable in late pregnancy and especially in early childhood. The implications for the many millions of children in the world who live in appalling conditions of endemic malnutrition are abundantly clear. Indeed, studies already indicate that as well as the short-term physical toll of malnutrition adverse long term consequences to learning and behaviour also exist.

Control of growth

The genetic message which directs growth is allowed its optimum expression through permissive influences of endocrine and nutritional factors which provide the appropriate milieu for growing organs and tissues. In their absence growth will continue although at a much slower rate (p.342). It is an intriguing fact that endocrine secretions have a far greater influence on growth after birth than during prenatal life (see also p.344).

Growth hormone

This single-chain polypetide, containing 191 amino acids and synthesised in the anterior pituitary gland, is required for normal growth from birth until final mature size is reached. Without growth hormone, adult height reaches only about 130 cm. Its mechanism of action is principally on the liver where it stimulates production of a group of hormones, the *somatomedins*, which act on the growing cells of the cartilage growth plate and muscle.

Thyroid hormones

The release of thyroxine and tri-iodothyronine is under the control of pituitary thyroid stimulating hormone (TSH). Like growth hormone, its release is regulated by hypothalamic releasing factors. Thyroid hormones have a major role in both fetal and postnatal life being responsible for cell differentiation and protein synthesis in the nervous system, mitotic activity of the cartilaginous growth plate and maturation of ossification centres.

Adrenal hormones

Glucocorticoids

Cortisol plays little part in regulating normal growth. However, in conditions of over-secretion (as might occur with adrenal hyperplasia or with pharmacological over-dosage of steroid therapy in children with conditions such as severe asthma, eczema, nephrotic syndrome and rheumatoid disease) corticosteroids can slow down the rate of growth by interfering with secretion of somatomedins by the liver and even perhaps by blocking the stimulant effect of somatomedins on the growth plate itself. The rate of osseous maturation is accelerated and closure of the epiphyses hastened.

Sex hormones

Androgens

There are a few closely related substances, of which *dehydroepiandrosterone* predominates, secreted by the suprarenal gland that closely mimic the actions of testosterone. The control of their release is through some as yet unidentified hormone of the anterior pituitary gland. They contribute significantly to the puberty growth spurt in boys and girls, and to some other secondary sex characteristics such as pubic hair and muscle bulk in boys. Androgens are also somehow involved in maturation of the skeleton and the eventual closure of growth plates.

Testosterone

In fetal life this male sex hormone along with dihydrotestosterone that is produced from it (see Chapter 15) is primarily responsible for the differentiation of the male genitalia. At puberty, testosterone is responsible in the male for the development of secondary sexual characteristics and accompanying physiological changes (*vide infra*).

Oestrogens

This is a collective term used for the female sex hormones produced by the ovary, the principal one being *oestradiol*. Before puberty the circulating levels are very low. At adolescence, levels increase under the influence of follicle stimulating hormone causing growth of the breast and uterus. Oestrogens also contribute in some way to the growth spurt.

Insulin

This hormone, whose principal action causes glucose to be taken into cells as a source of energy and stored as glycogen in the liver and muscle, is not believed to play a major role in influencing growth in childhood. However, the stunting of growth which can occur in badly controlled childhood diabetics, in whom there is little circulating insulin, suggests that its presence in physiological amounts does make some contribution to normal growth. In prenatal life insulin might somehow function far more as a growth hormone, this inference coming from the observation that in the exceedingly rare condition of neonatal diabetes mellitus the babies are invariably severely growth retarded (see also p.315).

Growth and development before birth

Embryonic period

This period, extending from conception to about 8 weeks, is the interval when the basic structure of the organs and tissues of the body are differentiated. It encompasses the formation of the three germ layers which emerge in the early weeks following conception. The conceptus enters the embryonic period as a primitive being, unrecognisable as human: it emerges with many of the essential features of a human baby in miniature (Fig. 17.4). The crown−rump length can first be measured soon after the end of the fourth week (about 4 mm). At this stage there is a large pericardial cavity which forms a bulge below the developing facial and pharyngeal regions, although the branchial arches are not yet all present. The neural tube is completely closed and the mesodermal somites are a prominent feature (Fig. 17.4a). Shortly after this the limb buds appear. The embryo is growing in length at about 1 mm per day and by the end of the embryonic period it has reached a length of about 30 mm. Thereafter (during the fetal period) the rate of growth increases to about 1.5 mm per day.

Early fetal period

This period, from 8-28 weeks, witnesses the very rapid growth of the body along with maturation of its tissues and organs. At 8 weeks, crown−rump (CR) length averages of 29 mm are recorded. At 28 weeks these measurements are 28 cm and weights of 1,000 g are recorded. Accompanying this rapid growth are profound changes in external form. At 12 weeks the human fetus has a disproportionately large head and the physiological umbilical hernia (caused by intestinal loops in the umbilical cord) has just re-entered the abdominal cavity: sex is easily identified. At 16 weeks the human appearance is even clearer with the eyes looking forwards rather than laterally, the ears much closer to their definitive positions at the sides of the head and the infra-umbilical region beginning to expand, so that the umbilicus lies relatively higher in the abdomen. At 20 weeks fine downy hair (*lanugo hair*) covers the whole body including the head and, at this stage, the mother becomes aware for the first time of *function* in her baby, due to movements caused by muscle activity in the arms and legs. This is called *quickening*. Between 24 and 28 weeks the appearance is that of a wizened old man caused by an almost total absence of fat in the subcutaneous tissue (Figs. 17.4 and 17.5). 28 weeks marks the end of the fetal period. This stage of demarcation has important legal implications since it marks the end of the period of *non-*

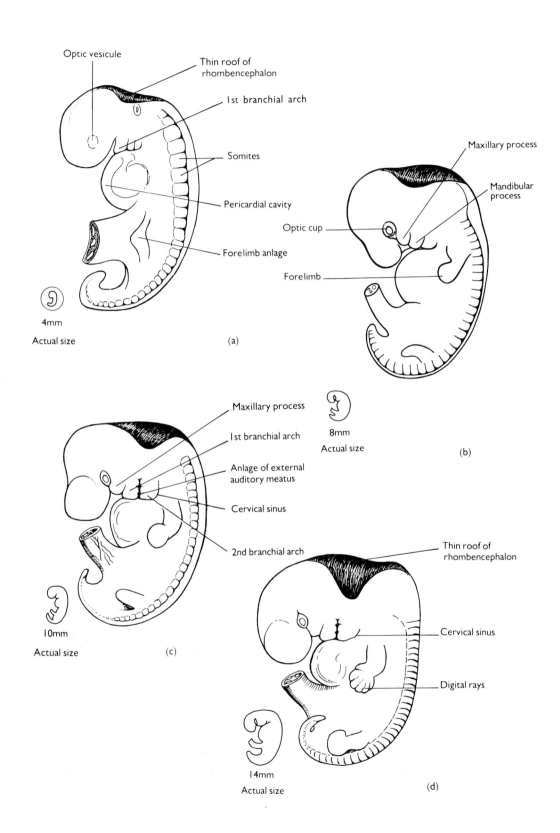

Optic vesicule

Thin roof of rhombencephalon

1st branchial arch

Somites

Pericardial cavity

Forelimb anlage

4mm

Actual size

(a)

Maxillary process

Mandibular process

Optic cup

Forelimb

8mm

Actual size

(b)

Maxillary process

1st branchial arch

Anlage of external auditory meatus

Cervical sinus

2nd branchial arch

10mm

Actual size

(c)

Thin roof of rhombencephalon

Cervical sinus

Digital rays

14mm

Actual size

(d)

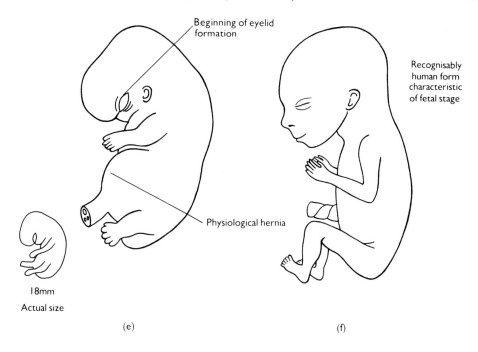

Fig. 17.4. Drawings of human embryos and fetuses at different stages of development. These are not to scale but the approximate actual size of each embryo is shown.
a. 28 days   4 mm   — O'Rahilly Stage 13
b. 35 days   8 mm   — O'Rahilly Stage 15
c. 37 days   10 mm   — O'Rahilly Stage 16
d. 40 days   13.5 mm — O'Rahilly Stage 16/17
e. 47 days   18 mm   — O'Rahilly Stage 19
f. 110 days 100 mm

viability when termination of pregnancy (in Britain and many other countries) is under certain circumstances allowed by law. However, with the advances which have been made in the care of the very prematurely born baby the whole issue of 'viability' must be re-evaluated since it is now possible for 'non-viable' babies born between 26 and 28 weeks to survive, many without long-term handicap. There is, therefore, a peculiar inconsistency that a baby born dead at 26 weeks is considered an abortion whose death does not require registration, yet if it is born alive and then dies it is included in statistical records such as perinatal and infant mortalities as a neonatal death. As can be imagined, very disturbing ethical dilemmas are now posed as the clinical harnessing of modern technology makes possible survival of babies born late in the period of non-viability.

Late fetal period

The second part of the fetal period commences when viability is reached between about 26 and 28 weeks. It is characterised by very rapid growth and continued

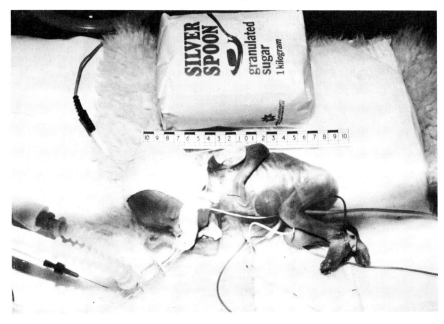

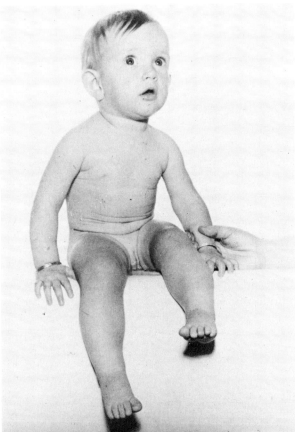

Fig. 17.5. A preterm baby born at 27 weeks of gestation. The bag of sugar provides a reference standard for size. The other photograph shows the same baby at 12 months.

changes in body form. At 28 weeks average body weight is about 1,000 g: at 40 weeks it is around 3,300 g.

The testes are never far from the deep inguinal ring and, by about 36 weeks, they have in most cases fully descended into the scrotum. In girls the labia minora become gradually obscured by the labia majora. The skin and superficial fascia become thicker and paler due to accumulation of fat in the subcutaneous tissues; the skin becomes less wrinkled and loses its lanugo hair but continues to be covered by *vernix caseosa* (p.128). Finger nails grow to reach the end of the digits by the time of birth. The eyelids are fused up to about 7 months, after which the eyes can be opened. Many organs such as the lungs and kidneys have not, however, developed fully either structurally or functionally.

Weight

Largely because of the relative ease of its measurement, weight is the most widely used single clinical indicator of growth. Weight is the sum of body fat and lean

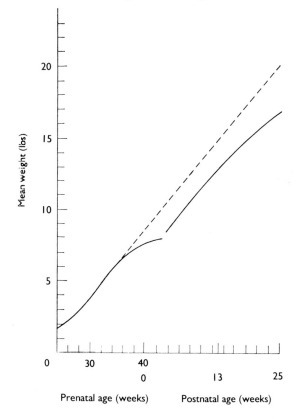

Fig. 17.6. Growth from the 25th week of prenatal life to 25 weeks after birth. The relative slowing down in the immediately prenatal period is clearly shown. (Modified after McKeown and Record. From *Textbook of Human Anatomy,* edited by W.J. Hamilton, Macmillan & Co. Ltd., 1956, Used by permission).

body tissue so that weight *gain* must represent the sum of increments of different body components, including muscle, skeleton, adipose tissue and water. For these reasons it is a rather non-specific measure of growth. To provide a more comprehensive assessment other measurements are needed: crown–heel length, head circumference and skinfold thickness are now being increasingly used. Notwithstanding this, weight is still an important measurement since, in the short term, it is a more sensitive index of ill-health and poor nutrition than either length or head circumference.

Many populations have now been studied for their intra-uterine weight gain. In the latter half of pregnancy the weight curve is S-shaped (Fig. 17.6). In the 28th week weight gain is about 107 g and this increases to a maximum of 240 g in the 34th week. The weight curve then begins to level off due, it is believed, to declining growth support from the intra-uterine environment, especially that coming from the placenta, since as soon as the newborn baby has become adapted to extra-uterine life weight gain for the next couple of months is similar to the intra-uterine rate before its deceleration. On average the fetus weighs about 3,000 g when the growth begins to falter (at about 36–37 weeks' gestation) but differences do exist between various infant populations.

Length

The accurate measurement of crown–heel length provides the best clinical measure of skeletal growth since, unlike weight gain, it is not influenced by the accumulation of water and fat. Total body length at birth is about 50 cm.

The pattern of linear growth is similar to that described by weight gain. In the 25th week the fetus grows 1.0 cm; the rate increases to 1.3 cm per week between 31 and 32 weeks at which it remains until, at 34 weeks, there begins a gradual deceleration to 0.5 cm in the 40th week. After birth the rate of linear growth soon returns to that achieved at about 32 weeks of intra-uterine life. This suggests therefore that, as with weight gain, the slowing down of growth in the latter part of the third trimester is due to diminishing growth support for the fetus, increased velocity after birth being viewed as 'catch-up' (p.330).

Head circumference

Although head circumference has been shown to correlate well with intra-cranial volume and brain weight, there is no simple relationship between *head circumference growth* and *brain growth*. The chief value of measuring the growth of head circumference is that it provides a clinical measurement of total *head growth*. Normal growth of external body dimensions is a harmonious process so that any significant deviation of head growth could point to an underlying growth disorder, whether or not it involves the brain. Head circumference is a measure of the maximum circumference around the supraorbital ridges and the occipital protuberance.

Head circumference growth in the latter part of pregnancy is also S-shaped. At 30–32 weeks of gestation when the weekly rate of increase is nearly 1 cm there is a gradual flattening of the curve as with weight gain and length until a rate of only about 0.5 cm exists in the 40th week. The average head circumference at birth is 34 cm.

The maximum head growth velocity of normal full term infants soon after birth reaches nearly 1 cm per day which is only slightly lower than the peak intra-uterine velocity, inferring that head circumference growth is also restricted during the last weeks of gestation. Using conversion formulae, the intra-uterine curve of brain weight in the last trimester, calculated from both head circumference and bi-parietal diameter measurements, is almost linear with little sign of terminal flattening. It closely agrees with the true curve of brain weight derived directly from post-mortem analyses over the same period. The fact that the brain does not exhibit a prenatal slowing of growth means that changes in external linear dimensions of the head cannot necessarily be correlated with changes in its intra-cranial content.

Subcutaneous skinfold thickness

About 80 per cent of body fat is contained in the subcutaneous tissues. A relative measure of this fat can be obtained with skinfold calipers and correlates well with other anthropometric indices of nutritional status, for example various weight-for-height indices. This measurement will be discussed in more detail on p.328.

Disorders of growth *in utero*

Embryonic period

It is in this period that the embryo is especially vulnerable to teratogenic influences which interfere with organ and tissue differentiation. Some of these are known, such as rubella (German measles) virus and the drug Thalidomide; most are unknown. Anomalies of growth and differentiation which have their origins in this highly vulnerable state constitute most of those structural abnormalities which have been discussed in the earlier chapters. The factors that may predispose to the development of anomalies in this period will be discussed in Chapter 18.

Early fetal period

Sandwiched as it is between the embryonic period with its particular vulnerability to teratogenic influences and the later 'viable' fetal period growth, less is known of growth disturbances which have their origins in the early fetal period. In this period spontaneous abortions ('miscarriages') continue to take place and termination of pregnancy for social and medical reasons is legal. The alteration in the abortion law has meant that the fetus can now be investigated for abnormality with a view to preventing birth at term by the termination of pregnancy.

Because fetuses which are born prematurely in the early fetal period are, in most instances, non-viable much less is known of anomalies of growth which might originate in this period. Two conditions are of interest in this connection. The first is the very small head and later mental subnormality in some of those babies who were exposed to radio-activity *in utero* following the dropping of the atomic bomb in Japan in 1945. This is believed to have been due to interference with neuronal multiplication between about 10 and 20 weeks. The second group constitute infections with certain viruses, principally rubella. Although most widely recognised as causing anomalies when maternal infection occurs in the embryonic period, infections with these, and other viruses, can cause significant stunting of skeletal and brain growth and chronic inflammatory responses in the liver when infection occurs in the early fetal period.

Late fetal period

The relation of weight to gestational age at birth is widely used to assess the normality, or otherwise, of a newborn infant's size. For clinical purposes it is important to recognise patterns of atypical* intra-uterine growth since they can hinder adaptation to extra-uterine life and, especially in the case of very small babies, may even have some bearing on future growth and neuro-psychological development. There is no universally accepted definition for atypical size at birth, the most likely explanation for this being the considerable influences of racial, geographical and socio-cultural factors on the rate of intra-uterine growth. Two standard deviations above or below the mean with allowances for the three important physiological influences on the rate of intra-uterine growth — maternal height and parity (number of pregnancies) and the sex of the infant — are the most commonly used limits of normality in Britain.

Most 'heavy-for-dates' infants (i.e. babies who are heavier than expected from the calculated duration of pregnancy), are fat and long with big heads. Babies weighing 4.5 kg and over at birth (*macrosomia*) will often have about 20—25 per cent of their weight as fat. Unlike their small baby counterparts (*vide infra*) pathological influences in the mother or fetus account for only a very small proportion of abnormally big infants. Women who give birth to the majority of big babies constitute a distinctive biological group compared with women who have infants of normal birth weight. They are often older, taller, heavier, of higher parity and sometimes show excessive weight gain during pregnancy.

---

*The term 'atypical' is used in preference to the more widely used 'abnormal'. Many babies who are born might well be of a size which is beyond the statistical definitions of 'normal' (i.e. +/−2SD from the mean) simply through genetic influence. We are disinclined to call these babies abnormal yet, at the same time, recognising that in these statistical categories there will be some whose unusual size is due to pathological influences.

Most big babies are one extreme of a normal continuum of size at birth. Several exceedingly rare conditions are associated with macrosomia at birth but only one relatively common pathological 'variant' is described here, namely infants of diabetic mothers.

Maternal diabetes increases the likelihood of excessive birthweight through an above-normal rate of intra-uterine weight gain over the last 12 weeks or so of pregnancy. Heaviness at birth is due mainly to the intra-uterine deposition of excessive amounts of fat in subcutaneous tissue probably resulting from an increased rate of fetal insulin secretion from β-cell hyperplasia in response to maternal hyperglycaemia. Infants of diabetic mothers used to weigh an average of about 500 g more than control infants, the distribution of birth weights being normal but set at a higher level. However, babies of diabetic mothers are now not as heavy as they were in the past, a trend believed to be due to the now more rigorous control of blood glucose during pregnancy. Another interesting developmental problem of infants of diabetic mothers is their threefold increase in congenital abnormalities and spontaneous abortion. This is believed to be due to the abnormal metabolic *milieu* of the developing fetus which might be provided by mothers whose diabetes is inadequately controlled rather than to any intrinsic fault in the fetus' own metabolism.

'Light-for-date' babies are almost the exact mirror image of heavy babies, being small in all their physical dimensions. Pathological influences in either mother or fetus are also far more prevalent. While intra-uterine infections (e.g. rubella, cytomegalovirus), congenital abnormalities and chromosome anomalies are sometimes associated with, and in some way are probably responsible for, some infants who are very small at birth, most appear normal being differentiated mainly by the extent to which they show external signs of intra-uterine undernutrition. Thus, while some show unmistakable signs of wasting with loss of subcutaneous fat and muscle bulk together with dry skin (the syndrome of 'placental insufficiency'), others have been described as 'perfect miniatures', i.e. small in all dimensions. The explanation for this diversity in external appearance is likely to be found in the two main mechanisms which regulate the rate of fetal growth. Wasted infants, which account for about 70 per cent of all 'light-for-dates' babies are likely to be due to inadequate growth support while the 'perfect miniatures' are small probably for genetic reasons. In practice there is likely to be considerable overlapping between these variants.

Deformations

In the last section it has been learnt that harmful influences in the fetal supply line, such as hypertension or rubella in the mother, can retard prenatal growth in the latter half of pregnancy and, in the case of maternal diabetes, even accelerate it. Another type of disordered growth in the late fetal period has its origins in the immediate intra-uterine environment, namely abnormal mechanical forces which act on parts of the musculo-skeletal system that were previously normally formed.

The resulting abnormalities are termed *congenital postural deformations* and they have been estimated to occur in approximately 2 per cent of babies born. Those most well recognised (which will be described in further detail) are *talipes, postural scoliosis, arthrogryposis multiplex, congenital dislocation of the hip, plagiocephaly, mandibular asymmetry* and *Potter's syndrome.*

The theory to account for congenital deformations is that the natural posture and movements of the rapidly growing fetus in the latter half of pregnancy are constrained by abnormal extrinsic forces thereby causing growth of that part of the body exposed to this force to become distorted. Hippocrates was the first to write about the problems over 2000 years ago: '. . . infants become crippled in the following way: where, in the womb, there is narrowness at the part where the crippling is produced it is inevitable that the body moving in a narrow place shall be crippled in that part'.

Growth constraint

Growth constraint can occur in three principal ways.

1. Small volume of amniotic fluid (oligohydramnios)

The ratio of amniotic fluid volume to fetal mass falls during pregnancy. At 12 weeks the ratio is 3:1; at 28 weeks 2:1 and, at 40 weeks, it has fallen to 1:1 and continues to fall for as long as gestation continues. In the latter part of pregnancy much the greater part of the amniotic fluid is derived from fetal urine (p.103) which complements the fluid produced by the amnion itself. Indeed, the major role of the kidneys in intra-uterine life is to maintain normal amniotic fluid volume, not to preserve the fetal *milieu intérieur* which is controlled by means of placental transfer of solute and water. As the volume of liquor gradually falls the fetus is normally able to resist the resulting external pressure from the uterine wall because of its rapidly calcifying skeleton and slower rate of growth, making it less vulnerable to deforming forces. Certain conditions accelerate the process of diminishing amniotic fluid volume thereby making possible congenital deformities. Notably amongst these are (i) placental insufficiency — often caused by hypertensive disease in the mother; (ii) bilateral renal agenesis (one component of Potter's syndrome) causing lack of urine flow into the amniotic cavity, and (iii) prolonged leakage of amniotic fluid from prematurely ruptured membranes.

2. Position of the fetus

The fetus lying in the *breech* position, particularly with legs extended over the abdomen, will have its movements severely restricted since the breech forms an angular pole resting in the pelvis acting as a splint to discourage kicking movements and allow intra-uterine forces to act. It is not surprising, therefore, that postural deformities are more common in breech born babies, especially congenital dislocation of the hip.

Transverse, face and *brow presentation* increase the likelihood of distorted facial and skull growth. On rare occasions a primary fetal neuromuscular abnormality (anterior horn cell disease, congenital myotonic dystrophy) can lead to abnormal fetal positions thereby allowing extrinsic forces to deform part(s) of the body. It is, therefore, important always to be aware of the possibility of the existence of intrinsic fetal disease when assessing multiple deformities.

3. Uterine and pelvic abnormalities

These structural anomalies can distort the shape of the amniotic cavity. Bicornuate uterus (p.275), large uterine benign growths (*fibroids*) and a prominent sacrum can all markedly limit intra-uterine space and interfere with the accommodation of the fetus. One important feature shared by many congenital postural deformities is the capacity of the distorted part of the skeleton to recover its normal structure when it has been released from constraints on growth — a type of 'catch-up' growth. This is in marked contrast with earlier errors in morphogenesis with their origins in the embryonic period when natural recovery does not take place (see Chapter 18).

Specific types of congenital postural deformities

Potter's syndrome

This is an extreme example of cranio-facial and limb deformities due to the severe oligohydramnios resulting from fetal *anuria* (failure to secrete urine). Babies with this condition have absent, or severely hypoplastic, kidneys and are usually stillborn or die within a very short time of birth. The intra-uterine deforming forces give rise to a characteristic set of features — squashed face, large low-set ears flattened against the head, hooked flattened nose, loose skin, compression of arms and legs, dislocation of the hips, talipes and arthrogryposis multiplex (*vide infra*). There are also restrictions to the growth of the thoracic cage which results in secondary lung hypoplasia. In the rare event of these babies surviving birth, death soon takes place due to respiratory insufficiency. Potter's syndrome is an excellent example of a malformation (*renal agenesis*) being responsible for multiple deformations.

Arthrogryposis multiplex

This clinical label is given to babies who are born with a stiffness of several joints (*contractures*) with secondary muscle wasting. The condition is the end result of a wide spectrum of abnormalities of which oligohydramnios is only one. Intrinsic neuromuscular disease (anterior horn cell disease, congenital myotonic dystrophy) can have the same end result in limiting fetal movement. Local lesions, such as meningomyelocele can also cause arthrogryposis of the lower limbs (p.161).

Scoliosis

Lateral curvature of the spine is sometimes detected at birth. This is often due to growth constraint from a transverse lie of the fetus during late gestation. Spontaneous recovery usually takes place in the first year after birth. Many cases of scoliosis, however, are of unknown origin and begin to develop at puberty.

Congenital dislocation of the hip

This deformity, in which the head of the femur fails to articulate normally with the acetabulum, is more common in the female. It should be diagnosed soon after birth when the newborn baby is given its first examination. The occurrence of hip dislocation, which has an incidence of about 2/1000 live births, is dependent on two predisposing and one precipitating factor. Laxity of connective tissue of the joint capsule and sloping angulation of the acetabulum are the important predisposing factors, which are often under genetic influences. The precipitating factor is uterine constraint. More than 50 per cent of dislocations are found in breech deliveries (the extended breech being especially vulnerable), its abnormal position forcing the loosely articulating head of the femur out of its joint. Early detection with subsequent treatment of a dislocated, or unstable, hip is essential if the child is later to walk correctly and to prevent osteoarthrosis developing in the joint. The object of treatment is to reduce the dislocation by returning the hip into the acetabulum and retaining it for 3−6 months by means of a plaster splint. Operative reduction is occasionally resorted to if conventional treatment is unsatisfactory.

Plagiocephaly

This skull deformity consists of an abnormal protrusion of one frontal bone and retrusion of the other. The corresponding occipital bones exhibit a mirror image abnormality. It is believed to be due to intra-uterine constraint of the head in an oblique plane. The effect is often made worse by ischaemic changes taking place in the middle part of the sterno-mastoid muscle leading to fibrosis and contraction (*wry neck* or *torticollis*). The underlying brain is not usually affected by the abnormal pattern of skull growth. Recovery is almost invariably spontaneous, although surgery to a shortened sterno-mastoid muscle is sometimes indicated. In severe forms of plagiocephaly a helmet will need to be constructed to restrain growth of the prominent parts of the head, allowing the shallow parts to grow.

Congenital talipes equino-varus ('club foot')

Plantar flexion (*equinus*) of the whole foot, inversion (*varus*) and adduction of the forefoot makes up this relatively common abnormality (1−2 per 1000 live births). Secondary wasting of the calf muscles will occur (*disuse atrophy*) and the affected foot is always smaller. Although this anomaly can be caused by 'intrinsic disease' (meningomyelocele, neuro-muscular disease) it most commonly occurs from uterine constraint acting on the folded legs splinting the foot (as, for example, if the legs are flexed and folded across each other at the level of the ankle) or as part of a wider syndrome of multiple joint deformities as with Potter's syndrome. Treatment is by daily manipulation of the deformity beginning as soon as possible after birth with correction maintained by splintage. However, surgical correction is needed in over 50 per cent of cases if conservative therapy fails, usually involving lengthening of the Achilles tendon, with release of the tibialis posterior, flexor hallucis longus and flexor digitorum longus.

Mandible deformation

A small chin (*micrognathia*) may be caused by compression against the chest or against the uterus as in a brow presentation. Mandibular asymmetry, with a laterally tilted mandible, can occur if the shoulder is thrust up under the mandible. After birth there is invariably recovery of normal form. It should be remembered that the mental protuberance of the mandible is normally under-developed at birth (Fig. 17.7).

Changes in body composition
during intra-uterine growth

The rapid increase in size of the fetus in the last trimester of pregnancy is accompanied by marked changes in body composition, a knowledge of which will help in understanding the nutritional needs of preterm infants who are born early in the third trimester. The principal changes include:

Fat

Little fat is laid down early in pregnancy except for the structural phospholipids of cell membranes. Up to 20 weeks only about 1 per cent of body weight is made up of fat. During the second half of gestation white fat, derived from glucose and fatty acid precursors transported across the placenta, is rapidly laid down in specialised connective tissue cells in the skin and around the internal viscera. As a result of these physiological processes at 26 weeks the fetus has 2−3 per cent fat in its body; at 35 weeks 8 per cent and, in a full term baby of 3.5 kg about 15 per cent.

Of this fat 80 per cent is in subcutaneous tissues and provides, along with valuable thermal insulation, an important energy store to cover the period after birth when feeding is becoming established.

Brown adipose tissue, so named because of its macroscopical appearance, also develops in the latter part of gestation around the great vessels of the thoracic inlet and aorta and surrounding the kidney and adrenal gland. The activity of this tissue is indicated by the high density of mitochondria in its cells. Its major function is to produce extra heat in response to cold stress. Heat generated by the hydrolysis of brown fat is disseminated by the blood stream to the remainder of the body. After birth brown cells lose much of their fat — although it now seems possible that somehow they continue to play a metabolic role, especially in later obesity.

Water

One of the characteristics of mammalian development is the fall in the percentage of water in fat-free body tissue which takes place with time. The smallest human fetuses that have been analysed weighing about one gram contain 93–95 per cent water (mainly extra-cellular fluid). At 1000 g (<28 weeks) the percentage has fallen to about 85 per cent and, at term, to 82 per cent. The amount of water continues to fall after birth until, at maturity, 72 per cent of fat-free tissue is water. The distribution of body water between the different fluid compartments also changes with a gradual contraction of the extra-cellular water and an expansion in intra-cellular water associated with increasing cell number and size.

Nitrogen and minerals

Accompanying the growth of the various organs, tissues and extra-cellular fluid compartments, there is a progressive increase of nitrogen, potassium, calcium, phosphate and magnesium. With the decreasing ratio of extra- to intra-cellular water there is a steady fall in the sodium and chloride concentrations, with the concentration of sodium falling less quickly than chloride owing to its deposition in growing bone.

Function during intra-uterine growth

Accompanying the increase in size and constantly changing body composition of the rapidly growing fetus physiological changes take place in the organs and tissues of the body which prepare the fetus for the difficult transition which lies ahead at birth when its comfortable environment is suddenly changed for one far more hostile. The essential body functions which require to be established at birth are those performed in fetal life by the placenta. Especially important are the following:

Respiration

The exchange of oxygen and carbon dioxide between fetal and maternal circulations provides the basis of fetal respiration. The lungs in the latter half of pregnancy mature rapidly with the Type II alveolar cells acquiring the capacity to synthesise *surfactant* (p.240). An assessment of this lung maturation can be made by removing a small volume of amniotic fluid by *amniocentesis* (sampling the amniotic fluid with a needle) and estimating a lecithin/sphingomyelin ratio. A ratio >2:1 reflects maturity of mechanisms required for surfactant synthesis. This information will often be of help to the obstetrician when deciding whether to end pregnancy in the event of the mother having severe hypertensive disease or other medical problems which might endanger both herself and her unborn baby if the pregnancy were to be allowed to continue (see also Chapter 18). It is now also becoming increasingly evident that secretions from the lungs themselves during intra-uterine development serve somehow to stimulate their own growth. Conditions such as early rupture of membranes leading to chronic loss of amniotic fluid (part of which is derived from the lungs) causes lung hypoplasia. In parallel with this 'peripheral' preparation of the lungs the respiratory centre in the medulla matures in order that the appropriate respiratory drive will emerge at birth.

Nutrition

Maturation of the digestive system (including the liver) takes place in the late fetal period whilst the fetus is deriving a perfect balance of intravenous nutrients from its mother delivered across the placenta (see Chapter 16). After birth these nutrients, together with immune substances to protect the newborn baby against certain infections (particularly gastro-enteritis) are contained in milk synthesised and made available in the mammary glands (p.113).

Homeostasis

Before birth the fetus can be viewed as being haemodialysed by the placenta to maintain an extra-cellular environment free of waste products and of optimum osmolar balance, but the fetal kidney is mature enough at birth to immediately take over the function of the placenta in maintaining the *milieu intérieur* (p.253).

Maintenance of body temperature

The warmth provided prenatally by the mother remains essential for normal fetal metabolism after birth at which time it has to be provided by the baby's metabolic processes. Formation of brown fat for generating heat and white fat for conserving it are fundamental developments taking place in the later part of pregnancy to prepare the baby for birth.

If birth occurs around the expected time the functional changes, which have been taking place over the later months of pregnancy, allow in most instances for a smooth and efficient adaptation to the extra-uterine environment. Premature delivery on the other hand renders the newborn baby especially vulnerable, the extent of this being proportional to the degree of prematurity. Irregular control of breathing (respiratory centre immaturity), the need to feed milk into the stomach by feeding tube (due to immature sucking and swallowing mechanisms), jaundice (immaturity of the liver with low glucuronyl-transferase activity), hypothermia (little brown fat to generate heat and lack of thermal insulation) are commonly encountered problems. However, the most threatening single problem results from the lack of surfactant leading to difficulty in breathing and impaired exchange of oxygen and carbon dioxide — the syndrome of *hyaline membrane disease* which, in severe cases, will require assisted ventilation and which is responsible for about one half of infant deaths in the neonatal period. Indeed, hyaline membrane disease is the single most common cause of death in childhood, accounting for 10 per cent of the total. However, so successful is modern intensive care that, under optimum conditions in babies of 1–1.5 kg at birth (28–31 weeks' gestation) who are born without congenital malformations, survival is in the order of 95 per

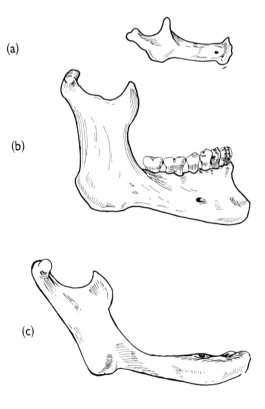

(a)

(b)

(c)

Fig. 17.7. Age changes in the mandible. (a) At infancy. (b) In the adult. (c) In old age.

cent (Fig. 17.5). At the same time it must be pointed out that a percentage (fortunately small—about 5 per cent) of these survivors will develop cerebral palsy or other types of neuro-developmental handicap (epilepsy, hydrocephalus, visual and hearing defects and learning problems). There is, therefore, a cost to being born too early. The principal aim of neonatal care is to ensure maximum survival with minimum handicap.

The anatomy of the infant

Characteristically, an infant's face is very small compared to the size of the cranium. This is easily seen in a fetal skull and is due in large part to the very rudimentary state of the maxillary antrum and the underdeveloped tooth-bearing part of the jaws (Figs. 17.7, 17.8). For about a week after birth there is often evidence of considerable 'moulding' of the bones constituting the vault of the skull. These often overlap each other to some degree when the head is subjected to the pressure of childbirth. The bones move at the unossified regions between them which, for the most part, persist as cranial sutures of the adult. Meanwhile the brain is protected by prominent reduplications of the dura mater known as the *falx cerebri* and *tentorium cerebelli* which hold its various parts in place. At about

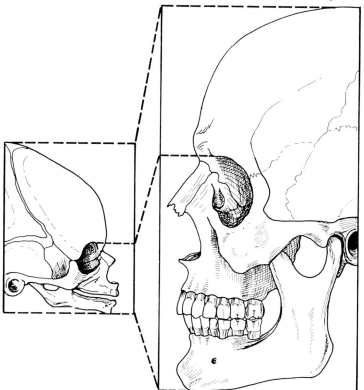

Fig. 17.8. Diagrams of neonatal and adult skulls to show the increasing relative size of the face during postnatal growth.

three months the *posterior fontanelle* (a membrane-filled gap between the parietal and occipital bones at the site of the future lambda) disappears. At about the same time the two halves of the lower jaw unite in the midline at the *symphysis menti*. During the first year the external auditory meatus is short and entirely fibro-cartilaginous and the facial nerve runs a very superficial course after leaving the skull. Towards the end of the infantile period the upper and lower incisors have erupted and suckling becomes uncomfortable for the mother. The anterior fontanelle (p.125) closes at about 18 months.

Infants have characteristically chubby cheeks due to the presence of a buccal pad of fat lying on the masseter and buccinator muscles. This is sometimes quite wrongly called the 'sucking pad'. In fact, it is merely a part of the general layer of subcutaneous fat and plays no active part in sucking. The tongue is, however, important although it is less mobile than in the child. It acts during suckling merely to raise and lower the floor of the mouth thereby effecting a change in buccal pressure and its pointed tip is only developed when its other functions begin later in life. Many operations were performed in the past to cut the *frenulum*, a fold of tissue attached to the lower surface of the tongue because an infant was thought to be 'tongue tied'. They were done because the form of the infant's tongue was not properly appreciated.

The central nervous system develops enormously during infancy and will be discussed later.

Infants' necks appear to be very short but this is because the shoulder girdle is high in position, the epiglottis is also high and there is a short trachea which correspondingly affects the position of the lungs. The chest is round in transverse section, the ribs are more or less horizontal and *respiration is entirely diaphragmatic*. The heart is relatively large compared to the adult and, indeed, it has more work to do because the metabolic rate is higher and an infant's small size means that it has a greater surface area relative to its mass and is subject to greater heat loss. An important anatomical feature of the infantile period is the presence of a relatively large thymus gland (p.178) with two large lobes extending from the thyroid above to the roots of the great vessels (where it is overlaid by the lungs) below.

In the abdomen the kidneys are still lobulated and the suprarenals very large due to incomplete involution of the fetal cortex (p.249). From the practical point of view perhaps the most important feature is the fact that the bladder is almost entirely an abdominal organ because the cavity of the true pelvis is still rudimentary. The distended bladder is thus very liable to injury.

Post-natal growth

Size attained and velocity growth

The characteristics of growth and development after birth can be best understood by viewing growth as a journey whose destination is adult size and sexual

maturity. At any one time this journey, which in day-to-day practice is represented by the curve of growth, can be described in terms of distance travelled
(attained size) and the speed of travel (rate (velocity) of growth). Of the two, the
rate of growth is the more sensitive measure of current growth performance:
attained size reflects previous events (see also p.302). A French naturalist, Guenau
de Montbeillard in the 19th Century was the first to provide a complete set of
longitudinal height data from measurements of his own child taken every six
months from birth to the age of 18. The growth curve from these plots is illustrated
in Fig. 17.9 and is remarkably similar to those drawn today. Examination of the
velocity curve of height reveals four well defined periods of growth in childhood:
First: extends from the time the newborn infant has recovered from the terminal
intra-uterine slowing of growth, between 1 and 3 weeks, until the age of about

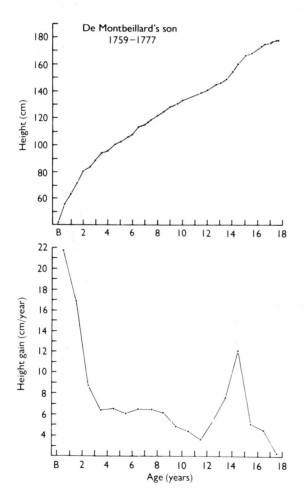

Fig. 17.9. Growth in height of the Count de Montbeillard's son from birth to 18 years (1759–1777).
Above: height attained. Below: growth velocity. Published by permission.

2 years. The prominent feature of this period is a steady deceleration in growth rate.

Second: this period is characterised by much slower deceleration (which, in actual practice, is taken as an almost constant rate of growth) which lasts about 10 years.

Third: the *adolescent growth spurt*. When this is complete the child enters the

Fourth: and final phase, that of growth deceleration until, at maturity, growth in height ceases.

A striking feature of the human growth curve is the long pre-adolescent phase, a phenomenon peculiar to primates, which reaches its maximum expression in man. This long period of relative quiescence might be seen as providing the brain with ample opportunity to prepare for an adulthood where survival depends more on higher cerebral function than on primitive and instinctive qualities of aggression seen in other animals.

Growth patterns

The growth of the whole body is the result of the growth of its constituent organs and tissues, each having unique growth characteristics. The following growth patterns have been described (Fig. 17.10).

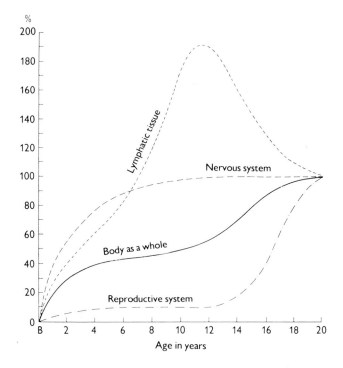

Fig. 17.10. Differential growth in three body tissues compared to the body as a whole. (From *The Measurements of Man* by J.A. Harris et al., University of Minnesota Press, 1930).

Visceral type

The internal organs, lungs, liver, pancreas, kidney and spleen follow the same general course as that for height and weight.

Neural type

The brain, together with its covering membranes, spinal cord, eyes, auditory mechanisms and skull vault, undergoes the most rapid period of its growth in the last part of fetal life and the first few years of post-natal life (p.304).

Lymphoid type

This is represented also not only by lymph nodes but by structures such as the thymus and tonsils. All show similar characteristics — rapid gains in size

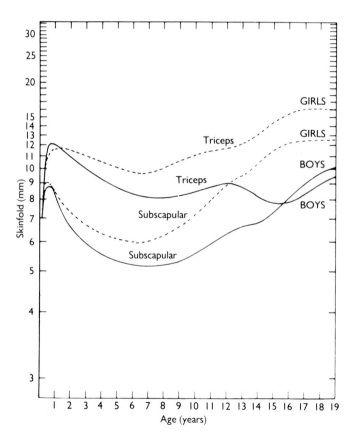

Fig. 17.11. Growth of subcutaneous tissue (50th centile for British children) measured by a skinfold caliper over the back of the arm (triceps) and beneath the scapula (subscapular). Published by permission.

throughout infancy and childhood to reach, at puberty, a peak which greatly exceeds the final adult dimensions. This growth pattern is due probably to the constant exposure of the child to micro-organisms over this period with accompanying reactive changes taking place in lymphoid tissue. After adolescence there is a progressive decline in lymphoid mass.

Genital type

This type of growth is very different from those preceding. It is represented by growth of the prostate gland, testes, epididymis, seminal vesicles in the male and by the ovaries and uterus in the female. In these organs there is a slight spurt in infancy, a long period of consistently slow growth until puberty at which time there is extremely rapid growth to attain full sexual maturity.

During the prenatal stage of growth this diversity in growth patterns is much less evident. With few exceptions (notably the brain), organ and tissue growth closely follows the curve of total body growth. Infancy is the transition period in which the organs and structures of the body depart one by one from the very simple style of growth characteristic of the fetus.

Adipose tissue type (Fig. 17.11)

Most of the fat in the body is contained in subcutaneous tissue. A measure of its amount can be gained by picking up a fold of skin and measuring its thickness with a specially designed caliper. Two sites are most commonly used, the skin over the triceps and subscapular regions. From 30 weeks of prenatal life until about 1 year postnatal life there is an increase in skinfold thickness. Thereafter there is a gradual loss of fat (the loss being greater in boys) until about the age of 6−8 years when the thickness of subcutaneous fat increases again, particularly in girls. Puberty accelerates the rate of fat accumulation in girls.

Developmental age

Children grow to sexual maturity at differing rates which are largely genetically determined. The size of a child at any given age is not a reliable marker of developmental maturity. Thus a child might be tall through inheriting genes for tall stature from its parents yet still have a slow rate of development. Alternatively, this given height could be reached over a shorter period of time through an accelerated rate of maturity. Likewise, a child might be small for genetic reasons or because of a slow tempo of maturation.

Skeletal maturity

The measure of developmental maturity most widely used in clinical practice is that of osseous maturation, the *bone age*. To estimate this an X-ray is taken, usually of the wrist and hand (under 18 months the legs and feet are more widely used), in order to examine the appearance of various ossification centres of the wrist, carpus and digits. A quantitative measure of maturity can be made either by comparisons with reference standards, as in the method of Greulich and Pyle (whose radiological atlas of North American children in the 1930s continues to be widely used), or by using a complicated but more reliable method in which about 20 individual bones of the wrist and hand are scored according to their maturity. The sum total of the scores are converted into a *bone age* which is simply the chronological age for which the given score is the arithmetic average of all the scores recorded. Boys and girls pass through the same stages of skeletal maturity but boys pass more slowly averaging only about 80 per cent the bone age of girls at any one time.

Estimating skeletal maturity is an important clinical tool in the investigation of various growth problems, especially short stature, since it will help to determine

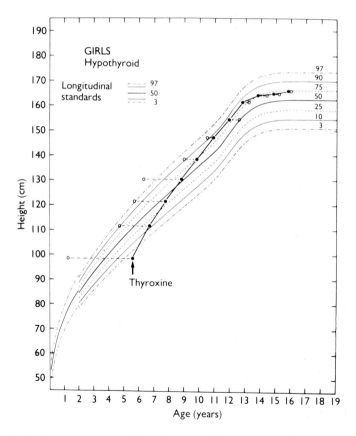

Fig. 17.12. Retarded osseous maturation ('bone age') in a child with hypothyroidism. ●....● Bone age. O----O Chronological age. With treatment, the bone age gradually gains on chronological age. The numbered curves are 'centiles'. Textbooks of paediatrics should be consulted for the significance of these. Published by permission.

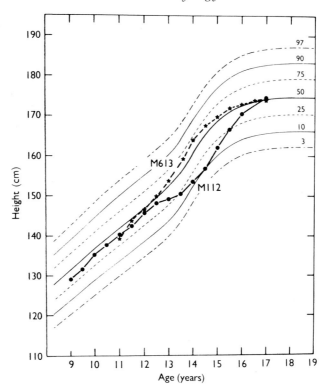

Fig. 17.13. Height growth of two boys. One (M 613) has an early adolescent growth spurt, the other a late spurt. Between the ages of 13 and 16 the former is taller but by the age of 17 the heights attained are the same. Published by permission.

whether genetic or pathological causes are primarily responsible. Disease such as growth hormone deficiency, hypothyroidism, malnutrition (see also p.339) will not only slow down growth but also significantly retard osseous maturation (Fig. 17.12). In economically developed countries it is unusual to find a pathological cause for short stature. In genetically small children an estimate of osseous maturity will help to predict the age at which the puberty growth spurt will begin since, as has been already explained, this more closely correlates with maturity than with absolute age. For example, if the bone age of a small child lags behind its chronological age the pre-adolescent period of growth will usually be longer giving rise to a later adolescent growth spurt. In this way the child will be seen to 'catch-up' (and sometimes even overtake) his peers who were taller at a younger age (Fig. 17.13). Another example of the clinical value of bone age, this time at the other extreme of growth range, is the very tall girl of 10 whose parents are worried that she will continue growing for several more years to become far too tall. If her bone age is in advance of her chronological age an early growth spurt can be anticipated leading to early cessation of growth. There now exists a formula which will reliably determine the final mature height of a child to within a few centimetres which takes into account existing height, skeletal maturity and genetic potential as indicated by mid-parental height. This height prediction has a social application as well as a clinical one: thus, in girls wishing to enter ballet school where a uniform height of a *corps de ballet* is desirable an estimate of bone age is often required as a condition for admission in order that an estimate of mature height can be made.

Physical maturity and psychological development

Children who are more advanced in their physical maturity tend on average to score slightly, but consistently, better in tasks of mental and physical ability than those of the same age and of lesser physical maturity. This might well underlie some of the differences which exist in the school performances of girls and boys. To what extent these differences are due to intrinsic differences in brain matura-tion or to the social and physical accompaniments of early maturity (confidence, greater physical strength, etc.) is not known. No area of development biology illustrates more vividly the complex interactions between biological roots and the environment. Under normal circumstances nothing can be done to alter the tempo of development. It is important, therefore, that those who are responsible for teaching children are aware of the influence on school abilities of differing levels of maturity and, where appropriate, make special and sensitive allowances.

Growth in infancy and early childhood

This period extends from birth until about the end of the second year. For the first 9–12 months or so the baby is normally breast fed. The term *extero-gestate fetus* describes the extension of the baby's complete dependence on the mother for its nutrition and immunological protection in these early and highly vulnerable post-natal months. After this period the young infant soon learns to stand upright and develops the beginnings of manipulative skills, language and various aspects of social behaviour.

After birth, growth rates for weight gain and growth rates in length and head circumference accelerate to reach maximum velocity between 4 and 6 weeks (Fig. 17.14) and then decline over the next few years (Fig. 17.9).

Factors influencing growth in infancy

Genetic factors

As discussed earlier (p.307), intra-uterine growth is largely regulated by maternal influences but, at birth, the infant is released from these and grows under the direction of its own genetic machinery. The infant's own growth curve may deviate from the 'normal' growth curve but there is always a tendency to return to this. Thus many underweight infants can regain the 'normal' curve by 'catch-up'

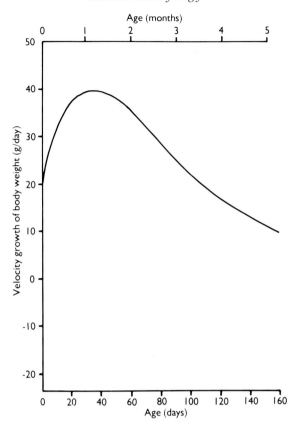

Fig. 17.14. Daily velocity weight gain (curve of growth rate cf. Fig. 17.1(b)) in infants over the first 5 months of life. Published by permission.

growth (p.330) while overweight babies also tend to approach 'normality' for reasons as yet poorly understood.

Nutritional influences

In healthy infants the type of early nutrition has remarkably little effect on the rate of growth. Infants who are fed milk formulae based on cow's milk constituents gain weight at approximately the same rate as breast fed infants. It used to be widely held that the early introduction of solid foods causes an acceleration in the rate of weight gain but this has now been shown not to be the case.

In under-privileged communities and in economically developing countries the *most important influence in retarding infant growth is malnutrition* (p.342).

Growth in later childhood

Childhood 'proper' is the longest of the three periods between birth and maturity. It extends from the end of the early phase of rapid growth deceleration (at about the age of two) until the beginning of the adolescent growth spurt (Fig. 17.9). The rate at which the healthy child grows in this period is remarkably constant, 5–6 cm in height and 2–2.5 kg in weight per year. The period lasts about 10 years and may be seen as a relatively quiescent phase between the more dramatic growth changes of infancy and adolescence and as providing opportunity for the acquisition of intellectual skills in preparation for adulthood.

Certain patterns of growth can be identified. The rate of growth of the skull vault, accompanying the steady deceleration of the brain growth spurt, is now much slower. The fontanelles become ossified by about 18 months to 2 years. The capacity of the skull increases thereafter by a process of deposition of bone beneath the pericranium and removal of bone from the inner table. At the same time the vertical diameter of the skull is also increasing through the growth of the mandible and maxilla which have to accommodate the primary dentition (20 milk teeth) and later the beginnings of secondary dentition (6 years onwards). As the permanent teeth erupt the paranasal sinuses begin to develop. The external auditory meatus becomes longer and the mastoid process appears at about the age of two years with the outgrowth of air cells from the tympanic antrum. As a result of these changes, which continue until puberty, the relative sizes of the cranium and the face alter, the facial skeleton becoming relatively larger (Fig. 17.8).

The curvatures of the spinal column, typical of the adult, become apparent during infancy and early childhood. They are easily straightened at first but become permanent with differential bony growth particularly in the lumbo-sacral region. *In utero* the fetus lies in a flexed position and the spinal cord is concave anteriorly. At 3 months post-natally, when the infant begins to raise its head, a ventrally convex curvature of the cervical spine appears and just before the age of

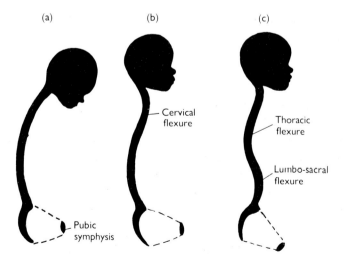

Fig. 17.15. Showing the development of the curvatures of the spine. (a) Fetal condition (b) Development of the cervical flexure (c) Development of the lumbo-sacral flexure and forward tilting of the pelvis.

one year, a second ventral curvature in the lumbo-sacral region develops as the child begins to sit up and then to walk. These changes are illustrated in Fig. 17.15 and are associated with a forward tilting of the pelvis.

In the toddler the centre of gravity is high so that stance has a wide base; it also lies more anteriorly than later because the shallow pelvis fails to accommodate the abdominal viscera: all this leads to an exaggeration of the lumbar lordosis in order to bring the body into a vertical position. By the age of 5 the pelvis has become deeper, allowing the bladder and other abdominal viscera to descend. The lumbar lordosis is reduced and posture becomes that of a young adult. Accompanying these postural changes are those of stance — at 18 months the baby is often bow-legged; at the age of 3 often 'knock-kneed' at the age of 6 the legs assume a normal pattern although there exist considerable variations in form.

These various patterns of growth accompany, and indeed in large part are responsible for, changing proportions of the body. At 18 months the head is about one quarter of the total length of the body. During the childhood period the contribution of the head to total body length becomes less so that, at the onset of adolescence, it is a little over one-eighth the body length. The legs (heel to perineum) of the young infant constitute about one-third of his body length; at puberty this ratio is nearly one-half due to the relatively greater growth of the lower segment of the body compared with the trunk. The human, therefore, changes from being short-limbed with a relatively large head to long-limbed with a relatively smaller head (Fig. 17.3). Increase in size is coupled with the development of more angular features compared with the rounded contours of infancy. This results from a steady decrease in the amount of fat contained in the subcutaneous tissues until, at about the age of 6–8 years, it begins to increase once more. Girls tend to lose less fat from the subcutaneous tissues of both trunk and limbs.

Adolescence*

Adolescence, during which reproductive capacity is attained, is a term used to describe the changes which take place in the period of life which links childhood and adulthood. It is characterised by three harmoniously inter-related processes — namely, (i) a rapid increase in body size; (ii) profound changes in the endocrine system; (iii) important psychological changes. These will now be discussed in detail.

The adolescent growth spurt and changes in body proportions

There is considerable variation in the age at which the adolescent growth spurt

*In this section 'adolescence' is used as synonymous with 'puberty'. In other texts a distinction is sometimes made — 'adolescence' referring to the psychological events and 'puberty' to the physical changes of this link period between childhood and adulthood. There is no unanimous agreement about this however — which is why we use 'adolescence' and 'puberty' synonymously.

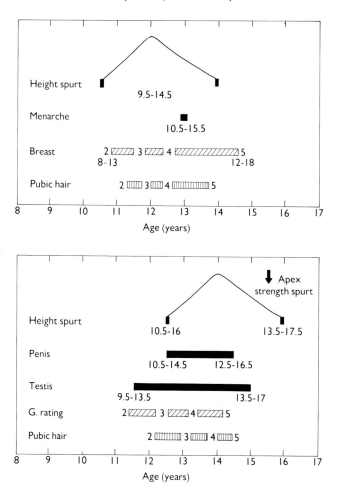

Fig. 17.16. The sequence of events at puberty in girls (above) and boys (below). Rating numbers indicating onset and relative development interrupt bars for breast, pubic hair and G. rating (Tanner, 1978). Published by permission.

(Fig. 17.9) begins. There are also marked sex differences. Girls on average begin their growth spurt at around 10 years, about 2 years sooner than boys (Fig. 17.16). In both sexes the mean duration of the spurt is about 3 years. The peak growth velocity is greater in boys than in girls but is reached later, about 14 years for boys and 12 years for girls. The amount of height gained by boys is greater — 7 cm in the first year of the spurt, 9 cm in the second and 7 cm in the third, compared with values of 6, 8 and 6 in girls. Accompanying this adolescent spurt are periods of accelerated growth of abdominal viscera including liver, kidneys, pancreas, lungs and heart.

The longer pre-adolescent period of growth (by about 2 years), the higher peak growth velocity and greater gain in height during the spurt (about 28 cm in boys and 25 cm in girls) account for the greater ultimate stature of adult men over women of about 13 cm. Growth in height very largely ceases when the epiphyses close, usually before the age of 18 in boys and 16 in girls. There is, however, an approximate 2 per cent increase in growth into the mid-20s through continued vertebral column growth. The explanation for the slowing down and eventual cessation of activity of the cartilaginous growth plate remains to be established, although it is likely to be genetically determined and mediated by a complex endocrine *milieu* in which growth hormone, androgens and sex hormones all play important roles.

Consideration of the curve of total body growth alone during puberty conceals subtle differences which exist in the growth patterns of individual parts of the skeleton. In these there is a well-defined sequence with the feet and hands being the first parts to undergo their spurt, followed by calf and forearm, thigh and arm, hips and shoulders and finally chest. Last to undergo its growth spurt is the trunk. During adolescence growth of the trunk through the vertebral bodies is relatively greater than that of the legs which have undergone much of their growth in the pre-adolescent period. These non-uniform, though harmonious, patterns of skeletal dimensions account for the well recognised day-to-day obser- vations in adolescents that hands and feet appear for a short time relatively larger and out of proportion giving often a rather ungainly appearance being a frequent source of embarrassment. Reassurance can be given that, eventually, the hands and feet will be, if anything, a little smaller in proportion to the arms and legs. With leg length being the first dimension to reach its peak growth, the adolescent boy will grow out of his trousers before his jacket.

In its early stages the adolescent growth spurt is initially linear. Lateral growth takes place towards the end of the spurt predominantly through the continued growth of the clavicle, the last bone in the body to stop growing and one which thrusts the shoulders from the trunk. The shoulder width spurt is greater in boys due to the influence of testosterone. In girls, through oestrogen activity, the pelvis becomes wider, especially at the inlet. The head does not participate in the growth spurt, its growth mostly having been completed in early childhood. Continued, but slow, growth in adolescence is made up mostly by some 15 per cent increase in thickness of bone, development of brow ridges and frontal sinuses and slight enlargement of the middle and posterior cranial fossae. It is likely however that the brain continues to grow at a very slow rate, together with increasing organi- sation and complexity of its neuronal connections. The face undergoes marked changes during adolescence, especially in boys (in girls there is often very little change in facial dimensions). The forehead becomes prominent, maxilla and man- dible are thrust forward and the facial muscles develop.

Sexual dimorphism during adolescence, which must be seen as an acceleration of a process which has begun in pre-natal life, is reflected in changes in body composition as well as in the extent of the growth spurt. The thickness of bone cortex is greater in boys who also show a much greater increase in muscle bulk, thereby allowing them to become stronger than girls. By maturity men have a much more lean body and skeletal mass than women. In order to cope with more extensive body growth in boys, there is a greater increase in heart and lung size than in girls, a higher systolic blood pressure, a lower resting heart rate, a greater oxygen carrying capacity in the blood through a greater red cell mass and haemoglobin, (at mid-adolescence mean haemoglobin in the male is 16.0/100 ml compared with 14.0/100 ml in girls). These physiological adaptive changes in the male are all believed to be under the influence of testosterone and adrenal androgens and are presumed to have evolved in order to help the male acquire the qualities of strength and endurance required for the tasks of hunting, fighting and manipulating heavy objects for food gathering, all concerned with a primitive primate role for survival of the species. Both sexes gain in total body fat but boys on average lose subcutaneous fat at adolescence, more so on the limbs than on the trunk. The time at which least fat is present coincides with the peak growth velocity. A similar, but a quantitatively smaller, effect is seen in girls in whom fat is deposited in areas of secondary sexual distribution — breasts, hips, axillae and neck. At maturity women have twice as much body fat as men.

Development of the reproductive system (gonads and secondary sex characteristics)

During the adolescent growth spurt the reproductive organs and secondary sex characteristics grow and mature to reach their adult status (Fig. 17.16). In analysing these it is important to recognise the considerable variation which exists in the ages at which these events occur in individual children.

The earliest sign of puberty in boys, at a median age of about 11.5 years, is testicular enlargement (accompanied by changes in colour and texture of the scrotal skin) resulting from growth in length and tortuosity of the seminiferous tubules. These external changes begin approximately one year before the onset of the growth spurt. Growth of the penis, together with prostate gland, seminal vesicles and bulbo-urethral glands, commences about a year later under the influence of testosterone, now being produced by the Leydig cells of the testes, and adrenal androgens. Sperm frequently appear in the first morning sample of urine from spontaneous leakage into the urinary tract at a median age of about 14 years.

In girls the earliest sign of puberty is the formation of the breast bud which appears at a median age of 11 years. Breast development is influenced by oestrogens secreted by the ovary and is a very sensitive indicator of oestradiol secretion. Growth of the uterus and vagina develop simultaneously with the breasts. In some boys there is a brief period of breast enlargement which can be a source of considerable embarrassment. When marked, this is termed *gynaecomastia* but it usually regresses of its own accord within a few years of its onset. If it fails to do so the condition can be alleviated by removal of subareolar fat.

The development of body hair has received rather little attention. Pubic hair appears relatively early in the onset of the pubertal growth spurt, slightly earlier in girls than boys (Fig. 17.16). Axillary hair and, in boys, facial hair and 'breaking' of

the voice due to a greater degree of laryngeal growth than in girls, develop after
the peak of the growth spurt. Hair elsewhere on the body appears later still.

Menarche

The first menstrual period is a late event in puberty representing the time when
the concentration of oestradiol is sufficient to cause endometrial hyperplasia to
break down when oestrogen concentration falls in cyclical fashion (p.51). It occurs
after the peak of the growth spurt has been passed; only about 6 cm of height is
gained after this time. Menarche is easily recognisable and better remembered
than any of the male characteristics of maturity, hence its value as a marker of
examining trends in maturity. The average age of its appearance in European girls
is 13 years with a range such that in 95 per cent of girls menarche will be reached
between 11 and 15 years.

There is a misconception that girls reach *sexual maturity* before boys. Certainly
the growth spurt begins 2 years sooner and breast development is more evident
than increase in testicular size. In boys, the readily apparent secondary sexual
characteristics, development of facial hair and breaking of the voice do not occur
until the genitalia are approaching maturity towards the end of the growth spurt.
*However sexual maturity as measured by ovulation and spermatogenesis are reached at
approximately the same age between 14 and 15 years.*

Endocrinology of puberty

The complex hormonal changes which underlie the events of adolescence are still
incompletely understood. The following description presents current opinion.

In pre-pubertal life there is relative quiescence in the activity of the ovaries
and testes, their sex hormones being secreted in only very small amounts under
the control of follicle stimulating hormone (FSH) and luteinizing hormone (LH).
These gonadotrophins are produced by cells in the adenohypophysis in response
to hypothalamic gonadotrophin releasing hormone (GnRH) reaching the anterior
pituitary gland via the hypothalamic pituitary portal circulation. These hormones
are, however, produced in sufficient quantities to operate the feedback inhibitory
system. With maturation of the nervous system, hypothalamic receptors lying in
close proximity to the cells which synthesise and secrete GnRH are less susceptible to inhibition by circulating levels of gonadal hormones. Ultimately, the
gonadotrophins FSH and LH are secreted in larger quantities by the adenohypophysis causing a surge in secretions of the gonads and adrenal gland. A new
feedback equilibrium of the hypothalamic-pituitary-gonadal axis is re-established
with higher circulating levels of sex hormones and gonadotrophins. This system
is described in more detail in Chapter 4.

Rising levels of FSH in the female cause the ovarian follicles to develop and
secrete oestradiol. In the male FSH causes maturation of the seminiferous tubules
and spermatogenesis, feedback possibly being through the hormone Inhibin.

LH causes the Leydig cells in the testes to enlarge and manufacture testosterone. Oestrogens are responsible for growth of the female secondary sexual characters — breasts, uterus and vagina. Pubic, axillary and facial hair in boys is mainly under the influence of testosterone. In girls, androgens from the suprarenals are responsible for axillary and pubic hair.

These endocrine mechanisms, as far as they are known, have been established by using radio-immunoassay techniques which are now giving more and more information. Testosterone, growth hormone and adrenal androgens act synergistically but their individual roles are not yet fully understood. Sex steroids are primarily responsible for changes in the vertebral column and the width of shoulders and hips. Growth of the legs is predominantly under the influence of growth hormone. A current hypothesis is that in males growth hormone continues to be secreted in the same amounts as in the pre-adolescent period — contributing about 4–5 cm per year; testosterone and other androgens produced in the gonadal spurt superimpose on this an additional 5–6 cm per year. In females, the mechanisms underlying the adolescent growth spurt are less well understood, especially the reason for the earlier height spurt. Perhaps the low levels of oestrogen act synergistically with growth hormones. Adrenal androgens produced under the influence of a pituitary factor (likely not to be ACTH) then have a superimposed role. Muscle increase and width of bone cortex is caused by adrenal androgens in both sexes, with testosterone in the male responsible for their greater increase. Loss of subcutaneous fat in boys might be under the same influence. Oestrogens are responsible for the characteristic distribution of fat in girls.

Psychological changes

Adolescence is often a period of psychological stress. Understanding the physical changes which are taking place in the body; adjusting to the acquisition of sexual maturity; the need to seek independence; increasing social pressures, many encouraged by the media, fear of unemployment etc. all combine to make life difficult for many adolescents. Early and late onset of puberty will often be a source of embarrassment and interfere with educational achievement.

Factors which influence growth in later childhood

Many factors account for the considerable variations which exist in the rate of growth and size attained in later childhood (p.328). Conventional practice is to consider these in two principal categories — genetic and environmental (nutrition, infection, climate, socio-economic conditions). They may also be appropriately considered in two principal groups according to whether the origins of these variations are physiological or pathological.

Genetic factors

The size and body proportions of a child, together with the tempo of its growth and therefore the onset of puberty, are all under the influence of many genes contained on several chromosomes which are switched on and off at pre-determined times. These polygenic influences are allowed full expression only if the internal metabolic environment provided for the growing organs and tissues is optimal. The heritability of stature is high, as indicated by the degree of corre-lation existing between close relatives. It is likely, although not easily proven, that social class effects on stature, also partly of genetic origin, are established as early as 2 years of age.

Genetic factors account for many of the physical differences in size and deve-lopment which exist between the various groups of mankind. For example, babies of African stock are more mature at birth and acquire motor milestones (such as sitting, crawling and walking) sooner than do those of Caucasian origin. As adults, men of African descent — although of similar height — have longer legs in relation to sitting height; this is perhaps an example of the persistence of an adaptive phenomenon evolved to facilitate heat loss. In contrast, the thick-set body and short legs of the 'mongoloid' peoples, particularly the Chinese, are adaptations for the conservation of heat in a cold environment.

Genetic factors also account for the differences in physical and developmental characteristics between males and females. This sexual dimorphism, although most marked from the onset of puberty, even exists in prenatal life. At 20 weeks of gestation the osseous maturation of the skeleton is already about 3 weeks more advanced in girls. By the time of birth this gap has widened to 5—6 weeks, although they are on average about 150 g lighter than boys due to a slightly slower rate of weight gain *in utero*. Their pelves are also more capacious. Accompanying this prenatal skeletal precocity is likely to be advancement of physiological sys-tems (for example, synthesis of surfactant) which partly accounts for the reduced mortality in the perinatal period of girls compared with boys. In childhood, girls reach the major motor milestones concerned with the attainment of upright posture and free mobility (sitting, crawling, standing, walking) sooner, acquire bladder control earlier and more rapidly and learn the skills of fine co-ordination which are required, for example, in being able to write. Their understanding and use of words is also more advanced at equivalent ages. Throughout childhood the tempo of growth as already mentioned proceeds about 10 per cent more rapidly in girls which is reflected in their reaching half their mature stature at an average age of 1.75 years compared with 2 years in boys. Just as girls are ahead in skeletal maturity, they also lead in the time of eruption of secondary dentition. Until puberty there is little, or no, significant difference in body size for age between the sexes although in terms of body composition girls, even before puberty, have more subcutaneous fat.

Seasonal effects

In Western Europe there is seasonal variation in the rate of growth. On average, children grow faster in spring and summer than in the colder autumn and winter months. During the relatively stable period of childhood, between 5 and 10 years, a child in its fastest quartile of growth might grow at three times the rate of its slowest quartile. These observations are of practical importance for example when investigating the possibility that growth retardation in a child is due to some endocrine cause such as growth hormone deficiency. Thus, any period of less than a year is insufficient to provide an accurate and reliable measure of growth rate. The explanation for the seasonal effect is incompletely understood. The fact that it appears to be less evident in blind children suggests that, as with its influence on breeding cycles in some animals, a nervous system response to light might somehow influence growth.

Disorders of growth in later childhood

Contrary to widespread clinical belief, retarded growth and short stature are not always synonymous. Certainly in some children who are abnormally short for their age there will be a pathological explanation but, in most instances, genetic reasons predominate for this smallness. Likewise, there are some children whose size is within the normal range yet who might still be failing to grow adequately. This section provides a brief introduction to ways in which pathological influences can retard growth.

Primary growth failure

In these disorders the primary fault is within the cells of growing organs and tissues, particularly of the skeleton. The cellular defect might be determined at, or very soon after, conception (as with chromosome abnormalities and various genetic defects) or very early in fetal life.

Genetic abnormalities

Most conceptuses with an abnormal karyotype are aborted very early in pregnancy. Of those who survive, the most common chromosome anomaly to be associated with a disturbance of growth of many tissues and organs, including the skeleton, as judged from distribution of weight, height and head circumference at birth is *Down's syndrome* (Trisomy 21), a condition better known for its associated mental retardation. Mean birth weight is reduced by 400 g and length by about 2 cm. There is a general reduction in size of all the organs due to a reduced number of parenchymal cells. The average height of the adult male is 158 cm; for females the mature height is about 140 cm.

Turner's syndrome — gonadal dysgenesis provides another example of genetic growth failure. In this condition mean birth weight is about 2.80 kg with a mean birth length of 48 cm. The slower than average growth rate, which begins in prenatal life, continues through childhood (especially from the age of about 4 years) and into adolescence, which does not contain any growth spurt. The ultimate height attained in these girls is only about 140 cm although, in contrast with Down's syndrome, there is a correlation with mid-parental height. Deprived of secondary sexual characteristics and manifesting permanent infertility, girls with gonadal dysgenesis must be seen as considerably disadvantaged, although being mentally quite normal.

Many primary defects in bone and cartilage exist in isolation or together with growth defects in other organs and tissue systems, as syndromes of unknown aetiology. *Achondroplasia*, due to a dominant mutation of a single gene, is an excellent example. In this condition abnormalities include short upper arms and thighs, together with a normal length trunk and a large head with a characteristic face. The syndrome can be explained by abnormalities in growth of bone originally laid down as cartilage (Fig. 9.11).

However diverse their aetiology and presentation, disorders in which the growth failure is due to a primary defect in cell function have two features in common. Firstly, growth deficiency begins in the prenatal period, a point which is often overlooked since the size at birth of these babies is often within the 'normal distribution' (substantiating the point made above that normal size does not preclude abnormal growth). Secondly, there is no effective therapy to recover the deficit of growth rate since the genetic machinery controlling growth is abnormal from the outset. The growth failure is therefore progressive, the child's height falling steadily further from the normal during childhood.

Secondary growth failure

In the disorders included in this category *growth potential* is normal but this is not allowed complete expression because of adverse environment influences which:
1 deprive growing cells of substances essential for growth (food, hormones and oxygen);
2 interfere with cell function through abnormal extra-cellular homeostasis (as in kidney failure);
3 damage growing cells (toxins and infectious agents).

Under-nutrition

In prenatal life, maternal hypertensive disease, due to its effect on placental vessels and thus by interfering with placental transfer of nutrients, will often restrict growth of the fetus as well as depriving it of oxygen and thereby increasing the risks of intra-partum asphyxia. Affected infants are underweight for their length (which is also diminished) and, unless they are adequately fed, are likely to have hypoglycaemia during the neonatal period, attributable to low reserves of liver glycogen (Fig. 17.17). Somewhat surprisingly, perhaps, under-nutrition in the mother during pregnancy does not apparently result in significant fetal growth retardation. The fetus is an extremely effective parasite when it comes to protecting its own growth.

In post-natal life short illnesses have only a temporary effect on growth. Repeated or chronic illnesses can have an irrecoverable effect on growth, a fact particularly relevant to two-thirds of the world's children who suffer severe and prolonged protein and calorie malnutrition. Many die but even more suffer the long-term consequences of malnutrition. The condition usually begins after weaning when the little food available is of poor nutritional value and likely to be contaminated. As already mentioned, growth curves of children in developing

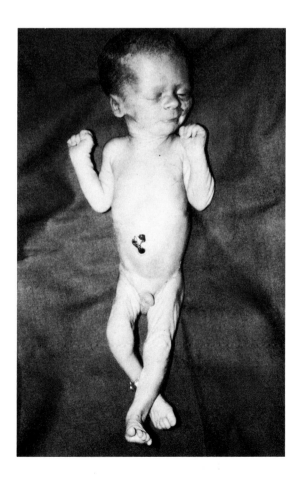

Fig. 17.17. Prenatal under-nutrition in a baby born at term to a mother with severe hypertensive disease. Note the florid wasting.

countries fall well below those in developed countries where primary nutritional deficiency is uncommon in post-natal life. When it occurs it is most commonly due to early lactational failure. Secondary under-nutrition, such as might occur in the course of systemic illness, though more common, is quite rare. It is met, for example, in young infants with severe congenital heart disease who are in heart failure; they are just unable, because of fatigue, to take in enough food. Part of the psycho-social deprivation syndrome (*vide infra*) might also be mediated through poor appetite due to emotional trauma.

Several syndromes of malabsorption result in a failure of nutrients to reach growing tissues. Of these, gluten enteropathy or coeliac disease, an abnormal reaction of the gut to the wheat protein gluten, cow's milk protein intolerance and cystic fibrosis (in which, as part of widespread exocrine gland malfunctions, there is malabsorption of fat due to pancreatic insufficiency) are most common. Severe primary malnutrition will in itself also cause secondary malabsorption.

With malnutrition, regardless of cause, the primary type of growth disturbance is failure of weight gain (failure to thrive) followed by skeletal growth retardation; infants are, therefore, underweight for their height. With chronic malnutrition, or long-standing gastro-intestinal disease, there is progressive stunting of linear growth.

In all the conditions in which there is a failure of nutrient delivery to growing cells, growth failure must be seen as an essential adaptive function. If growth were to continue normally in the face of diminished resources of available energy and protein, children would be deprived of essential substances for metabolic processes required for survival. Growth might, therefore, be seen as a luxury which can be afforded only when basal maintenance needs have been satisfied.

Endocrine deficiencies

Growth hormone deficiency leads to children with this condition ending up as adults only about 130 cm tall. They fall into two categories.

First, children in whom there is idiopathic growth hormone deficiency, occuring in about 1/10,000 live births, either isolated or associated with other anterior pituitary hormone deficiencies — *hypopituitarism*. In these children there is no obvious growth deficit in prenatal life. It is most commonly diagnosed at about the age of 5 or 6, when children start school and are noted by their parents to be extremely small compared with their friends. In their external features children with idiopathic growth hormone deficiency appear doll-like with an increase in subcutaneous fat, normal skeletal proportions, small penis and often undescended testes. Intellectually they are normal.

Second, children in whom growth hormone deficiency can develop, form a group where the hypothalamus or anterior pituitary has been destroyed as, for example, by a *cranio-pharyngioma* (a cystic mass derived from Rathke's pouch, (p.149)), other malignant infiltrations or by cranial irradiation for leukaemia.

Suspicion of growth hormone deficiency may, at first, be aroused because of poor height gain velocity and is later confirmed by demonstrating failure of insulin-induced hypoglycaemia to cause an adequate rise in growth hormone. Treatment is the regular administration of growth hormone (together with other hormones if indicated, such as thyroxine, corticosteroids and androgens) for the whole duration of childhood and adolescence until growth is complete. This replacement therapy with growth hormone results in rapid catch-up growth, although at maturity these children remain very small (perhaps indicating a permanent deficit), a fact which has provided the impetus for detecting these children at a much earlier age in the hope that with treatment instituted sooner the genetic potential for stature will be attained.

In view of the fundamental role of thyroid hormones in brain growth and protein synthesis in the skeleton, it is not surprising that deficiencies of these hormones will cause growth failure in both fetal and post-natal life (*cretinism*). The origin of the thyroid abnormality is either dysmorphogenesis (maldevelopment of the thyroid gland) or metabolic errors in the synthesis of thyroid hormones. In older children thyroid deficiency can be a secondary disorder due to destruction of a previously normal thyroid gland by circulating antibodies. The age onset is usually between 8 and 15. In these children there is growth failure associated with delayed bone maturation and abnormal appearance of the epiphyses. With treatment there is complete catch-up and no residual mental disorder.

Other endocrine disorders, some iatrogenic (i.e. the result of medical treatment), may lead to disorders of growth. Cortisone, and its derivatives, are widely used in the treatment of various disorders in childhood, including asthma and renal or rheumatoid disease. Although cortisone itself has little role in regulating growth its excess can slow down growth quite markedly, probably by interfering with the action of somatomedins on the cartilage growth cells. There is also some evidence that the synthesis of somatomedins is interfered with in the liver by excessively high levels of cortisone. Rarely, excess hydrocortisone can be produced by an adrenal tumour or hyperplasia. This results in *Cushing's syndrome* with growth deceleration and increase in adipose tissue especially in the trunk and nape of the neck and cheeks.

Miscellaneous causes

Lack of oxygen

Included in this category are children with severe cyanotic heart disease, such as Fallot's Tetralogy (p.229) and chronic lung disease as, for example, in fibrocystic disease and even in asthma where an association has been described between height and the severity of the respiratory symptoms. These conditions can be shown to be independent of their incidental treatment with growth retarding drugs, such as steroids, in causing delayed skeletal maturation and late puberty.

Renal failure

Reasons why chronic renal failure should cause poor growth are still not understood but, in part, they are likely to be related to failure to excrete organic acids
and other waste substances which accumulate in the extra-cellular *milieu* thereby
'poisoning' growth processes; vitamin D metabolism is also affected in chronic
renal failure because of impairment of the secondary stage of cholecalciferol
hydroxylation (at the 1 position) to 1,25-dihydroxycholecalciferol and this might
well be partly responsible for slow bone growth as well as inadequate calcification
of bone matrix (renal rickets).

Psycho-social influences

These are well recognised as associated with stunting of growth. Usually these
children are living in very poor social conditions and are emotionally deprived.
They are most frequently aged between 3 and 8, although no age is beyond all
risk. In many instances there is global retardation in growth with retention of
infantile proportions of the skeleton (e.g. short legs in relation to the rest of the
body). Reasons for psycho-social growth failure are complex. They include poor
food intake from a blunted appetite, together with an overall depression of
endocrine function reflected in depressed growth hormone levels: indeed, the
features are more typical of an adaptation to malnutrition rather than to primary
endocrine disease.

Secular trends in growth

Secular trends in body size refer to changes in height and weight which take place
over a period of time in the same population. Since the earliest collection of
growth data from Western Europe and North America in the 19th century it has
become evident that the height of children at equivalent ages has progressively
increased. For example, the difference in children's height in Sweden between
1883 and 1938 is equivalent to about 1.5 years of growth. Ten-year-old Swedish
children in 1883 (the first large scale documentation of children's size) had a mean
height of 121 cm compared to 140 cm in the present generation. At the age of
18 average heights were respectively 160 and 175 cm. As well as changes in size,
secular changes have similarly occurred in the tempo of development. Using the
age of menarche as an objective measure of sexual maturity, data from Finland
shows that whilst in 1860 menarche occurred at a mean age of about 17 years, in
the early 1970s it occurred at about 12.5 years (Fig. 17.18). What is quite fascinating
is that, over the same period as these secular changes have taken place in the size
of children and the tempo of development, there appears to have been much less
difference in final attained adult height. What has altered is the *age* at which this
mature adult height is reached which is now about twenty years compared with

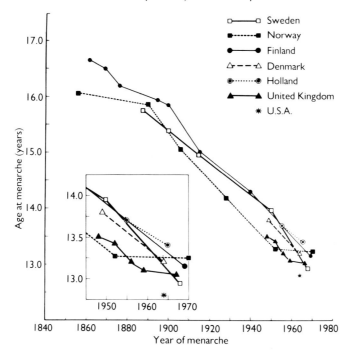

Fig. 17.18. Secular changes in the age of menarche, 1860–1970. Published by permission.

25 years early this century. Thus, the secular change in the size of children is likely to relate to an acceleration in the tempo of growth. There is now evidence that the trend towards increasing size and maturity in developed countries has not continued since the 1950s.

Many factors have been proposed to account for these secular trends including environmental influences, particularly improvements in nutrition and reduction in infection through social and therapeutic means which will allow the rate of growth to proceed unhindered, fulfilling the growth and development potential. The hypothesis that genetic and climatic factors have also played a role in secular changes in growth has not been substantiated. There have been hints that childhood obesity may also have shown a secular trend in the last few decades in Britain with improved living standards. The impression again is largely unsubstantiated.

Further reading

Falkner, F. and Tanner, J.M. (Eds.) (1977). *Human Growth: Vol. 1, Principles and Prenatal Growth; Vol. 2, Postnatal Growth.* Ballière Tindall, London.

Goss, R.J. (1978). *The Physiology of Growth.* Academic Press, New York.

Marshall, W.A. (1977). *Human Growth and its Disorders.* Academic Press, New York.

Roberts, D.F. and Thomson, A.M. (Eds.) (1976). The biology of fetal growth. *Symp. Soc. Study Hum. Biol;* **15**.
Sinclair, D.C. (1978). *Human Growth after Birth*, 3rd ed. Oxford University Press.
Smith, D.W. (1977). *Growth and its Disorders.* Saunders, Philadelphia.
Tanner, J.M. (1978). *Fetus into Man; physical growth from conception to maturity.* Open Books, London.
Thompson, D'Arcy. (1966). *Growth and Form.* Cambridge University Press.

18
Embryopathy and Prenatal Diagnosis

Introduction

Abnormal development ends in one of four ways.

1 Death

The embryo dies either before or after implantation. In the former case *resorption* occurs and the mother is probably not aware of her lost pregnancy. After implantation embryonic and fetal death are usually followed by *abortion*. The mortality level during pregnancy is difficult to estimate precisely. Most authorities suggest a pre-implantation death rate of about 30 per cent mostly due to chromosomal abnormalities in the embryo but, in some cases, a result of maternal factors. Abortions and stillbirths, often associated with abnormalities of the conceptus, account for a loss of a further 20 per cent so that *perhaps 50 per cent* of all human pregnancies are unsuccessful.

2 Congenital malformation

The birth occurs of an infant with *anatomical congenital malformations*. Here, again, the incidence is difficult to define, partly because abnormality rates differ geographically and temporally and partly because there is no generally accepted boundary between the extremes of variation and frank abnormality. The 'best estimate' figure is that between *2 and 5 per cent* of all live births are born with at least one serious malformation; at the end of the first year of life this figure is even higher because some abnormal children do not manifest their malformation until some time after birth.

3 Failure to thrive

There may be a transient or permanent 'failure to thrive'. This is usually due to a *functional deficit* in the neonate, often caused by adverse circumstances encountered relatively late in gestation or even in the perinatal period. At this stage, major organogenesis is complete and the fetus is in the stage of histogenesis and functional maturation. Possibly one of the most significant examples of functional deficit is mental deficiency without any apparent physical or genetic cause.

4 Under-sized, under-weight children

The birth of under-sized and under-weight children can also be the end result of an abnormal pregnancy. Often this is completely recoverable, having perhaps been due to relative placental inefficiency, malnutrition or an unbalanced diet during pregnancy. Recently low birth weight has been associated with maternal smoking (see Chapter 17). Sometimes the *growth retardation* is associated with functional deficit in which case the effect may be permanent.

Discussion of the causes and treatment of abortion and stillbirth, as well as intra-uterine growth retardation belongs to the study of obstetrics and, apart from the features described in Chapter 17, will not be further considered. The causes of functional deficit have, as yet, been little investigated and incompletely characterised. We shall, therefore, confine ourselves to a discussion of anatomical congenital malformations. Specific examples have been given throughout the text in relation to their developmental background. It is now appropriate to study the problem in its entirety.

Congenital malformations

Up to perhaps 70 per cent of congenital malformations in man are of unknown causation. Their aetiology may be complex and, in the vast majority, probably involves multiple environmental factors acting on a polygenic sensitivity. This may not mean that they are beyond eventual treatment. It is quite possible that one factor (perhaps something like folic acid deficiency) may be a very important component of the aetiological mix in certain cases. Its elimination would then abolish the condition in spite of the persistence of a remaining predisposition.

About 20 per cent of malformed births (see Chapter 2) are of known genetic transmission (e.g. achondroplasia) and perhaps 5 per cent are due to chromosomal aberration as, for example, in Down's syndrome (see Chapter 17). A small proportion of the total are among the few known environmental causes of congenital defect in man.

Certain infectious diseases cause malformations. Rubella (German measles) was identified as a *teratogen* by Gregg in 1941. Maternal infection causes the embryo to become secondarily colonised by the virus which causes cataracts, cardiac defects, deafness, abnormalities of the teeth and mental retardation. The exact pattern of malformation depends upon the time of infection (*vide infra*). Less than 50 per cent of offspring are affected but the incidence of defect depends upon the strain of virus. As one would expect, prematurity and abortion are also manifest.

Another virus infection — *cytomegalovirus* — also causes fetal infection, frequently with resultant malformation. The virus is like that of herpes simplex and the maternal infection usually passes unnoticed though recently serious effects on the immune system have been suspected. If infection occurs early in pregnancy it is thought that it may well cause embryonic death. Later in gestation, and in the neonatal period, severe effects include microcephaly, hydrocephalus, intracerebral calcification and jaundice associated with hepatosplenomegaly. Although infection is thought to take place in the 3rd or 4th month of gestation its asymptomatic nature means that it is impossible to define critical periods for the various types of malformation.

It is possible, but not proven, that other virus infections — such as herpes simplex, measles, ECHO, Coxsackie and influenza viruses may cause a small number of malformations. If so, the malformation rate must be very low indeed.

Infection with *toxoplasmosis gondii*, a unicellular parasite, is teratogenic. It causes — among other defects — hydrocephalus, microcephaly, cerebral calcification and chorioretinitis. Like cytomegalovirus it is difficult to localise the time of maternal infection, which is usually asymptomatic, so that critical periods cannot be determined.

Bacterial infection with syphilis has been known for many years to affect the fetus. A great variety of manifestations may be present at birth following infection between 20 weeks of gestation and birth.

On present evidence, few chemical agents responsible for environmental teratogenesis have been identified. This is because of the multifactorial nature of the process. Thalidomide, a drug used in the 1960s for morning sickness and as a sleeping tablet, produced dramatic effects on the unborn. Depending upon the time of its administration it caused gross limb defects (phocomelia, etc.), facial and other abnormalities. The effect was almost universal if the drug was administered between approximately 20 and 36 days after conception. Though usually without damaging effect in the young adult, Thalidomide is now never prescribed.

The anticonvulsants used for epilepsy and *petit mal* are, unfortunately, almost certainly teratogenic in a small but significant proportion of women. It seems that cleft lip and palate, as well as digital hypoplasia and heart lesions, are among a spectrum of malformations encountered. Perhaps the most dangerous of the antiepileptic drugs is Hydantoin, though Trimethadone — used for *petit mal* — also has an effect. Discontinuance of drug therapy during pregnancy is, however, often more dangerous than the risk of congenital malformations.

Some steroid hormones, in particular *androgens* and *progestogens*, are teratogenic if taken at the critical period of maturation of the genitalia. Cortisone, though teratogenic in mice, is innocuous in man. Other known human teratogens are the anticoagulant warfarin and the folic acid antagonist aminopterin. Indeed, mild folic acid deficiency is currently suspected as being responsible for neural tube defects. Treatment with polyvitamins seems to lower the incidence of this malformation in mothers who have previously conceived a child with such a defect. Interest has also focused on alcohol consumption and it is widely believed that maternal alcohol intake at a level not yet defined can lead to a series of relatively minor physical defects associated with mental retardation in the so-called 'fetal alcohol syndrome'. The undoubted connection between ionising radiation and congenital malformations is now so well recognised that the dangers from therapeutic and diagnostic X-rays have been virtually eliminated. Accidental irradiation from radioactive materials or atomic explosion remains a hazard. Diabetes mellitus is associated with congenital defects, particularly involving the sacral region in the so-called 'caudal regression syndrome' as well as 'heavy-for-dates' babies that have been discussed in Chapter 17. The defects probably result from transient hyperglycaemia because there is evidence that well controlled diabetics are less often affected. Metals, such as mercury and lead, are of proven embryotoxicity and a number of other chemicals, e.g. aspirin, LSD and unidentified factors relating to the operating room environment are increasingly suspect.

Fetal deformations (Chapter 17) are often considered in the same context as congenital malformations. The reader is referred to p.315 for a consideration of these conditions.

The action of teratogenic agents

Wilson (1973) has devised a generalised format for the mechanisms underlying teratogenesis and their secondary effects which is useful in the present rudimentary state of our knowledge. He postulates that the numerous environmental factors, often acting together upon a receptive genotype, are responsible for certain basic *teratogenic mechanisms*. Examples of these are mutation, chromosome breaks, alteration of nucleic acid, altered energy sources and osmotic imbalance. Mechanisms of this nature result in a relatively restricted number of *pathogenic manifestations* — such as excessive cell death, failed cellular interaction, impeded morphogenic movement or mechanical disruption. The pathogenic features result in the production of too few cells or cell products to support complete functional maturation and this, in turn, leads to one of the four *embryopathic* entities mentioned at the beginning of this chapter. They are embryonic or fetal death, congenital malformation, failure to thrive or insufficient growth before and after birth.

Armed with the concept of a *modus operandi* for teratogens, it is possible to consider a few basic principles regarding the circumstances of their action. Four of these are of particular importance.

Stage of development at which the teratogen acts

The stage of intra-uterine development at which a teratogen acts often determines the susceptibility of the conceptus and the types of malformation produced. This is clearly a consequence of the developmental process itself. By and large each organ *anlage* will pass through a critical stage, or stages, at which it is sensitive to specific teratogens. Usually the embryo in its pre-gastrulation stages is insensitive because, for practical purposes, if non-lethally damaged it can 'regulate' itself by virtue of the fact that its cells are relatively uncommitted. During the immediately-following embryonic period, however, the embryo is highly susceptible because the massive tissue movements and their precisely timed interactions can easily be disturbed by relatively minor external stimuli. A good example of this principle has previously been mentioned when it was pointed out that thalidomide caused phocomelia only if taken between the 20th and 36th days of pregnancy. Outside this period the drug did not produce limb defects.

Nature of stimulus

We have seen that the timing of a noxious stimulus is important in determining the nature of a malformation. The nature of the stimulus itself is, however, just as important. Clearly, the underlying mechanism and pathogenesis will depend upon the mode of action of the teratogen. The toxicology and pharmacology of potential teratogens often depend upon their ability to cross the extra-embryonic membrane to reach the embryo.

Genotype of embryo

The basic genotype of the embryo will often modify the action of a teratogen. Some genotypes are particularly sensitive and others relatively resistant to specific agents. This is well shown in experimental animal studies where differential strain sensitivity can often be demonstrated. Sometimes the maternal genotype is also crucially important — often because of the intra-uterine environment provided.

Dose/response curve

A dosage/response curve can be constructed as the result of the action of most teratogens. It is important to be aware of this because very many substances can be shown to have a teratogenic effect under experimental conditions though the serum levels are far higher than would ever happen naturally or therapeutically. In addition there is thought to be a 'cut-off' dose for most teratogens below which they are ineffective.

Prenatal diagnosis

It is usually possible to offer women whose pregnancy is complicated by a severely malformed child the choice of a medical termination if they wish it. Early and accurate prenatal diagnosis is therefore imperative. The clinician is often put on his guard by a family history of abortion or of congenital malformations. He will also be especially vigilant with elderly mothers or with mothers who seem to have an excess of amniotic fluid (hydramnios), this being a condition often associated with deformed offspring. New methods are increasingly becoming available for fetal diagnosis. The following are now widely used:

1 *Radiology* can often detect fetal abnormality in the last trimester of pregnancy. The risks from irradiation resulting from a straightforward X-ray of the abdomen are small enough to be negligible. Anencephaly and limb defects are the most common anomalies diagnosed by this method.

2 *Sonography* (ultrasound) enables the clinician to obtain an image of the embryo using ultrasonic waves. The diagnosis of an empty gestational sac — a common condition — may be made in the second month of pregnancy while after 12 weeks anencephaly is not difficult to see.

3 *Amniocentesis* (i.e. amniotic fluid sampling) has some dangers. In about 1 per cent of cases abortion results from irritation due to passage of the needle to withdraw fluid. Examination of the fluid is so useful, however, that the procedure is often carried out. The clinical criteria for proceeding with it are outside the scope of this book but it is never performed until after blood tests and other physical methods, such as sonography, have been done.

Following amniocentesis, amniotic fluid cells may be cultured and chromosome abnormalities, such as Down's syndrome, diagnosed. Certain metabolic defects may also be identified from amniotic cell culture. The biochemistry of the fluid is of importance. It is possible to estimate the viability of the fetus by calculating the lecithin/sphingomyelin ratio arising from pulmonary surfactant (p.321). Levels of amniotic α-fetoprotein (AFP) are also important. Normally these levels are low but, if there is a surface loss of epithelium, the exposed wound results in the leakage of this fetal protein into the fluid. Anencephaly and spina bifida are by far the commonest causes of raised AFP. This is often accompanied by a small rise of AFP in the maternal blood but usually this is so slight that it fails to be a reliable diagnostic sign.

Further reading

Carter, C.O. (ed.) (1975) Human congenital malformations. *Brit. Med. Bull.* **32**. 21–26.

Smithells, R.W. (1978) The Prevention and Prediction of Congenital Malformations. In: *Scientific Basis of Obstetrics & Gynaecology*, ed. McDonald, R.R. Churchill Livingstone, Edinburgh.

Wilson, J.G. (1973) *Environment and Birth Defects.* Academic Press, New York.

Wilson, J.G. & Fraser, F.C. (eds.) (1977) *Handbook of Teratology*, Vols. 1–4, Plenum Press, London and New York.

19
Interacting Systems Operative During Development and Differentiation

Chapters 5, 6 and 9–16 of this book are concerned with the detailed organogenesis of the main systems in man. We shall now consider some general embryological principles associated with the differentiation of the tissues within these systems. In a single short chapter we can only treat this complex subject very superficially and the interested reader is referred to the textbooks of developmental biology recommended for further reading.

Early mammalian development

During the last ten years scientists have begun a study of the physiological determinants involved in mammalian development. They have worked almost entirely with the mouse and it is quite likely that many of the observations are species specific. This body of work can now be added to previous observations on lower vertebrates.

In sub-mammalian species development before the formation of the primitive streak is under the control of an RNA of maternal origin present in the egg before fertilization. There is evidence that, in the mouse, expression of the paternal genome commences during cleavage which is well before this stage. The first sign of differentiation probably occurs at compaction when the trophectoderm cells become *determined* (see also Chapter 5, p.73). By 'determination' we mean that cells are irreversibly committed to a developmental line. Their fate cannot be changed even under experimental conditions. For example, if they are transplanted to other regions of the embryo their differentiation is unchanged — they develop *selfwise* rather than *neighbourwise*. Later in development the cells which make up the primitive knot (p.82) also become determined. The biochemical reasons for such *self determination* are unknown. In some lower forms, though not in mammals, it may be caused by specific cytoplasmic factors which become localised in particular regions as a result of earlier cell division (see p.73). Experimental evidence from lower vertebrates suggests that the cell nuclei remain flexible because it has been shown that nuclei transplantated from fully differentiated tissues (e.g. neurons) are stimulated to divide and sustain normal development if transplanted into an enucleated zygote.

Organizers

Chapter 6 described the formation of the primitive streak and the primary germ

355

layers. This stage of development involved morphogenetic movements that brought cells, which had previously been widely separated from one another, into close proximity. The causes of cell movement at gastrulation are not understood, but the consequences cannot be over-estimated. New micro-environments are created, thus allowing cell interaction to play a part in the continuing process of differentiation. For the first time, the process of *induction* is involved in development and certain areas, such as the notochordal process, are known to act as *organizers*, that is to say the cells modify adjacent cell regions. Thus, as well as exercising an influence on adjacent endoderm and mesoderm, the notochordal process induces the overlying ectodermal zone to form the neural tube. Cells which come under the influence of organizers must be *competent* to react to the *evocator* produced by the organizing zone. Experiments have shown that induction is chemically mediated and does not require cell-to-cell contact. The nature of the chemical(s) involved under natural (as opposed to experimental) conditions is in doubt and possibly varies in different organizer systems; suffice it to say that directly, or indirectly, the evocator probably influences the genome of competent cells and causes them to undergo *dependent differentiation*. The latter term implies that, in the absence of the organizer, the specific differentiation normally evoked by it would not have occurred, i.e. presumptive neural tube ectoderm would develop into ordinary epithelium in the absence of the notochordal process but *having once been subjected to the action of the latter* it becomes irrevocably destined to form neural tube.

The primitive knot, which is homologous with the dorsal lip of the blastopore in lower forms, is sometimes referred to as the *primary organizer*. Similar systems are common in a variety of embryonic regions developing after gastrulation. They have been extensively analysed, both *in vivo* and *in vitro*, and their characteristics are found to vary quite extensively. A frequently recurrent theme is that of interaction between two closely related tissues. For example, the apical ectodermal thickening in the region of a limb bud induces the underlying mesoderm to proliferate and form the musculo-skeletal system of the limb. Removal of the ectodermal thickening prevents this process and, in this sense, the ectoderm acts as the limb organizer. However, experiments with limbless mutant chicks have shown that the underlying mesenchyme produces a 'maintenance factor' without which the ectodermal thickening cannot survive in its normal form. Meso-ectodermal interaction rather than straightforward induction is, therefore, operative in this system.

Finally, we must consider the question of how the various parts of an induced organ are produced appropriately to form a composite, and often highly complex structural whole. It is not enough, for instance, to postulate that the notochordal process induces the formation of the neural tube; we must also explain how the neural tube becomes organized into the highly specialised regions of the brain and spinal cord. There is evidence that regional differences are inherent in the inductor and, indeed, separate regions of the amphibian notochord are sometimes classified as the head inductor, trunk inductor, etc. This explanation, however, only begs the question of how the various parts of an organizer differ. One possible explanation based on findings in amphibia has been proposed. It is suggested that the primary organizer produces at least two separate chemical substances which form gradients along its length. The so-called neuralizing substance, which may be a ribonucleoprotein, is thought to be present along the whole length of the organizer while another agent, a mesodermalizing substance possibly protein in nature, begins to be emitted at the cranial limit of somite formation and increases in concentration in a caudal direction. The balance of materials produced by the notochordal process could, therefore, account for the cranio-caudal organization of neural, mesodermal and endodermal structures.

Positional information

It has become increasingly clear recently that adjacent cells in certain tissues may have considerable power of direct communication by virtue of permeable 'tight junctions' between their plasma membranes. This has led to the concept that a cell may possess *positional information*, i.e. that the system is constructed so that cells are able to 'sense' their position in it. Various suggestions concerning the process of differentiation have been put forward based upon this concept. Essentially they establish the self-regulatory nature of certain developmental systems and, in some instances, replace or amplify the organizer hypothesis by one based upon the positional information available to a cell. The details of these concepts are beyond the scope of this book but the interested reader is referred to a review by Wolpert (1969) for further information.

Some other systems of importance during embryogenesis

Tissue aggregation and differentiation

An important characteristic of embryonic tissues is their capacity to aggregate into specific patterns and to adopt consistent positions relative to each other if they are mixed. When a variety of cell types (even if they originate from different species) are cultured together in rotating flasks so that they are *suspended* in the culture medium they are able to sort themselves out into a sort of hierarchical order so that, for example, cells of epidermal origin will come to surround those of medullary plate origin. Many factors undoubtedly regulate morphogenetic movements and only a few of these are beginning to be understood. Thus the chemical and physical organization of the substratum over which the cells move is one relevant factor in the creation of certain specific patterns. Another is the inability of some cells to move over each other (at least in culture conditions); this is known as *cell contact inhibition* and results in certain cell types repelling each other. Motility and the surface properties of cells change during embryogenesis so that adult cells have often lost the capacity for specific reaggregation inherent in their embryonic counterparts.

Tissue aggregation is often followed by differentiation, when a critical concentration of cells is reached. For example, chick myoblasts, when plated out in culture, form small 'nests' of cells or clones, each derived from a single ancestor. When these clones have reached a certain size, the local concentration of specific chemicals necessary for their further development into striated myotubules is reached, and they become histologically differentiated.

The role of cell death

Although apparently the antithesis of development, cell death in fact constitutes an integral part of embryogenesis. The phenomenon is said to occur in three biological situations, though the distinction between them is somewhat academic.
1 *Morphogenetic cell death* is a basic factor in tissue remodelling and occurs in structures as diverse as the retina and the sclerotome as each changes shape during development.
2 *Phylogenetic cell death* occurs when degeneration of a functionless structure, usually the expression of evolutionary recapitulation, takes place; an example is the disappearance of the pronephric rudiment in mammals (or, indeed, of most of the mesonephros in the female).
3 *Histogenetic cell death* occurs when functional tissues become isolated by morphogenetic movement; the disappearance of epithelia in the leading edges of fusing palatal shelves (p.189) is a good example, as is the elimination of the cervical sinus (p.176).

This chapter is not concerned with the utility or mechanisms of embryonic cell death since much controversy still surrounds these topics. Nevertheless, it is clear that a disturbance of this process may easily lead to the genesis of congenital malformation.

Growth and regeneration

Factors controlling the relative growth of various organs and system are ill-understood but undoubtedly exist. Some, such as a nerve growth factor which acts upon the sympathetic nervous system, have been identified as chemicals which stimulate growth while others, known as *chalones*, may act as anti-mitotic agents to regulate the stimulatory action of specific hormones or enzymes. Compensatory hypertrophy (overgrowth) of some organs occurs, even in adults, in response to increased demand and is probably controlled by unidentified substances, possibly regulatory peptides, in the circulation; thus when one kidney is surgically removed the other normally enlarges. Regenerative and regulatory powers are severely curtailed after embryogenesis in mammals. Generally speaking, only scar tissue (consisting of collagen) will repair a wound or other area of tissue destruction. Post-natal growth is the subject of Chapter 17.

Differentiation

Differentiation is a much used and, until recently, little understood word. It implies that the functional part of the genome has a certain inherent stability. When, and if, differentiated cells divide they give rise to others of the same type and in certain cases (as in the neurone) the power of cell division has been lost completely. In molecular terms, therefore, it seems that parts of the genome are normally repressed during differentiation. Tissue culture experiments and other observations have led to the conclusion that the function and morphology of a cell is not as rigidly fixed as it would appear at first sight to be. Monolayer cultures, (i.e. a single layer of cells usually cultured in petri dishes from outgrowths of organ rudiments), result in the reversion of almost all cells into three basic types and it is clear that the cell genome is, to some extent, still under the control of its environment. It is wiser to think of cells as being relatively differentiated rather than 'differentiated' and 'undifferentiated'.

Conclusions

In a very superficial way, we have discussed some of the more important physiological factors operative during embryogenesis. The aim and scope of this book is such that it would not be appropriate to study others and to construct complex models to explain the development of various systems. We should, however, be aware of the sequential and interdependent nature of all the factors which make up ontogeny. Thus the primary organizer cannot function unless nucleocytoplasmic interaction and the appropriate morphogenetic movements have taken place. In turn, the laying down of the body axis allows secondary organizers to act. Tissue remodelling occurs and so, by a host of hierarchial processes, processes differing qualitatively and quantitatively in various parts of the embryo, development proceeds to completion.

Further reading

Balinski, B.I. (1975) *An Introduction to Embryology*, 4th edn. W.B. Saunders & Co., Philadelphia, London & Toronto.

Gurdon, J.B. (1968) Transplanted nuclei and cell differentiation. *Sci. Am.*, **219,** 24.

Hinchcliffe, J.R. & Johnson, D.R. (1980) *The Development of the Vertebrate Limb*. (Clarendon Press, Oxford.

Newth, D.R. (1970) *Animal Growth and Development*. The Institute of Biology's studies in Biology, No. 24 Edward Arnold, London.

Oppenheimer, J.M. (1940) The non-specificity of germ layers. *Quart. Rev. Biol.* **15**, 1.

Saunders, J.W. (1966) Death in embryonic systems. *Science, N.Y.* **154**, 604.

Slack, J.M.W. (1983) *From Egg to Embryo*. Cambridge University Press, London.

Wolpert, L. (1969) Positional information and the spatial pattern of cellular differentiation. *J. Theor. Biol* **25**, 1.

Index

Muscle *continued*
  myometrial 40, 45, 111
    in pregnancy 111
  ovarian smooth 64
  stylohyoid 175
  stylopharyngeus 175
  thoracic wall 123
  uterine 40, 45, 111
Mutations
  chromosome 22, 27
  frameshift 23
  point 22, 24
Myocardium 195
Myometrium 40, 45, 111
Myotome 119, 127

Naevi 134
Nares, anterior 188
  posterior primitive 188
Neck 175
Neo-cerebellum *see* Brain
Nephrogenic ridge 246
Nephron/s 251
Nerve/s
  cervical 128
  chorda tympani 174, 180, 186
  cranial 142, 174
  facial 142, 174, 186
  glossopharyngeal 174, 186
  hypoglossal 127, 186
  intercostal 127, 240
  laryngeal 174, 213
  optic 156
  phrenic 128, 240
  pretrematic 174
  spinal 120, 128
  thoracic 127
  trigeminal 174, 186
  vagus 174
Neural
  crest/s 138, 143
  groove 82
  plate 82
  tube 82, 138
Neuraminidase 65
Nipple, inverted 130
Notochord 84, 121
  fate of 122
Nucleus/nuclei
  caudate 148
  cranial nerve 141
  lentiform 148
  pontine 151
  pulposus 122
  red 151
Nutrition
  effects of poor 342
  embryonic 91, 92
  haemotrophic 92
  histiotroph(ic) 91
  via placenta 104 *et seq.*

Odontoblasts 186
Oesophagus 237, 278
  atresia of 290
Oestradiol *see* Hormone/s
Oestrogens *see* Hormone/s

Oestrus 46
Olfactory placodes 187
Oligohydroamnios 316
Olivary complex 151
Omentum
  greater 281
  lesser 282
Oocyte 42, 65
  primary 41
Oogenesis 41
Oogonia 41, 261
Ootid 66
Opercula 149
Operations, Procedures, etc.
  Rashkind 222
  shunt, Taussig-Blalock 229
    Waterston 229
Optic
  cup 155
  nerve *see* Nerve(s)
  stalk 156
  vesicle 153, 155
Organ, enamel 186
Organizers 355
Ostium
  primum 208
    defect 227
  secundum 208
Otocyst 146, 180
Outgrowth
  hepatic 283, 284
  pancreatic, dorsal 283
    ventral 283
Ovary/ies
  at puberty 338
  development 260
  endocrine functions of 45, 46, 306
  in pregnancy 115
Ovotestes 273
Ovulation 63
Ovum 42, 44, 63
  nutrition 74
  transport of 64

Pachytene 11
Palate 187
  cleft 189 *et seq.*
  hard 189
  primitive 188
  soft 189
Pancreas 283
  annular 294
Pars basalis and functionalis (of
    endometrium) 50
Parthenogenesis 67
Parturition 116
Patent ductus arteriosus (PDA)
    see Ductus
Penis 265
  anomalies 270 *et seq.*
  at puberty 337
Pericardium 86, 89, 117, 195, 234, 239
Periderm 128
Peritoneum 89, 234, 239
  relation to ovary 41
Phaeochromocytes 143
Phallus 265
Pharynx 170, 280